Ducarmelle D.

Diabetes Mellitus:
Diagnosis and Treatment

Diabetes Mellitus:
Diagnosis and Treatment

Mayer B. Davidson, MD

Director, Diabetes Program
Cedars-Sinai Medical Center
Professor of Medicine
UCLA School of Medicine
Los Angeles, California

A Wiley Medical Publication
John Wiley & Sons
New York/Chichester/Brisbane/Toronto

Acknowledgments: I gratefully acknowledge Margo E. Blackburn for her excellent secretarial skills in producing this book, and Jane Lehan, RD, for her help with the sections on exercise and sick-day rules in chapter 7. I also thank James Anderson, MD, for his help on the section on high-fiber diets.

To Roseann: With much gratitude for her loving support.

Library of Congress Cataloging in Publication Data

Davidson, Mayer B
   Diabetes mellitus, diagnosis and treatment.

   (A Wiley medical publication)
   Includes index.
   1. Diabetes.   I. Title.   II. Series. [DNLM:
1. Diabetes mellitus. WK 810 D253d]
RC660.D37   616.4'62   81-84
ISBN 0-471-09506-0 (v. 1)   AACR2
ISBN 0-471-09542-7 (v. 2)
ISBN 0-471-09543-5 (combined)

Printed in the United States of America

10 9 8 7 6 5 4 3 2 1

Preface

Diabetes mellitus has a tremendous impact not only on the health of individuals but also on the health care system in the United States. According to the National Commission on Diabetes, this disease now affects 5% of the population of this country (approximately 10 million people), and it is estimated that a similar number of cases remain undiagnosed. Because the incidence of diabetes is increasing by 6% per year, the size of the diabetic population will double in 15 years. In 1974 (the last year for which statistics were available when the National Commission made its report), 38,000 deaths in the United States were directly attributable to diabetes mellitus. Since vascular complications are so common in diabetic patients, it was estimated that this disease was responsible for 300,000 deaths annually—a figure making it the third leading cause of death. Diabetes is the leading cause of new cases of blindness in this country. Compared with nondiabetics, diabetics are 25 times more likely to develop blindness, 17 times more likely to develop renal disease, 20 times more likely to develop gangrene, and twice as likely to develop heart disease or suffer a stroke. Over 80% of the major amputations performed in the United States occur in diabetics. Fourteen percent of diabetic patients (usually the elderly) are bedridden for an average of 6 weeks per year. The total annual economic impact of diabetes mellitus was estimated at more than 5 billion dollars in 1974 and at approximately 8 billion dollars in 1979.

Although the importance of diabetes mellitus is finally being recognized, considerable controversy currently exists with regard to the diagnosis and treatment of this syndrome. As is often the case in medicine, physicians are called upon to make decisions that are based on fragmentary and inconclusive evidence and that may have a profound influence on patients. Of these decisions, those related solely to the diabetic component of care fall into only a few areas. In other words, most of the clinical judgments required in the care of diabetic patients are not very different from those required in the treatment of non-diabetics. Problems associated with infection, heart disease, renal disease, cerebral vascular disease, neuropathy, and so on are similar in diabetics and nondiabetics. Although the onset and clinical course of some conditions (such as bacterial and fungal infections) may have certain distinctive features in diabetic patients, the basic decisions regarding diagnosis and treatment do not differ appreciably.

On the other hand, several types of clinical judgments are limited to the treatment of patients with diabetes. Some obvious examples are insulin therapy, prescription of diabetic diets, education of the patient and the patient's family about diabetes, prescription of sulfonylurea agents, and treatment of diabetic ketoacidosis. As heretical as it may sound, my feeling is that much of the information in textbooks and review articles on diabetes mellitus is not pertinent to these kinds of clinical decisions. For instance, the facts that insulin increases glucose transport in muscle tissue, has an independent effect on glycogen synthesis, does not affect glucose transport in the liver, but does affect the rate-limiting enzymes of glycolysis and gluconeogenesis in a way that limits hepatic glucose production and enhances glucose utilization do not really help the physician to decide how to use insulin in a diabetic patient. Other examples of data that contribute to an understanding of the pathogenesis and ramifications of diabetes mellitus but are not important (yet) in the actual care of diabetic patients are those involving cell-mediated immunity, histocompatibility antigen (HLA) typing, basement membranes, and mechanisms of insulin secretion.

The purpose of this volume is to offer guidance in making those clinical decisions that are necessary only in the treatment of diabetic patients. My personal approach, which has evolved during 15 years of caring for these patients, is presented. Where scientific data are available that permit a fuller understanding of the problem and/or provide support for the approach used, they are briefly discussed and referenced so that interested readers can avail themselves of more information. In many instances, however, there are no firm data on which to base a decision about the superiority of one method over another. In these situations, my personal reasons for using a particular approach are presented.

Two excellent dietitians, Marian Susuki and Pauline Nelson, with whom I have had the pleasure of working at the UCLA Center for Health Sciences for a number of years, have joined me in writing the chapter on dietary therapy. Two dedicated and superb diabetes educators, Roz Morgan, RN, and Mary Pearce, RN, with whom I work in the Diabetes Program at Cedars-Sinai Medical Center, have collaborated with me to produce a chapter for allied health professionals involved in the care and education of diabetic patients. We hope that both dietitians and nurses will benefit from these chapters without having to refer to other parts of the book. Finally, the chapter on the emotional aspects of living with diabetes has been written entirely by Jay Skyler, MD, and his colleagues Wendy Citrin, MSW, and Gary Kleiman from the University of Miami.

In chapter 10, I have presented an approach to the diagnosis and treatment of hypoglycemia. A widespread misconception seems to exist about the prevalence of bona fide hypoglycemia and the clinical symptoms that hypoglycemia can cause. Although hypoglycemia is not a common disorder, it can be a manifestation of serious disease processes, and a careful evaluation of the problem is important. I hope that the information in this chapter will provide the physician with a logical approach to the patient with "hypoglycemia."

This book is intended primarily for physicians and other professionals who provide care for patients with diabetes mellitus. Although scientific background has been provided wherever possible to support the clinical approaches suggested, I recognize that the potential audience is an extremely busy group of people. Therefore, I have included a practical summary at the end of most chapters. I hope that these summaries will provide the reader with a concise, ready reference for the specific problem being considered, and that as such they supplement the full discussions in the chapters proper.

Contents

Chapter 1

Diagnosis of Diabetes Mellitus

Definition

Diabetes mellitus is a syndrome involving both metabolic and vascular abnormalities. Alterations in carbohydrate, lipid, and protein metabolism are caused by a relative or absolute lack of effective insulin action. Two kinds of vascular lesions are found: a microangiopathy that is characterized by a thickening of capillary basement membranes and is clinically manifested as diabetic retinopathy and/or glomerulosclerosis, and a macroangiopathy that does not differ in pathological or clinical terms from atherosclerosis in nondiabetic individuals, except that it usually appears earlier and may follow a more malignant course. Various neuropathies are also associated with the syndrome of diabetes mellitus, but it is not entirely clear whether the underlying abnormalities are metabolic or vascular. In the final analysis, both types of lesions will probably be revealed.

Currently, the presence of abnormally high glucose levels in the blood is the only criterion on which a diagnosis of diabetes mellitus may be based. If the fasting glucose concentration is higher than normal, there is little disagreement concerning the diagnosis. However, if glucose levels are normal or nearly normal after an overnight fast, the diagnosis must be based on an evaluation of glucose disposal after administration of a carbohydrate load. The current practice is the administration of an oral challenge with a simple carbohydrate solution (rather than a test meal). This oral glucose tolerance test (OGTT) is more sensitive than the intravenous glucose tolerance test (IVGTT), which should be used only in special circumstances (see *Gastric Surgery*). However, a number of factors affect the results of the OGTT, and a spirited controversy exists (1) concerning not only what levels of glucose should be considered abnormal, but also what combinations of abnormal values should determine the diagnosis of diabetes mellitus. Thus, the interpretation of the OGTT requires a careful evaluation of many factors.

3

Factors Affecting the OGTT

Methodology

The glucose oxidase method determines the true glucose concentration since it uses an enzymatic reaction involving the glucose molecule itself. Other methods are nonspecific and yield values 5 to 10 mg/100 ml higher than those from the glucose oxidase method. These differences are not important clinically. However, the older Folin-Wu method can give values 20 to 40 mg/100 ml higher than those obtained with the glucose oxidase method and therefore should no longer be used.

Whole Blood versus Plasma or Serum

The glucose concentration measured in plasma or serum of a given sample is approximately 15% (not 15 mg%) higher than the concentration in the same sample before separation of the cells. The reason for this discrepancy is that 35% to 45% of the volume of whole blood (depending on the hematocrit) is composed of red blood cells. Approximately 35% of the red blood cell is hemoglobin, and glucose is not distributed in this part of the cell. Therefore, for example, glucose is excluded from 15% of a blood sample with a hematocrit of 43% (0.35 × 43). In other words, only 85% of the volume used for the assay contains glucose, but the results are expressed for the entire volume. Thus, values obtained with whole blood are approximately 15% lower than with plasma or serum, in which glucose is distributed throughout the entire volume.

Sample Site

Arterial glucose levels are higher than venous concentrations because the peripheral tissues have not yet had the opportunity to extract the hexose. Capillary blood contains a mixture of arterial and venous blood and is often obtained for sampling during the OGTT by sticking of either the ear lobe or the pads of the fingers. If these areas are warmed or stimulated in order to increase blood flow, the arterial contribution to the sample is enhanced. In the fasting state, peripheral tissues (with the exception of red blood cells and the brain) do not use glucose; hence, there is little difference between capillary and venous samples. However, after a glucose challenge, depending on the amount of hexose administered and the time of sampling, there are appreciable differences between capillary and venous values (2). As would be expected, the more glucose given and the earlier the interval at which the sample is obtained, the greater the difference. For instance, 1 hour after the ingestion of 100 g of glucose, capillary values are 30 to 40 mg/100 ml higher than venous levels (2).

Diet

In the absence of adequate carbohydrate intake, the results of the OGTT are often abnormal (3). This phenomenon is termed starvation diabetes. Although the amount of dietary carbohydrate necessary in order to avoid starvation diabetes has not been determined, 150 g per day is probably sufficient if the diet is normal and the subject's weight is stable (4). Some experts recommend ingestion of at least 250 to 300 g of carbohydrate during each of the 3 days preceding the test (3). The effect of diet on the OGTT in the elderly is a particular problem (see *Age*).

Activity Level

Physical inactivity can be associated with an abnormal result in the OGTT. This problem is also particularly important in the elderly (see *Age*).

Bed Rest

Glucose tolerance decreases in subjects who have been confined to bed for several days. This factor is independent of inactivity per se since, even if subjects exercise while lying down, glucose disposal is impaired (5).

Chronic Illness

Patients who are chronically ill often have abnormal results in the OGTT. Poor diet, physical inactivity, and/or lying down most of the time may account in large part for this abnormality. However, patients with liver disease commonly have abnormal OGTT (3), and it seems unlikely that these 3 factors provide a sufficient explanation in these patients.

Diurnal Variation

If a glucose tolerance test is performed in the afternoon, the resulting values are higher than those obtained for the same individual in the morning (6). If relatively sensitive criteria for making the diagnosis of diabetes mellitus are used, an OGTT done late in the day often gives abnormal results. The mechanism underlying this diurnal variation in OGTT results is unknown, but the differences probably reflect diurnal variations of certain hormones.

Medication

Four commonly prescribed drugs adversely affect the OGTT: diuretics (usually thiazides), which cause potassium depletion; glucocorticoids; synthetic estrogens; and diphenylhydantoin (Dilantin). Potassium depletion impairs glucose-stimulated insulin release and thus may obviously affect the OGTT. Unfortunately, potassium concentrations in serum can be normal even though a patient has a total-body deficit of potassium. Therefore, patients who are taking diuretics should be given potassium supplementation before an OGTT is performed.

Glucocorticoids are potent insulin antagonists and may have profound effects on glucose disposal. Many patients being treated with these agents have a normal OGTT, but only at the cost of increased insulin secretion. The higher the dose and the longer the period of administration, the more likely it is that the result of the OGTT will become abnormal. If treatment with glucocorticoids is discontinued, it may be weeks before normal glucose tolerance returns. An abnormal OGTT often persists in these patients.

The most common sources of synthetic estrogens are the oral contraceptive agents. Decreased glucose tolerance is commonly observed after women begin to take oral contraceptives. In the vast majority of women, the results of the OGTT return to the "prepill" status within several months but, as with glucocorticoids, at the expense of increased insulin secretion. It is commonly believed that glucocorticoids and estrogens are more likely to precipitate diabetes mellitus in individuals with a genetic predisposition for the disease. The only evidence for this statement is the clinical impression that a positive family history is more common in such patients.

Diphenylhydantoin directly affects the pancreatic β-cell, inhibiting insulin secretion. This inhibition may cause profound glucose intolerance that is often reversible on cessation of treatment with the drug (7).

Several other agents may also influence OGTT results. Nicotinic acid (niacin) is sometimes used in high doses (3 to 6 g per day) for the treatment of hyperlipoproteinemia. Many months of therapy with this agent can produce an abnormal OGTT (8). Although ethanol is an important cause of fasting hypoglycemia (see chapter 10), chronic ingestion of alcohol can be associated with impaired glucose disposal (9). Finally, chronic ingestion of salicylates and monoamine oxidase inhibitors (especially the hydrazine derivatives) are associated with hypoglycemia (see chapter 10) and therefore may *lower* glucose levels after an oral challenge. These agents have been shown to stimulate insulin secretion, a characteristic that would account for their effect on the OGTT. Because the effects of the monoamine oxidase inhibitors (at least on central nervous system function) can last for weeks, glucose tolerance testing should be delayed for at least a month after the discontinuation of these agents.

Glucose Load

In normal subjects the glucose concentration after an oral dextrose challenge with 50 g is similar to that after 100 g. This result is explained by the increasing insulin responses as larger amounts of glucose are ingested (2, 10). However, many patients who manifest glucose intolerance after receiving 100 g of dextrose have a normal OGTT result after 50 g (11). In these individuals, a slower insulin response to the larger load of glucose (compared with the response in normal subjects) is postulated to account for the different glucose responses to the two amounts of dextrose. The form of the oral carbohydrate does not seem to matter clinically, as similar glucose concentrations are achieved after ingestion of the simple sugar itself and after ingestion of more palatable solutions of oligopolysaccharides, which must be hydrolyzed to monosaccharides in the gastrointestinal tract before absorption (12).

Reproducibility

Sampling every 30 to 60 minutes during an OGTT usually produces a curve that gradually rises from a basal level, peaks at 30 or 60 minutes in normal subjects (and usually later in diabetic subjects), and then falls to baseline values or below. However, if samples are taken every 10 minutes, a more accurate picture of the disposal of oral glucose is obtained (13). This point is illustrated in Figure 1-1. Each graph in the figure depicts OGTT results for one normal subject. The upper curve represents the glucose concentrations, and the lower curve represents the insulin responses. It is clear that a simple rise and descent of each parameter does not occur. Rather, the pattern is one of several increases and decreases similar

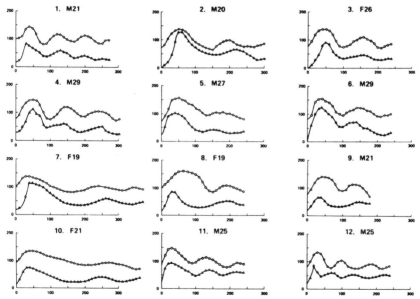

Figure 1-1. Patterns of response to oral administration of glucose (50 g) in 12 normal subjects. Upper curves represent blood glucose (mg%). Lower curves show serum immunoreactive insulin (μU/ml). The time scale is in minutes. Graph headings indicate subject number, sex, and age. (Reprinted with permission from Kraegen EW, Young JD, George EP, Lazarus L: Oscillations in blood glucose and insulin after oral glucose. Horm Metab Res 4:409-413, 1972.)

to two or three sinusoidal curves over the course of 4 to 5 hours. A close inspection of each graph reveals that an initial increase in glucose levels is followed closely by an increase in insulin concentrations. This insulin response results in a leveling off and then a fall in glucose values. Insulin levels tend to diminish as the glucose concentrations stop rising. This pattern is consistent with the recent observations in experiments with the artificial pancreas that the β-cell responds mainly to a change in glucose concentrations rather than to the absolute glucose level (14). When insulin concentrations approach baseline values, glucose levels start to increase again. The peaks of the subsequent increases are lower than the peaks of earlier increases, so that there is an overall fall in glucose concentrations. However, from the graphs in Figure 1-1, it is easy to see that the actual time of sampling has an important influence on the glucose value obtained. Furthermore, the "periodicity" of these sinusoidal curves differs among individuals; samples obtained at the same time after glucose ingestion may represent a nadir value in one person and a peak level in another. Finally, these kinds of oscillations explain the occasional OGTT in which there is a late increase in glucose concentrations.

There are undoubtedly other factors that influence the variability of results in the OGTT. However, even when the conditions of the OGTT are standardized as much as possible with regard to dietary preparations, length of fasting, time of day, glucose load, exercise, and other environmental conditions (e.g., smoking), reproducibility is poor when the test is repeated for the same normal individual within 48 hours (15). This point is illustrated in Figure 1-2, in which both the

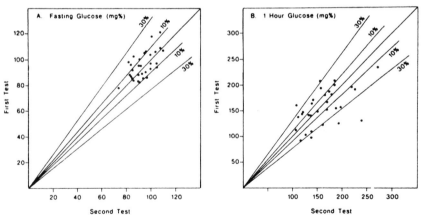

Figure 1-2. Reproducibility of glucose concentrations after an oral challenge (40 g/m^2 of body surface) in normal subjects. The value for the first test is on the vertical axis; the value for the second test (given 48 hours later) is on the horizontal axis. A 45° identity line has been drawn for comparative purposes. Points that lie outside the 10% and 30% deviation lines indicate observations that deviate by more than 10% and 30%. (Reprinted with permission from Olefsky JM, Reaven GM: Insulin and glucose responses to identical oral glucose tolerance tests performed forty-eight hours apart. Diabetes 23:449-453, 1974.)

fasting and the 1-hour glucose concentrations for two tests given within 48 hours are compared. If identical values were obtained in the two tests, they would fall on the 45° identity line. The 10% and 30% lines delineate variations of 10% and 30% between the two tests. Most of the fasting glucose concentrations are within 10% of each other. On the other hand, the majority of the 1-hour values lie outside the 10% deviation lines, and indeed many differ from each other by close to 30% or even more.

Large variations also occur in the results of OGTTs for patients with mild diabetes. In one study (16) (Fig. 1-3), two tests were given within 1 week. The left end of each line in Figure 1-3 represents the value obtained during the initial test, and the right end depicts that found during the second test of the same subject. In agreement with the results for nondiabetic subjects, fasting glucose concentrations were fairly constant. However, after oral challenge, marked variability was noted.

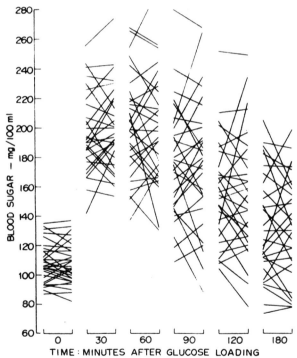

Figure 1-3. Reproducibility of 100-g OGTTs in subjects with mild diabetes. The test was repeated for the same individual within 1 week. The left end of each line represents the result of the first test, and the right end represents that of the second test of the same subject. (Reprinted with permission from Kosaka K, Mizuno Y, Kuzuya T: Reproducibility of the oral glucose tolerance test and the rice-meal test in mild diabetics. Diabetes 15:901-904, 1966.)

Table 1-1. Modified Criteria for the OGTT During Pregnancy[a,b]

Subject's Status	Glucose Concentration (mg/100 ml)[c]			
	Fasting	1 hr	2 hr	3 hr
Nonpregnant	125(110)	195(170)	140(120)	125(110)
Pregnant	105(90)	190(165)	165(145)	145(125)

[a]Reprinted with permission from O'Sullivan JB, Mahan CM: Criteria for the oral glucose tolerance test in pregnancy. Diabetes 13:278–285, 1964.
[b]See data for USPHS in Table 1–3 for interpretation of criteria.
[c]Values for plasma are limited, with corresponding values for whole blood in parentheses.

The randomness of the deviations in both normal and diabetic subjects is evident from Figures 1-2 and 1-3 and from the fact that the mean glucose concentrations of the two tests were virtually identical in both studies (15, 16). Although this finding may be valuable to the investigator, who can study large populations, it is disconcerting to the clinician, who must decide on the basis of only one (or at the most several) OGTTs whether the patient indeed does have diabetes mellitus.

Special Circumstances Affecting the OGTT

Regardless of the criteria used to make the diagnosis (see *Criteria for Diagnosis*) there are three types of subjects for whom special considerations are warranted: pregnant women, patients who have had gastric surgery, and older subjects.

Pregnancy

In pregnancy, carbohydrate homeostasis is changed in two ways. First, because of fetal demands for maternal glucose, the fasting glucose concentrations in the mother are decreased. Secondly, the disposal of a glucose challenge is retarded somewhat, probably because of a substance produced by the placenta (called either human chorionic somatotropin or human placental lactogen) that interferes with the action of insulin. Therefore, the usual criteria must be changed to allow for the lowered fasting glucose levels and the higher values late in the OGTT during normal pregnancy. A modification for the pregnant patient of the criteria adopted by the US Public Health Service (USPHS) is shown in Table 1-1 (17).

Gastric Surgery

An OGTT cannot be used to diagnose diabetes mellitus in patients who have undergone gastric surgery. The relation between the stomach and duodenum has been altered in such a way that the orally administered carbohydrate load passes quickly into the small intestine. This event leads to rapid absorption and to levels of glucose that are much higher than normal soon after ingestion of the carbohydrate. Insulin secretion is enhanced by these elevated concentrations of glucose, and the markedly elevated insulin levels often lead to hypoglycemia (see chapter 10). Therefore, elevated glucose concentrations early in the OGTT are to be expected and cannot serve to diagnose the patient as diabetic. However, an increased fasting glucose level in these patients continues to be the basis for diagnosing diabetes mellitus. If the fasting glucose concentration is normal or nearly normal, the only way to diagnose diabetes mellitus is to perform an IVGTT, which is usually less sensitive than an OGTT.

Age

The effect of age on the results of glucose tolerance testing is profound (18). The fasting glucose concentration increases by approximately 1 mg/100 ml per decade of age—a change that is clinically insignificant. However, after oral administration of a glucose load, the increase in 1-hour values per decade of age ranges from 4 to 14 mg/100 ml (with a mean of 9.5 mg/100 ml); for 2-hour values, the increase ranges from 1 to 11 mg/100 ml (with a mean of 5.3 mg/100 ml). Many studies have found a disproportionate increase in subjects over the age of 50 years (18). The distribution of glucose concentrations after a carbohydrate challenge is unimodal rather than bimodal. This fact implies that there are not two separate populations—one normal and one diabetic—with a preponderance of diabetic subjects in the older age group responsible for the observed effect of aging on the OGTT. Thus, further difficulty is encountered in deciding what the cutoff should be between normal and abnormal glucose levels. If the usual criteria, which were based on studies in younger normal individuals, are used for evaluation of the OGTT in subjects over 50 years of age, approximately 50% of the tests given to the latter group will be considered abnormal.

The cause(s) of the effect of aging on carbohydrate metabolism remain(s) obscure (18). Delayed absorption from the gastrointestinal tract is not a factor. Five other possibilities have been proposed: poor diet, physical inactivity, decreased lean body mass in which ingested carbohydrate may be stored, altered insulin secretion, and insulin antagonism.

As discussed previously, the preparatory diet has an extremely important influence on the OGTT. Seltzer (3) compared the 2-hour glucose concentration (after a 100-g load) before a 3-day high-carbohydrate diet with the 2-hour concentration after 3 days of such a diet in 24 nondiabetic subjects over the age of 50 years. The preparatory diet lowered this value in 23 of the 24 individuals. Fourteen of these subjects had abnormal values (according to the more sensitive criteria) when tested before the preparatory diet.

However, diet cannot entirely explain the effect of aging on carbohydrate metabolism. Many of the studies reporting such an effect have paid careful atten-

Table 1-2. Effect of Diet and Physical Activity on the Percentage of Abnormal Results in the OGTT Among an Older Population[a]

Diet	Activity	Abnormal (%)
Poor	Low	53
Normal	Low	33
Normal	Normal	17

[a]Adapted from Seltzer HS: Diagnosis of diabetes. In *Diabetes Mellitus: Theory and Practice.* Edited by Ellenberg M. Rifkin H. McGraw-Hill, New York, 1970, pp 436–507. Copyright © 1970 by McGraw-Hill, Inc. Used with permission of McGraw-Hill Book Company.

tion to diet. By the same token, some reports have assessed the amount of physical activity of older subjects and have concluded that decreased activity is not a factor in altered carbohydrate metabolism. Seltzer (3) has summarized 11 published papers on the relationship between diet and physical activity with regard to the OGTT in subjects over the age of 50 years (Table 1-2). Although the results of proportionately fewer OGTTs were abnormal as the amount of carbohydrates in the diet and the amount of exercise were increased, a substantial percentage remained abnormal. Thus, impaired glucose tolerance in the older age groups would not seem to be explained fully by poor dietary habits and lack of physical activity.

Of the remaining three possibilities, most of the evidence favors the presence of insulin antagonism in aging populations. However, the effect of aging on carbohydrate metabolism is probably heterogeneous in nature. Some or all of the five possible factors may affect glucose tolerance in individual subjects in varying degrees. Alternatively, the impairment of glucose tolerance in older subjects may represent a heterogeneous group of separate disorders. Whatever the cause(s), the effect of age on the interpretation of the OGTT remains a problem for the clinician.

Criteria for Diagnosis

Having considered the many factors that influence glucose tolerance testing, let us now turn our attention to the criteria on which the diagnosis of diabetes mellitus should be based. Six different sets of criteria promulgated by various authorities are summarized in Table 1-3. The numbers listed are concentrations in plasma with the corresponding values for whole blood in parentheses. Unless stated otherwise, all of the glucose levels in any set of criteria must be exceeded before the diagnosis of diabetes mellitus can be made. Four sets of criteria are relatively sensitive: those of Fajans and Conn, the World Health Organization (WHO), the British Diabetic Association (BDA), and the University Group

Table 1-3. Various Criteria for the Diagnosis of Diabetes Mellitus

		Glucose Concentrations $(mg/100\ ml)^a$			
Study (reference)	Glucose Load	Fasting	1 hr	2 hr	3 hr
Fajans and Conn (19)	1.75 g/kg of ideal weight		185(160)	140(120)	
USPHS[b] (20)	100 g	125(110); 1 point	195(170); ½ point	140(120); ½ point	125(110); 1 point
WHO (21)	50 or 100 g			150(130)	
BDA (22)	50 g		185(160)	125(110)	
UGDP (23)	30 g/m² of body surface	⟵Sum of fasting, 1-, 2-, and 3-hour values, > 600(500)⟶			
ESGDE (24)	50 g		250(220)	175(150)	

[a]Concentrations exceeding the listed values are abnormal. Values for plasma are given, with corresponding values for whole blood in parentheses.
[b]A score of 2 points or more is sufficient for the diagnosis.

Diabetes Program (UGDP). The remaining two sets—from the USPHS and the European Study Group of Diabetes Epidemiology (ESGDE)—are less sensitive.

Importance of the Criteria Selected

As might be expected, the more sensitive the criteria used, the more patients will be labeled diabetic. In one study (25), 340 subjects who presented them-selves for testing at a diabetes detection center were given an OGTT with 75 g of glucose over a 5-hour period. They were instructed to eat at least 200 g of carbohydrate during each of the 3 days preceding the test. The results were analyzed by all six sets of criteria. The prevalence of diabetes mellitus, according to the various criteria, was found to be as follows: BDA, 51%; UGDP, 48%; Fajans and Conn, 45%; WHO, 41%; USPHS, 24%; and ESGDE, 18%. The preva-lence was approximately twice as high when one of the four sensitive sets of criteria was used as when one of the two less sensitive sets was applied. (The fact that the prevalence of diabetes mellitus in these 340 subjects was much higher than in the general population, regardless of the criteria utilized, was anticipated, since many of these individuals had reason to present themselves for testing.) In another study (26), 13% of 746 individuals who were first-degree relatives of diabetics and were given an OGTT were found to be diabetic according to the USPHS criteria, 29% according to the criteria of Fajans and Conn, and 26% according to the UGDP criteria.

The profound importance of the criteria used to diagnose diabetes mellitus is also apparent in unselected populations. Five per cent of the population of Sudbury, Massachusetts, were given an OGTT after appropriate dietary prepara-tion (27). Known diabetics were excluded from the study. The prevalences of diabetes mellitus according to the USPHS, Fajans and Conn, and BDA criteria were 1.2%, 5.6%, and 6.8%, respectively. In the Bedford survey (28), 15.7% of the population was considered to have diabetes mellitus if the selected cutoff point was a 2-hour glucose concentration of more than 120 mg/100 ml in capil-lary whole blood after a 50-g challenge. The prevalence was reduced to 6.6% if a 140 mg/100 ml cutoff point was used. Over one third (35.2%) were considered diabetic if a peak value exceeding 180 mg/100 ml was utilized as the sole diag-nostic criterion, but if both the peak value and a 2-hour level of 120 mg/100 ml were used, only 11.1% could be labeled diabetic. Clearly, the prevalence of diabetes mellitus varies widely depending on the diagnostic criteria selected.

A Prospective Approach to Validating Criteria

The major difficulty in deciding which patients really do have diabetes mellitus is that there are currently no criteria other than glucose concentrations to confirm the diagnosis. A prospective approach to resolving this problem might be as follows. Abnormal glucose levels would be established; the levels chosen would be high enough to permit little disagreement about their abnormality. Then a group of subjects with normal fasting glucose concentrations but impaired glucose tolerance (according to various criteria) would be followed in order to ascertain the rate at which they could be clearly labeled diabetic. The results of 12 studies based on such a design are summarized in Table 1-4. Both the criteria used to classify these subjects as suspect in terms of subsequent deterioration of carbohydrate metabolism and the criteria used to diagnose overt diabetes mellitus are listed. The follow-up period in these reports ranged from 1 to 28 years.

Only a minority of the subjects suspected of becoming diabetic developed overt diabetes mellitus, despite the long follow-up period in most studies. Nine studies (29-31, 36-40, 42) evaluated the eventual deterioration of carbohydrate metabolism in suspected diabetics who were classified as such by a single set of criteria. Of these 1,023 subjects, only 21.4% developed overt diabetes mellitus.

Three additional studies (32, 35, 41) compared various criteria for predicting eventual deterioration. The rate of decompensation over a 10-year period in one report (35) is depicted in Figure 1-4.[*] The criteria used by the USPHS and by Fajans and Conn to classify the subjects initially as suspected diabetics are listed in Table 1-3. The criteria of Mosenthal and Barry are the most sensitive of the three sets compared: whole blood glucose values exceeding 150 and 101 mg/100 ml at 1 and 2 hours, respectively, during an OGTT. The criteria for decompensation are listed in Table 1-4. Of the 352 subjects meeting the criteria of Mosenthal and Barry, 9% manifested overt diabetes mellitus 10 years later. Of the 263 subjects who initially met the criteria of Fajans and Conn, 27% decompensated during this period. Of the 159 suspected diabetics who met the more rigorous criteria of the USPHS, over half (52%) subsequently developed overt diabetes mellitus.

In the second study, which had a follow-up period of 14 to 15 years (32), the maximal glucose concentration in whole blood during the initial OGTT was used to classify the subject. Of 57 subjects who had values exceeding 170 mg/100 ml, 40% went on to develop overt diabetes mellitus; of 110 subjects who had values between 140 and 170 mg/100 ml, only 14% showed subsequent deterioration of carbohydrate metabolism.

The third study (42) highlights the importance of the 2-hour value compared with the 1-hour level during a glucose tolerance test in predicting the eventual development of diabetes mellitus. Of 145 subjects with 1-hour glucose concentrations exceeding 180 mg/100 ml, 31 had 2-hour values of more than 135 mg/100 ml and 114 had levels of less than 135 mg/100 ml. Almost half (14 subjects) of the former group but only 2 of the latter group developed fasting

---

[*]The values for decompensation to overt diabetes differ between Table 1-4 and Figure 1-4 because those in the latter are calculated by an actuarial life-table technique in order to estimate what would have been found if all the patients had been observed for the full duration of the study.

Table 1-4. Follow-up of Subjects with Abnormal Results in the OGTT

Reference	Type of Subject	No.	Criteria for Classification	Years of Follow-up
29	Suspected diabetics	133	Abnormal OGTT result or glycosuria	>10, with majority >15
30	Suspected diabetics	200	<2.5 hrs, >180 mg/100 ml;[a] > 2.5 hrs, > 120 mg/100 ml[a]	10-28
	Controls	200	<2.5 hrs, <180 mg/100 ml;[a] >2.5 hrs, <120 mg/100 ml[a]	
31	Suspected diabetics	33	Abnormal OGTT	5
	Controls	62	Normal OGTT	
32	Suspected diabetics	57	1-2 hrs, >170 mg/100 ml[a]	14-15
	Suspected diabetics	110	1-2 hrs, 140-170 mg/100 ml[a]	
	Controls	262	1-2 hrs, <140 mg/100 ml[a]	
33	Suspected diabetics	83	F, >110 mg/100 ml; 1 hr, >170 mg/100 ml;[b] 2 hrs, >120 mg/100 ml;[b] 3 hrs, >110 mg/100 ml[b] (requires both F and 3-hr *or* 3 of 4 values exceeded)	2
34	Suspected diabetics	27[c]	*Either* F, >120 mg/100 ml, and 1.5 hrs, >200 mg/100 ml;[b] *or* 1.5 hrs, >220 mg/100 ml[b]	1-2
35	Suspected diabetics	352	1 hr, >151 mg/100 ml;[b] 2 hrs, >101 mg/100 ml[b]	10

	Follow-up Result		
	Overt Diabetes		
Criteria for Diagnosis	*%*	*Risk Factor*	*Normal (%)*
"Frank diabetes"	29	Positive family history	
F, > 140 mg/100 ml; < 2.5 hrs, > 300 mg/ 100 ml;[a] > 2.5 hrs, > 140 mg/100 ml[a]	29	>50 years of age (>50% diabetic in first 5 years)	
	10	Most subjects diabetic 10-20 years later	
Markedly abnormal OGTT or treatment as diabetic	21		24
	1.5		
F, >140 mg/100 ml >200 mg/100 ml[a]	40	*Both* positive family history *and* obesity	
	14		
	3		
			28
			15
Either <3 hrs, >300 mg/100 ml;[b] *or* both <5 hrs, >180 mg/100 ml,[a] and F, >120 mg/100 ml	9	Obesity	

continued

Table 1-4 *(continued)*

Refer-ence	Type of Subject	No.	Criteria for Classification	Years of Follow-up
	Suspected diabetics	263	1 hr > 160 mg/100 ml;[b] 2 hrs > 120 mg/100 ml[b]	
	Suspected diabetics	159	F, > 110 mg/100 ml; 1 hr, > 170 mg/100 ml;[b] 2 hrs, > 120 mg/100 ml;[b] 3 hrs, > 110 mg/100 ml[b] (requires both F and 3-hr *or* 3 of 4 values exceeded)	
36	Suspected diabetics	46	ΣF, 0.5, 1, and 2 hrs, 501-650 mg/100 ml[b]	1
	Controls	32	ΣF, 0.5, 1, and 2 hrs, < 500 mg/100 ml[b]	
37	Suspected diabetics[d]	183	Glucose values > 2 SD above means for normal age-matched controls after oral glucose	10
38	Suspected diabetics	12	Normal fasting value but failure to return to base-line value 2 hrs after glucose	5
	Controls	32	Return to baseline value by 2 hrs after glucose	
39	Suspected diabetics	118	Σ1 and 2 hrs, > 300 mg/100 ml,[b] F, < 120 mg/100 ml	5
40	Suspected diabetics	94	Abnormal OGTT result	0.5-6 (mean, 2)
41[f]	Suspected diabetics	31	1 hr, > 180 mg/100 ml;[b] 2 hrs, > 135 mg/100 ml;[b]	10
	Lag storage	114	1 hr, > 180 mg/100 ml;[b] 2 hrs, < 135 mg/100 ml;[b]	
	Controls	193	1 hr, < 180 mg/100 ml;[b] 2 hrs, < 135 mg/100 ml[b]	

Follow-up Result			
Overt Diabetes			
Criteria for Diagnosis	%	Risk Factor	Normal (%)
	27		
	52		
ΣF, 0.5, 1, and 2 hrs, >650 mg/100 ml[b]	24		15
	3		
Glucose values >3 SD above means for normal age-matched controls after oral glucose	19	Obesity; increased diastolic blood pressure [after 2-5 years, no cases of diabetes[e]]	
"Clinical diabetes" (required treatment)	8		40
	3		
Σ1 and 2 hrs, >300 mg/100 ml;[b] F, >120 mg/100 ml	14		36
Not stated	28	Positive family history; <60 yrs, nonobese	36
F, >130 mg/100 ml	45		13[g]
	2		32
	1		

continued

Table 1-4 *(continued)*

Refer-ence	Type of Subject	No.	Criteria for Classification	Years of Follow-up
42[h]	Suspected diabetics	204	All values,[b] <200 mg/100 ml; and peak, >180 mg/100 ml; plus 2 hrs, >120 mg/100 ml; and/or 2 values, >180 mg/100 ml	5
43	Suspected diabetics	37	1 hr, $\geqslant 190$ mg/100 ml;[b] and/or 2 hrs, $\geqslant 140$ mg/100 ml[b]	5

Abbreviations: F, fasting concentration; SD, standard deviation.

[a]Postprandial.

[b]After a glucose challenge.

[c]Number of subjects with hyperglycemia 1 month after myocardial infarction who were followed for 1 to 2 years.

[d]A diet had been prescribed for 124 of these suspected diabetics.

[e]See Carlstrom S, Lundquist A, Lundquist I, et al: Studies in subjects with positive postprandial Clinistix test. III. Special studies and follow-up of cases with borderline glucose tolerance. Acta Med Scand 189:415–422, 1971.

[f]Results are modified to fit the three sets of criteria as follows: groups A and C are included in the controls; group B is included in lag storage; subjects who were originally unclassified are not included; lag storage and suspected diabetics who were designated as unclassified on follow-up are considered normal.

[g]An additional 19% reverted to lag storage (defined as undue hyperglycemia during the early part of an OGTT, but normal 2-hour glucose values).

[h]All glucose challenges were given in the afternoon; for follow-up they were administered every 6 months.

hyperglycemia during a 10-year follow-up period. Thus, as might be expected, the less sensitive the initial criteria (i.e., the more abnormal the glucose levels), the more likely the subjects were to develop overt diabetes mellitus.

Five of the studies already discussed (31, 36, 38-40) and three others listed in Table 1-4 (33, 34, 43) also evaluated the percentage of suspected diabetics whose glucose tolerance returned to normal. Of the 450 subjects in these reports, 31.1% had normal OGTTs when subsequently retested. Finally, five studies compared directly the propensity to develop overt diabetes mellitus in subjects who

	Follow-up Result		
	Overt Diabetes		Normal (%)
Criteria for Diagnosis	%	Risk Factor	
2 successive 2-hr values, >200 mg/100 ml;[b] or 3 nonsuccessive 2-hr values, >200 mg/100 ml;[b] or 2 hrs, >200 mg/100 ml[b] at 5 years; or "unequivocal signs or symptoms of diabetes"	13		
			46

had normal results in an initial OGTT with this propensity in those whose OGTT values exceeded relatively sensitive criteria (30-32, 36, 38). Of the 588 subjects with normal OGTT results, 5.3% subsequently developed diabetes; of the latter patients, the majority became diabetic 10 to 20 years later. Of the 401 suspected diabetics in the same five studies, 22.9% eventually developed overt diabetes mellitus, usually within 5 years. *Thus, although abnormal glucose tolerance clearly delineates a group of subjects who may eventually manifest overt diabetes mellitus, only a minority of these individuals will do so. An approximately equal number of this group will have a normal OGTT in subsequent tests.*

Recommendations Regarding Diagnosis

Given this situation as well as an appreciation of the many variables that have an important influence on the OGTT, the following approach is recommended. The diagnosis of diabetes mellitus is applied to a patient only if fasting hyperglycemia is noted (i.e., a whole-blood glucose concentration exceeding 120 mg/100 ml or a plasma glucose concentration exceeding 140 mg/100 ml) on at least two occasions. If an oral glucose tolerance test is performed (after appropriate dietary preparation), the upper limits of normal are taken to be a plasma glucose level of 185 mg/100 ml at 1 hour and 140 mg/100 ml at 2 hours. The corresponding values for whole blood are 160 mg/100 ml and 120 mg/100 ml, respectively. For each decade of age after the fifth (i.e., after the age of 50 years), 10 mg/100 ml is added to these values. If both the 1- and 2-hour values are

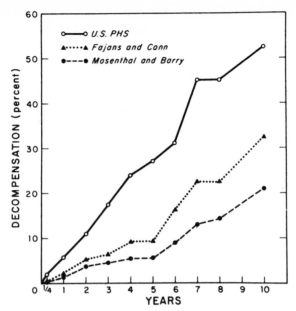

Figure 1-4. Rates of decompensated diabetes. All patients meeting each of the three graded criteria independently are included. Consequently, those with diagnoses based on standards of the US Public Health Service (USPHS)—the least sensitive criteria—are included in all three groups, and those meeting Fajans and Conn criteria—intermediate in sensitivity—are included in the Mosenthal and Barry group. (Reprinted with permission of the *New England Journal of Medicine* from O'Sullivan JB, Mahan CM: Prospective study of 352 young patients with chemical diabetes. N Engl J Med 278:1038-1041, 1968.)

exceeded, the patient is told that glucose intolerance has been found and is warned about the stress effects of obesity and infection (and pregnancy, if applicable). Appropriate dietary advice is given, especially if the patient is obese. Because of the social and occupational (44) as well as the insurance ramifications for a patient who is labeled diabetic, this diagnosis is avoided unless fasting hyperglycemia is found. It must be borne in mind that the majority of these patients will not progress to overt diabetes mellitus and that an appreciable number will have normal results on retesting.

These personal recommendations are in general agreement with the recent suggestions of the National Diabetes Data Group (45), who concerned themselves with the diagnosis and classification of diabetes mellitus and other categories of glucose intolerance. They proposed that the diagnosis of diabetes mellitus be restricted to those persons with (*a*) the classical symptoms of diabetes and unequivocal hyperglycemia, (*b*) fasting plasma glucose concentrations of more than 140 mg/100 ml on more than one occasion, or (*c*) fasting plasma glucose levels of less than 140 mg/100 ml but, on more than one occasion, glucose levels of more than 200 mg/100 ml both 2 hours after ingestion of 75 g of dextrose and at some other time point between 0 and 2 hours. They also proposed that a condition termed *impaired glucose tolerance* be defined for those individuals with the following values on an oral glucose tolerance test: fasting plasma glucose concentrations of less than 140 mg/100 ml, 2-hour plasma concentrations between 140 and 200 mg/100 ml, and one plasma level of more than 200 mg/100 ml between 0 and 2 hours. Finally, normal glucose tolerance (in nonpregnant adults) was defined as a fasting plasma glucose concentration of less than 115 mg/100 ml and a 2-hour level of less than 140 mg/100 ml, with no value of more than 200 mg/100 ml between 0 and 2 hours. Results that are above these normal values but that are below the criteria for either diabetes mellitus or impaired glucose tolerance would be considered "nondiagnostic." The National Diabetes Data Group did suggest that fasting plasma glucose concentrations between 125 and 139 mg/100 ml are probably abnormal. No suggestions were made concerning the adjustment of any of these criteria according to the age of the subject.

The utility of the fasting glucose concentration to establish the diagnosis of diabetes mellitus is supported by studies correlating the results of the OGTT and the development of specific diabetic complications. Diabetic retinopathy and proteinuria were limited to patients whose fasting plasma glucose levels exceeded 140 mg/100 ml (28, 46) and whose 2-hour glucose concentrations were more than 200 mg/100 ml (28) or more than 250 mg/100 ml (46). Since the presence of the microangiopathic complications of diabetes mellitus should serve as a specific marker for this syndrome, the criteria used to make the diagnosis in these particular patients should be relatively reliable.

Practical Summary

The diagnosis of diabetes mellitus should be made when the fasting glucose concentration in plasma exceeds 140 mg/100 ml or the fasting glucose level in whole blood is more than 120 mg/100 ml on more than one occasion. The National Diabetes Data Group would also make the diagnosis in subjects with fasting plasma glucose concentrations of less than 140 mg/100 ml if, on more than one occasion, the glucose levels (determined every 30 minutes for 2 hours) exceeded 200 mg/100 ml both 2 hours after ingestion of 75 g of dextrose and at some time point between 0 and 2 hours. If a glucose tolerance test is performed, subjects should be active and should have ingested 150 to 200 g of carbohydrate during each of the 3 days preceding the test.

The diagnosis of glucose intolerance should be made in subjects whose fasting plasma glucose concentrations are less than 140 mg/100 ml but whose 1- and 2-hour glucose levels during the OGTT exceed 185 and 140 mg/100 ml, respectively. For each decade of age after the fifth (i.e., after 50 years of age), 10 mg/100 ml should be added to these values. The National Diabetes Data Group terms this situation impaired glucose tolerance and recommends such a diagnosis for those subjects with fasting plasma glucose concentrations of less than 140 mg/100 ml, 2-hour plasma glucose levels between 140 and 200 mg/100 ml, and one plasma glucose value of more than 200 mg/100 ml between 0 and 2 hours. No adjustments are made for age.

References

1. Siperstein MD: The glucose tolerance test: a pitfall in the diagnosis of diabetes mellitus. Adv Intern Med 20:297-373, 1975
2. Forster H, Haslbeck M, Mehnert H: Metabolic studies following the oral ingestion of different doses of glucose. Diabetes 21:1102-1108, 1972
3. Seltzer HS: Diagnosis of diabetes. In Diabetes Mellitus: Theory and Practice. Edited by Ellenberg M, Rifkin H. McGraw-Hill, New York, 1970, pp 436-507
4. Wilkerson HLC, Butler FK, Francis JO'S: The effect of prior carbohydrate intake on the oral glucose tolerance test. Diabetes 9:386-391, 1960
5. Lipman RL, Raskin P, Love T, et al: Glucose intolerance during decreased physical activity in man. Diabetes 21:101-107, 1972
6. Aparicio NJ, Puchulu FE, Gagliardino JJ, et al: Circadian variation of the blood glucose, plasma insulin and human growth hormone levels in response to an oral glucose load in normal subjects. Diabetes 23:132-137, 1974
7. Malherbe C, Burrill KC, Levin SR, et al: Effect of diphenylhydantoin on insulin secretion in man. N Engl J Med 286:339-342, 1972
8. Berge KG, Achor RWP, Christensen NA, et al: Hypercholesteremia and nicotinic acid: a long-term study. Am J Med 31:24-36, 1961
9. Hed R, Nygren A, Rojdmark S, Sundblad L: Decreased glucose tolerance in chronic alcoholics after alcohol ingestion when fed a carbohydrate poor diet. Horm Metab Res 7:115-118, 1975
10. Peterson DT, Reaven GM: Evidence that glucose load is an important determinant of plasma insulin response in normal subjects. Diabetes 20:729-733, 1971
11. de Nobel E van 't Laar A: The size of the loading dose as an important determinant of the results of the oral glucose tolerance test. A study in subjects with slightly impaired glucose tolerance. Diabetes 27:42-48, 1978
12. Genuth SM: Plasma insulin response to an oral carbohydrate solution. Diabetes 18:434-436, 1969
13. Kraegen EW, Young JD, George EP, Lazarus L: Oscillations in blood glucose and insulin after oral glucose. Horm Metab Res 4:409-413, 1972
14. Albisser AM, Leibel BS, Ewart TG, et al: An artificial endocrine pancreas. Diabetes 23:389-396, 1974

15. Olefsky JM, Reaven GM: Insulin and glucose responses to identical oral glucose tolerance tests performed forty-eight hours apart. Diabetes 23:449-453, 1974

16. Kosaka K, Mizuno Y, Kuzuya T: Reproducibility of the oral glucose tolerance test and the rice-meal test in mild diabetics. Diabetes 15:901-904, 1966

17. O'Sullivan JB, Mahan CM: Criteria for the oral glucose tolerance test in pregnancy. Diabetes 13:278-285, 1964

18. Davidson MB: The effect of aging on carbohydrate metabolism. A review of the English literature and a practical approach to the diagnosis of diabetes mellitus in the elderly. Metabolism 28:688-705, 1979

19. Fajans SS, Conn JS: Prediabetes, subclinical diabetes and latent clinical diabetes. Interpretation, diagnosis and treatment. In *On the Nature and Treatment of Diabetes*. Excerpta Medica, New York, 1965, pp 641-656

20. Wilkerson HLC: Diagnosis, oral glucose tolerance tests. In *Diabetes Mellitus, Diagnosis and Treatment*. American Diabetes Association, New York, 1964, pp 31-34

21. McDonald GW, Hoet JP, Butterfield WJH: Diabetes mellitus: report of a WHO expert committee. WHO Rep Series no 310, 1965

22. Fitzgerald MG, Keen H: Diagnostic classification of diabetes. Br Med J 1:1568, 1964

23. The University Group Diabetes Program: Mortality. Diabetes 19(Suppl 2):789-830, 1970

24. European Association for the Study of Diabetes: A brief account of the European Diabetes Epidemiology Study Group recommendations and research. Diabetologia 6:453-454, 1970

25. Valleron AJ, Eschwege E, Papoz L, Rosselin GE: Agreement and discrepancy in the evaluation of normal and diabetic oral glucose tolerance test. Diabetes 24:585-593, 1975

26. Kobberling J, Creutzfeldt W: Comparison of different methods for the evaluation of the oral glucose tolerance test. Diabetes 19:870-877, 1970

27. O'Sullivan JB, Williams RF: Early diabetes mellitus in perspective: population study in Sudbury, Mass. JAMA 198:579-582, 1966

28. Jarrett RJ, Keen H: Hyperglycaemia and diabetes mellitus. Lancet 2:1009-1012, 1976

29. Rabinowitch IM: Diabetes mellitus. Am J Dig Dis 16:95-111, 1949

30. McCullagh EP, Fawalt WN: Significance of hyperglycemia without glucosuria. A ten to twenty-eight year study. JAMA 156:925-929, 1954

31. Walker JB, Brown PE: Early diabetes. A five year follow-up of diabetes in an English community. Lancet 2:246-248, 1964

32. O'Sullivan JB, Mahan C: Blood sugar level, glycosuria and body weight related to development of diabetes mellitus. The Oxford epidemiologic study 17 years later. JAMA 194:587-592, 1965

33. O'Sullivan JB, Hurwitz D: Spontaneous remissions in early diabetes mellitus. Arch Intern Med 117:769-774, 1966

34. Datey KK, Nanda NC: Hyperglycemia after acute myocardial infarction. Its relation to diabetes mellitus. N Engl J Med 276:262-265, 1967

35. O'Sullivan JB, Mahan CM: Prospective study of 352 young patients with chemical diabetes. N Engl J Med 278:1038-1041, 1968

36. Danowski TS: The evolution of diabetes from prediabetes. Postgrad Med J 46:125-130, 1970

37. Sartor G, Schersten B, Carlstrom S, et al: Ten-year follow-up of subjects with impaired glucose tolerance. Prevention of diabetes by tolbutamide and diet regulation. Diabetes 29:41-49, 1980

38. Strauss WT, Hales CN: Plasma insulin in minor abnormalities of glucose tolerance: a 5 year follow-up. Diabetologia 10:237-243, 1974

39. Kobberling J, Kattermann R, Arnold A: Follow-up of 'non-diabetic' relatives of diabetics by retesting oral glucose tolerance after 5 years. Diabetologia 11:451-456, 1975

40. Lubetzki J, Duprey J, Warnet A, et al: Borderline OGTT. Its evolution in correlation with some clinical and biological features. Study in 94 subjects (abstract). Diabetologia 12:407, 1976

41. Diabetes Survey Working Party: Ten-year follow-up report on Birmingham Diabetes Survey of 1961. Br Med J 2:35-37, 1976

42. Jarrett RJ, Keen H, Fuller JH, McCartney M: Worsening to diabetes in men with impaired glucose tolerance ('borderline diabetes'). Diabetologia 16:25-30, 1979

43. Genuth SM, Houser HB, Carter JR Jr, et al: Observations on the value of mass indiscriminate screening for diabetes mellitus based on a five-year follow-up. Diabetes 27:377-383, 1978

44. Knibbs S, Jackson JGL: Social and emotional complications of diabetes. In Complications of Diabetes. Edited by Keen H, Jarrett J. Year Book Medical Publishers, Chicago, 1975, pp 265-277

45. National Diabetes Data Group: Classification and diagnosis of diabetes mellitus and other categories of glucose intolerance. Diabetes 28:1039-1057, 1979

46. Rushforth NB, Miller M, Bennett PH: Fasting and two-hour post-load glucose levels for the diagnosis of diabetes. The relationship between glucose levels and complications of diabetes in the Pima Indians. Diabetologia 16:373-379, 1979

Chapter 2

Treatment—General Principles

Metabolic Principles

In the postabsorptive state, the plasma glucose concentration remains relatively constant and reflects the balance between glucose production by the liver and glucose utilization by peripheral tissues. The sources of hepatic glucose production are glycogenolysis (the breakdown of glycogen, the storage form of glucose) and gluconeogenesis (the synthesis of new glucose from noncarbohydrate precursors). After 8 to 12 hours without food intake, hepatic glycogenolysis ceases, and gluconeogenesis by the liver is the sole source of circulating glucose. At this time, glucose is utilized mainly by the brain and red blood cells, while the rest of the tissues use free fatty acids (FFA). The role of the basal insulin levels in the fasting state is to oppose the effect of glucagon on the liver and to restrain hepatic glucose production by modulating gluconeogenesis. Insulin does not affect peripheral glucose utilization by the brain or red blood cells.

Insulin is secreted in response to the carbohydrate and protein contents of a meal. Approximately 90% of the ingested carbohydrate traverses the liver, where the majority (55% to 60%) is stored as glycogen and the remainder released as glucose. In the 3-hour period after a meal, approximately 25% of the carbohydrate ingested is utilized by the non-insulin-dependent tissues (brain and red blood cells), while only 15% is metabolized by the peripheral insulin-sensitive tissues (muscle and fat). Less than 5% remains in the extracellular space.

Insulin increases the amount of glucose transported into muscle and fat tissues. Its effects on hepatic carbohydrate metabolism are complex. Essentially, insulin stimulates the utilization of glucose by enhancing its storage as glycogen, by diverting it into triglycerides, or by increasing glycolysis. Insulin also inhibits gluconeogenesis and glycogenolysis. The overall results of insulin action on the liver are an increase in glucose utilization after meals and a restraint on glucose production in the postabsorptive state.

Insulin also has a profound influence on fat metabolism. Ingested fat is stored in triglycerides in adipose tissue. Excess carbohydrate calories also form part of the triglyceride molecule. Insulin promotes triglyceride synthesis by helping the dietary fat to gain access into the fat cell and by stimulating the conversion of glucose to glycerol, the backbone of the triglyceride molecule. Once adipose tissue triglycerides are formed, insulin plays a critical role in inhibiting their breakdown. This effect is extremely important because the FFA released as a result of triglyceride hydrolysis (lipolysis) can be converted to ketone bodies in the liver. In fact, the most important determinant of the rate of formation of ketone bodies is the amount of FFA delivered to the liver. If excess FFA are released from adipose tissue, increased production of ketone bodies by the liver will follow. Although these ketone bodies can be utilized to some extent by peripheral tissues, they soon start to accumulate in the circulation and spill over into the urine.

The quantitative relation among the effects of insulin on selected aspects of carbohydrate and fat metabolism is depicted in Figure 2-1. Approximately 50 to 100 μU of insulin/ml is necessary to affect glucose metabolism by liver and muscle; 10 μU/ml is required to stimulate glucose uptake into fat. However, the inhibition of lipolysis requires only 1 μU of insulin/ml. Therefore, as the amount of effective insulin diminishes from normal, the first biochemical abnormality to develop will be postprandial hyperglycemia. Enough insulin will remain to maintain normal fasting glucose concentrations and to prevent ketosis. As the process continues, fasting hyperglycemia will develop but the patient still will

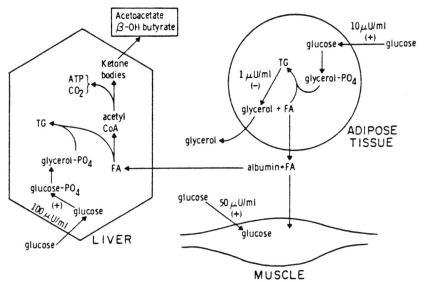

Figure 2-1. Pathophysiology of ketosis. ATP, adenosine triphosphate; (+), stimulation by insulin; (−), inhibition by insulin; TG, triglyceride; FA, fatty acid.

not become ketotic. Only when there is virtually no effective insulin available will ketosis occur. In other words, if an untreated diabetic does not manifest ketonuria, the pancreatic β-cells of that patient are still able to secrete some insulin. Alternatively, if a diabetic has ketonuria, very little, if any, effective insulin remains. (This discussion refers to diabetic ketosis and not to starvation ketosis, which will be discussed in chapter 7.)

Functional Classification of Diabetes Mellitus

The distinguishing of ketosis-resistant from ketosis-prone diabetics has important implications for therapy.* Since ketosis-prone diabetics have virtually no effective endogenous insulin, they require exogenous insulin. The need for insulin is not as imperative in ketosis-resistant diabetics, since without it they do not become ketotic and slip into acidosis. Ketosis-resistant patients may require insulin because sulfonylurea agents and/or diet fail to control hyperglycemia. However, in most cases, such patients can be treated with these other modalities for a while without undue risk before the decision regarding insulin therapy is made.

Ketosis-prone and ketosis-resistant diabetics differ in aspects other than the need for insulin therapy. These differences are summarized in Table 2-1. Ketosis-prone diabetes has classically been called juvenile-onset diabetes. This term is not accurate, however, because a small percentage of diabetics whose disease starts in adulthood may be ketosis-prone. Furthermore, an increasing number of patients in their teens or at the end of the first decade of life have been found to have ketosis-resistant diabetes. Patients who have ketosis-prone diabetes usually present with a short history of the symptoms of hyperglycemia (polyuria, polydipsia, lethargy, weight loss), and if their condition is not recognized quickly, it may develop into ketoacidosis.

Although the etiology of ketosis-prone diabetes is unclear, recent studies in epidemiology, virology, immunology, and genetics have suggested that an altered immune response to a viral assault on the pancreas in susceptible individuals may result in β-cell destruction. The amount of insulin remaining in the pancreas of ketosis-prone diabetics (if any does remain) is extremely small, and the fasting and stimulated insulin levels are also very low. Therefore, carbohydrate metabolism in these patients is extremely abnormal, leading to fasting hyperglycemia and a marked abnormality of glucose tolerance. The metabolic response to fasting (without insulin therapy) is ketosis and eventually ketoacidosis. Stresses such as infection or emotional upset may also lead to ketosis and possibly to ketoacidosis unless the insulin dosage is increased appropriately. Ketosis-prone patients are

---

*Since this chapter was written, a more formal classification of diabetes has been promulgated. In the terminology recently suggested by the National Diabetes Data Group (Diabetes 28:1039-1057, 1979), ketosis-prone patients have type 1 diabetes, and ketosis-resistant patients have type 2 diabetes.

Table 2-1. Functional Classification of Diabetes Mellitus[a]

Characteristic	Classification	
	Ketosis-Prone (type 1)	*Ketosis-Resistant (type 2)*
Synonyms[b]	Juvenile-onset diabetes, growth-onset diabetes	Adult-onset diabetes, maturity-onset diabetes
Age of onset	Usually during growth	Usually during maturity, increasing with age
Precipitating factors	Altered immune response to certain viruses (?)	Pregnancy, obesity, "stress" (e.g., infection)
Extractable pancreatic insulin	Low	Normal
Fasting insulin level	Absent or low	Low to normal (when adjusted for weight and glucose level)
Insulin responses to glucose	Little or none	Delayed and probably low when adjusted for weight and glucose levels in many (but not all) patients
Insulin antagonism	Absent	Present (independent of obesity)
Fasting glucose level	Markedly elevated	Often near normal
Carbohydrate intolerance	Severe	Moderate to severe
Response to prolonged fast	Hyperglycemia, ketoacidosis	Normal adjustment established
Response to stress	Ketoacidosis	Hyperglycemia without ketosis
Associated obesity	Absent	Commonly present ($\sim 80\%$)
Sensitivity to insulin	Quite sensitive	Relatively resistant
Response to diet alone	Negligible	Always present to some degree
Response to sulfonylurea agent	Absent	Present

[a]Reproduced with permission from Goodner CJ: Newer concepts in diabetes mellitus, including management. DM, September 1965, p 19. Copyright © 1965, Year Book Medical Publishers, Inc, Chicago.

[b]Although these terms have been used classically to refer to the two types of diabetes mellitus, they are inaccurate because some children and adolescents are ketosis resistant and some adults are ketosis prone.

usually sensitive to insulin, probably because they are generally not obese. Because ketosis-prone diabetics have an absolute requirement for insulin, they do not respond either to dietary therapy alone or to dietary therapy supplemented with sulfonylurea agents.

Ketosis-resistant patients are often called maturity-onset or adult-onset diabetics. As was stated previously, however, ketosis-prone diabetes can start in adults and ketosis-resistant diabetes (never progressing to ketosis) occurs in children. Nevertheless, the majority of cases of ketosis-resistant diabetes do begin after the age of 40 years. Pregnancy and obesity have been recognized as two precipitating factors, and occasionally an infection coincides with the diagnosis. In most ketosis-resistant patients, however, few or no symptoms herald the onset of diabetes mellitus. Insulin is present in the pancreas and the circulation. Whether these patients are insulinopenic is still an extremely controversial point. Most ketosis-resistant patients are obese, and elevated insulin concentrations are associated with obesity. Diabetic individuals also have higher glucose levels than do nondiabetic control subjects. When appropriate adjustments are made for these two factors, many (but not all) patients with ketosis-resistant diabetes are found to have diminished insulin secretion. Insulin antagonism, independent of obesity, has also been demonstrated in these patients. Whether the primary defect resides in low insulin secretion or insulin antagonism has yet to be determined. In all probability, ketosis-resistant diabetes represents a heterogeneous group of disorders, and more than one set of pathogenetic determinants will be uncovered.

Regardless of the cause(s), the carbohydrate abnormality in ketosis-resistant patients may be mild, with a nearly normal fasting glucose concentration and a moderately abnormal glucose tolerance test. In contrast to the situation in ketosis-prone diabetics, decreased food intake in the absence of drugs (insulin or sulfonylurea agents) results in improved carbohydrate metabolism in obese ketosis-resistant patients. Similarly, with rare exceptions, the response to stress is hyperglycemia without ketosis or ketoacidosis. If insulin is required relatively large amounts are necessary, probably because of insulin antagonism engendered by obesity. These patients always respond to some extent either to dietary therapy alone or to dietary therapy supplemented with sulfonylurea agents. Thus, the functional classification of diabetes between ketosis-prone and ketosis-resistant patients delineates certain metabolic characteristics with important clinical ramifications.

The prevalence of ketosis-prone and ketosis-resistant diabetes is shown in Figure 2-2. Of a hypothetical 100 diabetic patients, a small minority (5% to 10%) will have ketosis-prone diabetes. An unknown number, but certainly a small proportion, will be young (<20 years of age) ketosis-resistant diabetics. The great majority will have adult-onset diabetes; of these patients, most will be obese and ketosis-resistant. Normal-weight, adult-onset diabetics will be either ketosis-prone or ketosis-resistant. A minority of the ketosis-resistant diabetics (not necessarily those who are not obese) will require insulin (see chapter 5).

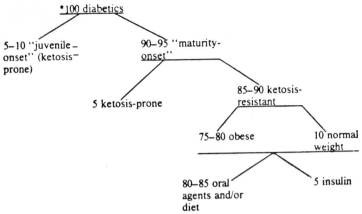

Figure 2-2. Distribution of ketosis-prone versus ketosis-resistant diabetes in a hypothetical population of 100 diabetic patients. Asterisk indicates that it has recently been recognized that ketosis-resistant diabetes occurs in older children and adolescents; the prevalence of this phenomenon is unknown at present.

Relation of Diabetic Control to Vascular Complications

The causes of death in the diabetic population changed drastically after the introduction of insulin therapy by Banting and Best in 1922 (Fig. 2-3). Today the vast majority of diabetic patients die from one of the vascular complications.

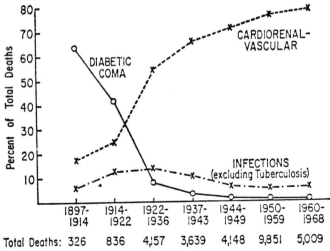

Figure 2-3. Causes of death in persons with diabetes monitored by the Joslin Clinic in Boston, Massachusetts. (Reprinted with permission from Diabetes 21 [Suppl 2]:632–636, 1971.)

These complications usually do not develop until many years after the onset of diabetes mellitus. Thus, there is ample time in which to prevent, or at least ameliorate, these complications. In recent years, accumulating evidence (1) from studies both of animal models of diabetes and of human diabetics has strongly suggested that good control of diabetes (as maintained by monitoring of the parameters of carbohydrate metabolism) is associated with a lessening or, in some instances, a reversal of diabetic microangiopathy, the clinical expression of which is diabetic retinopathy and glomerulosclerosis. However, few convincing data suggest that the macroangiopathy observed in diabetics (a condition causing accelerated vascular disease in the coronary, cerebral, and peripheral arteries) is influenced by control of diabetes. The relation between diabetic control and diabetic microangiopathy will be reviewed briefly here. [For a fuller discussion and complete documentation, see (1)].

Evidence from Studies in Animals

Glomerulosclerosis and retinopathy are found in all animal models of diabetes mellitus, whether occurring spontaneously or induced by chemical, viral, or dietary means. Specifically, glomerulosclerosis has been documented in monkeys with alloxan-induced diabetes; in dogs with diabetes occurring spontaneously, induced by alloxan, or induced by growth hormone (an insulin antagonist); and in rats rendered diabetic by streptozotocin, alloxan, a high-sucrose diet, or inoculation with encephalomyocarditis virus. Retinopathy occurs in rats made diabetic by streptozotocin, alloxan, or a high-sucrose diet and in dogs with spontaneously occurring or alloxan-induced diabetes. The morphologic hallmark of diabetic microangiopathy is increased thickness of the basement membranes surrounding capillaries, not only in the eyes and kidneys but in most other tissues throughout the body. Increased thickness of basement membranes of capillaries in muscular and glomerular tissues was demonstrated in monkeys with spontaneously occurring diabetes mellitus and in dogs with diabetes induced by alloxan or growth hormone. In monkeys (as in humans), the width of the basement membrane is related to the duration of the disease.

Reversion of the disordered metabolism to normal or nearly normal has a profound beneficial effect on the microangiopathic lesions in these animal models. In one study (2), glucose concentrations in diabetic dogs were well controlled (mean, 127 mg/100 ml) for 5 years (equivalent to 25 years of human life) with multiple daily injections of regular insulin; these dogs developed only mild cataracts and vascular changes in the eyes, kidneys, and muscles. Other diabetic dogs that were treated with suboptimal injections of intermediate-acting insulin and consequently had poorly controlled glucose concentrations (mean, 384 mg/100 ml) had severe cataracts and vascular changes.

Transplantation of pancreatic islets between genetically identical rats results in normalization of glucose and insulin levels in diabetic animals. Associated with this reversal of metabolic abnormalities is the regression of diabetic glomerulosclerosis and retinopathy. Transplantation of a kidney from a diabetic rat with glomerulosclerosis into a nondiabetic litter mate results in reversal of the vascular changes. Conversely, a normal kidney transplanted into a diabetic animal soon develops microangiopathic lesions.

Finally, decreased conduction velocity in motor nerves characterizes diabetic peripheral neuropathy and occurs soon after the induction of diabetes by streptozotocin in rats (mean glucose level, 539 mg/100 ml). If glucose concentrations are returned to normal (mean, 75 mg/100 ml) by twice-daily injections of long-acting insulin, the conduction velocity also returns to normal within 2 weeks. However, partial lowering of glucose levels (mean, 214 mg/100 ml) did not affect conduction velocity.

Evidence from Studies in Humans

Both indirect and direct evidence from studies in humans supports the idea of a relation between good control of glucose levels and fewer diabetic complications. Investigators who argue that the microangiopathic changes of diabetes mellitus are not caused by chronic hyperglycemia postulate that these complications follow an independent, genetically determined course. If this were true, patients whose diabetes mellitus is secondary to another condition would not have microangiopathic complications. However, the prevalence of both thickened glomerular basement membranes and the clinical manifestations thereof (retinopathy and glomerulosclerosis) in patients whose diabetes is secondary to pancreatitis, hemochromatosis, or carcinoma is similar to the prevalence in patients with genetic diabetes mellitus. By the same token, if the complications followed an independent, genetically determined course, it might be expected that microangiopathic changes would be present in some patients before metabolic abnormality developed. However, at the time of diagnosis in juvenile-onset diabetes, capillaries in the glomerulus, muscle, and ear lobes have basement membranes of normal widths, and the widths increase within several years. One report purports to show a slight but statistically significant increase in the thickness of basement membranes in the muscle capillaries of prediabetic individuals; however, this observation is not only unconfirmed but, in my view, has been amply refuted (3).

Direct evidence in humans for the relation between well-controlled glucose levels and diabetic complications is the appearance within several years of diabetic vascular changes in kidneys transplanted from normal donors into diabetic recipients. Conversely, vascular lesions cleared completely within 6 months after diabetic kidneys were inadvertently transplanted into two nondiabetic recipients.

Retrospective Studies. Many retrospective and a few prospective studies attempting to relate diabetic control and complications in humans have also provided direct evidence for this relation. In 1964, Knowles (4) reviewed 300 retrospective studies from 85 different centers. Fifty of these centers concluded that poor control was positively correlated with vascular disease, 25 concluded that there was no relation, and 10 were undecided. Knowles himself felt that most of the data reported were inadequate to serve as a basis for any decision and therefore, that an association between control and vascular complications remained unproven.

The difficulty of achieving good control with the current methods of treatment presents a problem in the interpretation of retrospective studies. The criteria for good control espoused by the Joslin Clinic in Boston, outspoken advocates of strict regulation, are summarized in Table 2-2. At least 70% of all glucose concentrations in plasma and whole blood must be lower than the listed value in order to achieve a given rating. Any physician who has cared for diabetics will recognize the difficulty of achieving good control as defined by the Joslin Clinic (especially in the insulin-requiring patient). Even the clinic itself admits to a success rate of only 15% (5). Therefore, most retrospective studies have compared patients whose diabetic control has ranged between fair and poor. Since it takes a number of years for microangiopathic complications of diabetes to become clinically manifest and since during this period diabetic control no doubt varies in each patient, it may be unrealistic to expect meaningful data from studies of small groups of patients. Furthermore, isolated measurements of glucose concentrations, qualitative urine tests, or even quantitative measurements of 24-hour urinary glucose excretion may not be accurate reflections of a patient's control during a given period.

Even with these limitations, one unique retrospective study deserves special comment. Johnsson (6) compared the prevalence of retinopathy and nephropathy in two series of diabetics whose diabetes was diagnosed in Malmö, Sweden, before they had reached the age of 40 years. Series I included those patients whose diagnosis was made between 1922 and 1936. During this period attempts were made to keep the urine sugar-free by means of a strict diet and short-acting

Table 2-2. Joslin Clinic Criteria for Diabetic Control

| Time | Glucose Concentration Required for Indicated Rating[a] | | |
	Good	Fair	Poor
Fasting	125(110)	150(130)	
1 hr postprandial	170(150)	205(180)	All higher values
2 hrs postprandial	150(130)	170(150)	
3 hrs postprandial	125(110)	150(130)	

[a]Concentrations required 70% of the time. Values for plasma are presented, with corresponding values for whole blood in parentheses.

insulin, the only preparation available. Series II included those patients whose diabetes was diagnosed between 1936 and 1945, a period during which long-acting insulin was available. At this time, diet restrictions were liberalized, and the importance of glucosuria was belittled as long as a patient had no polyuria or ketonuria. For the most part, the principles of treatment followed initially for patients in series I were maintained after 1936 in that group. Frequent reactions to insulin were much more common in series I patients. Thus, it seems reasonable to conclude that much better diabetic control for long periods was achieved in patients treated with short-acting insulin and a strict dietary regimen than in patients who were not encouraged to remain aglucosuric. After diabetes of 15 years' duration in both groups of patients, nephropathy (which was diagnosed if proteinuria was detected in more than half of all examinations during the preceding year) was seven times more prevalent in series II patients. Advanced retinopathy was six times more prevalent in series II patients even though the mean duration of their diabetes at the time of review was 15.9 years, compared with 26.5 years in series I patients.

Another major shortcoming of retrospective studies is related to the small number of subjects involved. Therefore, a recent report involving much larger numbers of patients is of special interest. Goodkin (7) followed 10,538 diabetics who applied for life insurance between 1951 and 1970. Mortality was reported after 10, 15, and 20 years of investigation. Applicants were classified as having poorly or "fairly well"-controlled diabetes on their initial examination. Poor control was defined as (a) excessive glucosuria (> 4%), (b) a 2-hour postprandial blood sugar level of > 250 mg/100 ml, (c) a recent history of high levels of blood sugar, or (d) a history of severe insulin reactions or onset of diabetic coma after the initial period of observation. The mortality among the poorly controlled group was approximately 2.5 times that among the fairly well controlled patients, despite the presence of a larger proportion of relatively young diabetics in the poorly controlled group.

Prospective Studies. Four recently published prospective studies also support a role for control in preventing or lessening the severity of diabetic complications. In one study (8), serial renal biopsies were taken in 23 patients whose fasting plasma glucose levels were measured every 2 weeks or more frequently. Good control was defined as values never exceeding 120 mg/100 ml, poor control as values of more than 150 mg/100 ml on "all or many occasions," and fair control as between good and poor control. The presence and degree of diabetic glomerulosclerosis in the biopsy specimens were evaluated independently by three nephrologists who had no knowledge of the patient's clinical course. Of 13 patients with poor control, 10 showed progression of nephropathy; 3 of 4 with fair control showed progression; but none of the 6 patients with good control showed progression. The duration of diabetes at the time of the first biopsy (~4.5 years) and the follow-up period (~4 years) were similar for patients whose lesions did not progress and for those showing progression. The age of onset (years ± SEM) of diabetes in the 13 patients whose nephropathy progressed was significantly lower (36.3 ± 3.9) than the age of onset of the 10 patients who showed no progression (52.6 ± 1.9). However, these results do not support the supposition that good control and a relative absence of glomerulosclerosis are associated only because the ketosis-resistant diabetic, in whom alteration of carbohydrate metabolism is less severe than in the ketosis-prone diabetic, has a genetic constitution that is less subject to nephropathy. In fact, 2 of the 4 adult-onset diabetics with poor control in this study showed progression of renal lesions.

In a second prospective study (9), the progression of retinopathy was correlated with fasting blood sugar levels over a 6-year period in 356 diabetics (mostly ketosis resistant). Degrees of control were defined as follows: good control, at least 80% of the fasting glucose levels of less than 140 mg/100 ml; poor control, >50% of the fasting glucose concentrations exceeding 170 mg/100 ml; and fair control, between good and poor control. Retinopathy was graded at least once per year after bilateral dilation of the pupils and examination with magnifying lenses by an ophthalmologist who had no knowledge of the metabolic status of the patient. Two, 4, and 6 years after the study began, the percentage of eyes in which new lesions appeared and old lesions progressed was lowest in patients with good control, intermediate in those with fair control, and highest in those with poor control. Conversely, the percentage of eyes in which old lesions improved was highest in patients with good control, intermediate in those with fair control, and lowest in those with poor control. After 4 and 6 years, proteinuria had progressed much less in patients with good control than in those with fair and poor control (10).

Patients with the following characteristics were included in a third prospective study (11, 12): (a) aged less than 60 years; (b) treated with less than 80 units of intermediate-acting insulin injected once per day; (c) affected by no life-threatening disease other than diabetes; (d) known for reliable attendance as an outpatient; and (e) experiencing an early stage of simple (not proliferative) retinopathy in the more diseased eye. Annual fluorescein angiography of the posterior pole was performed, and the number of microaneurysms was quantitated.

The patients were randomly allocated into two groups, one to continue receiving one injection of insulin per day and the other to receive multiple doses of insulin. The two groups had similar baseline characteristics, including duration of diabetes, age at both diagnosis of diabetes and onset of the trial, daily dose of insulin, urinary excretion of sugar (g/24 hours), and fasting blood sugar level. Twenty-one patients in each group were monitored for 2 to 5 years, with mean durations of follow-up of 49.1 months for the single-injection group and 51.1 months for the multiple-injection group. Most of the patients in the latter group received intermediate-acting insulin before breakfast and dinner. The fasting glucose concentration (mean ± SEM, mg/100 ml) during the study was significantly lower ($P < 0.05$) in the single-injection group (166 ± 9) than in the multiple-injection group (192 ± 8). Glucosuria (mean ± SEM, g/24 hours) decreased (by 5 ± 3) from baseline values in patients taking multiple injections, while in those receiving one injection it increased (by 5 ± 4). This difference was also significant ($P < 0.05$).

These modest differences in two parameters of diabetic control were associated with a 3-fold decrease in the rate of appearance of new microaneurysms in the eyes of patients taking more than 1 injection of insulin per day (Table 2-3). Although the number of microaneurysms fluctuated widely over time and some criticisms have been leveled at the statistical handling of the data (13), these results can be interpreted as another supporting link in the chain of evidence for an association between good diabetic control and a lessening of the severity of diabetic microangiopathy.

The fourth prospective study was a prodigious effort by a Belgian physician, Dr. Jean Pirart, and his colleagues (14). In 1947, Pirart began to enroll diabetics from two university hospitals (964 patients), a diabetic clinic (2,302 patients), and two private practices (1,132 patients) in a longitudinal study. One purpose of the study was to assess the relation between diabetic control and complications. The 4,398 patients in the study have been monitored closely by the same personnel for up to 25 years. The majority (2,795 patients) entered the study at the time of onset of their disease. The remaining 1,603 patients joined the study at various times after the diagnosis of diabetes had been made.

The patients were seen frequently, and much attention was paid to the accuracy of urine tests done at home at least daily but most often two to four times throughout the day. Blood sugar levels were measured at each office visit, and the time of sampling was purposefully varied in order to avoid a systematic bias because of the interval after eating and/or insulin injection. The criteria

Table 2-3. Development and Progress of Microaneurysms in Diabetic Patients Receiving Single or Multiple Injections of Insulin[a]

	No. of Microaneurysms (mean ± SEM) in indicated Group		
Parameter	Single-Injection	Multiple-Injection	P[b]
Baseline	13 ± 3	9 ± 3	NS
Last examination	55 ± 8	30 ± 7	<0.05
Difference	42 ± 7	21 ± 5	<0.02
Increase/year	9 ± 1	3 ± 1	<0.001

[a]Data adapted with permission from Eschwege E, Job D, Guyot-Argenton C, et al: Delayed progression of diabetic retinopathy by divided insulin administration: a further follow-up. Diabetologia 16:13–15, 1979.

[b]Determined by Student's t test between means. Significance accepted at the 0.05 level. NS, not significant.

Table 2-4. Criteria Used for Annual Ratings of the Degree of Control of Diabetes in 4,398 Patients Studied by Pirart[a]

Degree of Glycemic Control	Score[b]	Criteria for Scoring			
		Degree of Glucosuria During the Day	Postprandial Blood Sugar (mg/100 ml)	Fasting Blood Sugar (mg/100 ml)	Ketosis and/or Symptoms
Good	1	None or exceptionally few	$\leqslant 200$	$\leqslant 120$	None
Fair	2	Variable or constant but moderate	200-300	120-200	Rare and brief
Poor	3	Usually high and prolonged	$\geqslant 300$	$\geqslant 200$	Possible

[a]Reprinted with permission from Pirart J: Diabetes mellitus and its degenerative complications: a prospective study of 4,400 patients observed between 1947 and 1973. Diabetes Care 1:168–188, 1978.

[b]The score is based on the criteria in the last four columns.

used for assessing the annual degree of control are shown in Table 2-4. The records were reviewed each year and a score was assigned. There was excellent agreement between observers who judged the same record independently. A cumulative score estimating the degree of control during the entire period in which the patient was monitored was obtained by calculation of the arithmetic mean of consecutive yearly scores.

A neurologic and vascular evaluation of each patient was done at least yearly. A diagnosis of neuropathy was made if Achilles and/or patellar reflexes were lost in conjunction with a clear decrease in vibratory sensation. A patient was considered to have diabetic retinopathy if microaneurysms plus hemorrhages or exudates were found. In the absence of microaneurysms, hemorrhages and/or exudates were considered diagnostic of diabetic retinopathy only if major hypertension or thrombosis of a vein whose drainage area corresponded to the area of damaged retina was not discovered. Retinopathy was considered absent if neither eye contained microaneurysms, hemorrhages, exudates, or neovascularization. Retinopathy was graded as follows: grade 1, microaneurysms and/or small waxy exudates; grade 2, any hemorrhage and/or nonhypertensive soft exudates (even in the absence of microaneurysms or waxy exudates); and grade 3, areas of hemorrhage or exudates larger than the size of the disk. Proliferative retinopathy was diagnosed separately if even a slight degree of neovascularization was noted. Finally, a patient was considered to have diabetic nephropathy if unexplained proteinuria was discovered on several occasions.

The relations between cumulative diabetic control and the prevalences of neuropathy, retinopathy, and nephropathy are shown in Figures 2-4, 2-5, and 2-6, respectively. Three degrees of control are arbitrarily designated as follows, according to cumulative ($\bar{c}$) scores: 1.5 or less, fairly good control; 1.5 through 2, intermediate control; and more than 2, poor control. Since duration of diabetes

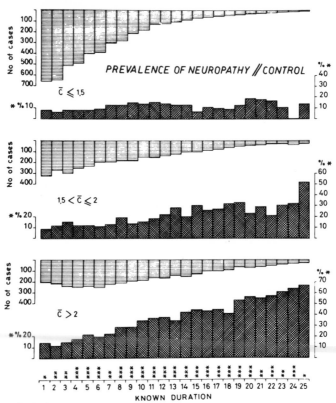

Figure 2-4. Relation between degree of diabetic control and the prevalence of neuropathy in a population of 4,398 diabetic patients monitored by one physician for up to 25 years. Light-colored bars represent the number of patients evaluated at each interval and who fall into the respective categories of control. Dark bars show the cumulative frequency (%) of a complication at each year of duration. $\bar{c}$, cumulative scores indicating degree of diabetic control. (Reprinted with permission from Pirart J: Diabetes mellitus and its degenerative complications: a prospective study of 4,400 patients observed between 1947 and 1973. Diabetes Care 1:168-188, 1978.)

has a marked effect on these complications, the prevalences of neuropathy, retinopathy, and nephropathy are also related to duration, which is shown on the abscissa of each graph. The frequency (in per cent) of a given complication at each year of duration is represented on the ordinate of each graph (dark bars). The number of patients evaluated at each interval and who fall into the respective categories of control (i.e., the denominator upon which the percentage of complications is calculated) is shown by the light-colored bars suspended from the top of the graphs. As would be expected, the number of subjects monitored decreases as the duration of diabetes increases. The slope of the histograms depicting prevalence (dark bars) represents the rate of increase of each complication.

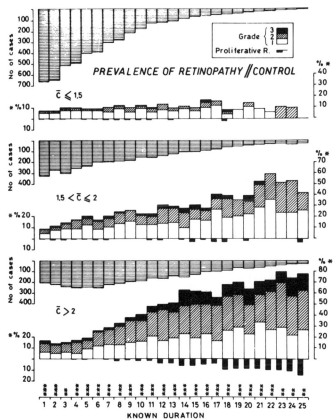

Figure 2-5. Relation between degree of diabetic control and the prevalence of retinopathy in a population of 4,398 diabetic patients monitored by one physician for up to 25 years. Light-colored bars represent the number of patients evaluated at each interval and who fall into the respective categories of control. Dark bars show the cumulative frequency (%) of a complication at each year of duration. $\bar{c}$, cumulative scores indicating degree of diabetic control. (Reprinted with permission from Pirart J: Diabetes mellitus and its degenerative complications: a prospective study of 4,400 patients observed between 1947 and 1973. Diabetes Care 1:168-188, 1978.)

The initial low prevalence of neuropathy (Fig. 2-4) did not change much as the duration of diabetes increased in the fairly well controlled group. In sharp contrast, the prevalence increased considerably over time in the other two groups, with the most poorly controlled patients experiencing a faster deterioration of peripheral neurologic function than did the intermediate group.

Similar observations were made with regard to retinopathy (Fig. 2-5). Only 15% or fewer of the patients in the best-controlled group had retinopathy, and of those who did, very few developed either grade 3 or proliferative changes. In the

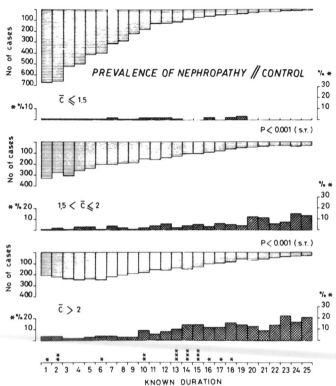

Figure 2-6. Relation between degree of diabetic control and the prevalence of nephropathy in a population of 4,398 diabetic patients monitored by one physician for up to 25 years. Light-colored bars represent the number of patients evaluated at each interval and who fall into the respective categories of control. Dark bars show the cumulative frequency (%) of a complication at each year of duration. $\bar{c}$, cumulative scores indicating degree of diabetic control. (Reprinted with permission from Pirart J: Diabetes mellitus and its degenerative complications: a prospective study of 4,400 patients observed between 1947 and 1973. Diabetes Care 1:168-188, 1978.)

intermediate group, the prevalence of retinopathy gradually increased to significant proportions, but the number with grade 3 or proliferative changes remained small. The poorly controlled group had the greatest increase in prevalence of retinopathy over time, and grade 3 and proliferative changes were not uncommon in this group.

Although the prevalence of nephropathy (Fig. 2-6) was much lower than the prevalences of the other two complications, the same relation between control and prevalence was found. Thus, the beneficial effect of good diabetic control in preventing or lessening the severity of diabetic neuropathy, retinopathy, and nephropathy seems to have been well established in this mammoth longitudinal study.

Evidence Not Supporting Relation Between
Diabetic Control and Microangiopathy

Two situations are not consistent with the view that good control has a beneficial effect on diabetic complications. An occasional patient presents with kidney disease that appears, on the basis of renal biopsy, to be glomerulosclerosis. The patient's glucose tolerance is only mildly abnormal or may even be within normal limits. The explanation usually given is that such patients have had undiscovered, probably intermittent hyperglycemia for various periods before renal disease became manifest. Indeed, it has been estimated that the actual onset of ketosis-resistant diabetes in adults precedes the diagnosis by approximately 10 years (15). Another theory, which has recently been supported by data from electron microscopic and immunofluorescent studies (16), is that other renal diseases are confused with diabetic glomerulosclerosis by light microscopy.

Conversely, a rare patient with a long history of poorly controlled diabetes mellitus develops no proteinuria and minimal retinopathy and/or neuropathy. These few patients remind us that other factors may affect the development of the microangiopathy of diabetes mellitus. However, in my view, the data from these patients do not begin to negate the considerable evidence relating good control to a lessening of microangiopathic complications.

Macroangiopathy

Although there is little evidence to suggest that the accelerated macroangiopathy associated with diabetes mellitus is influenced by improved diabetic control, cross-sectional studies have demonstrated a significantly positive correlation between glucose concentrations after an oral challenge and the presence of cardiovascular disease (17-19). One prospective study has related higher postprandial glucose levels to increased incidences of electrocardiogram abnormalities and retinopathy and to a shortened life expectancy (20). These data relating relatively mild impairments of carbohydrate metabolism to macroangiopathy may also be cited as evidence (albeit weaker than the results on microangiopathic complications) for a beneficial effect of good diabetic control on macrovascular disease associated with diabetes mellitus.

General Therapeutic Guidelines

Let us turn now to a practical consideration of the problem of treatment in diabetes mellitus. The glucose concentrations of nondiabetics range between 80 and 120 mg/100 ml throughout the day, and microangiopathy does not occur. Glomerulosclerosis, retinopathy, and neuropathy in diabetic animals can be prevented or reversed if normal or nearly normal metabolic conditions can be reestablished. Until the artificial pancreas or pancreatic transplantation become feasible in humans, however, glucose levels will remain significantly above normal in diabetics treated by current methods. Therefore, the crucial question is whether diabetic complications can be lessened in patients in whom glucose levels of approximately 120 to 250 mg/100 ml can be maintained consistently—day and night over many years—compared with patients whose glucose concentrations usually range between 200 and 400 mg/100 ml. This question cannot be explored either at the present time or, in all probability, in the foreseeable future (at least in humans). However, given that neither nondiabetic humans nor diabetic animals whose carbohydrate metabolism has been returned nearly to normal manifest microangiopathy, and given the relation between microangiopathic lesions and the indices of diabetic control discussed in this chapter, it seems to be an inescapable conclusion that lowering of glucose concentrations toward normal can only have an ameliorating effect on the complications associated with diabetes mellitus.

Although treatment will be discussed in much greater detail in subsequent chapters, some general guidelines are offered here. Minimal criteria for decisions concerning a therapeutic approach are depicted in Figure 2-7. Ketosis-resistant diabetics whose postprandial glucose concentrations during their usual diets are routinely less than 200 mg/100 ml should be treated by means of dietary therapy alone. If postprandial values are consistently above that level, a sulfonylurea agent should be added to dietary therapy. If fasting glucose concentrations

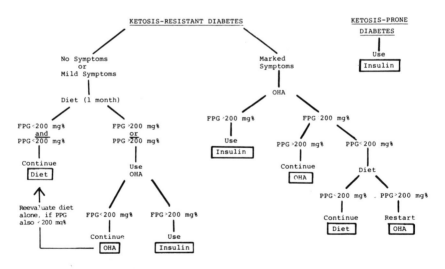

Figure 2-7. General guidelines for decisions regarding treatment of patients with diabetes mellitus. FPG, fasting plasma glucose concentration; PPG, 1- to 2-hour postprandial glucose concentration on usual diet; OHA, oral hypoglycemic agents.

usually exceed 200 mg/100 ml despite maximal doses of sulfonylurea agents, insulin therapy should be instituted. Finally, ketosis-prone diabetics must be treated with insulin for the reasons discussed earlier in this chapter. The therapeutic goal within each subset of diabetics is to lower glucose levels as much as possible without seriously disrupting a patient's usual activities.

Practical Summary

In the absence of treatment, a minority of diabetics have ketonuria, a condition that signifies the virtual absence of effective insulin. Ketosis-prone (type 1) diabetes usually, but not always, appears first in childhood or young adulthood. Although it is often called juvenile-onset diabetes, this term is not entirely accurate, since ketosis-prone diabetes can appear in adulthood. These patients secrete little, if any, insulin and respond to insulin normally. Obesity is extremely uncommon. In the presence of stress, infection, or inadequate insulin therapy, ketosis-prone patients become ketotic and eventually slip into ketoacidosis. Ketosis-prone diabetics must be treated with insulin.

Most diabetics have ketosis-resistant (type 2) diabetes, in which an absence of ketonuria in the untreated state signifies the presence of some effective insulin. This kind of diabetes has been called adult-onset or maturity-onset diabetes; however, these terms also are not accurate because some adults are ketosis-prone and some children and adolescents are ketosis-resistant. The great majority of ketosis-resistant diabetics are obese. Insulin secretion has been shown to be decreased, normal, or even increased in these patients compared with that in appropriate control subjects. This variation attests to the heterogeneity of type 2 diabetes. On the other hand, insulin antagonism (over and beyond that due to obesity) characterizes ketosis-resistant diabetes. In response to stress, ketosis-resistant patients will become hyperglycemic, but only rarely ketotic. Most of them, especially those who are obese, will respond to appropriate dietary therapy, and this modality of treatment should be used initially unless the patient is very symptomatic. If the fasting and postprandial glucose concentrations can be kept below 200 mg/100 ml, no further agents need to be added to the regimen. If either the fasting or the postprandial glucose values consistently exceed 200 mg/100 ml, then sulfonylurea agents should be introduced. If the fasting glucose level continues to exceed 200 mg/100 ml despite maximal doses, these agents should be discontinued and insulin prescribed.

There are two general kinds of vascular complications of diabetes mellitus: a microangiopathy, the clinical manifestations of which are nephropathy and retinopathy, and a macroangiopathy, which causes coronary artery disease, cerebral vascular disease, and peripheral vascular disease. The evidence that tight control of glucose concentrations will have a marked ameliorating effect on the large-vessel diseases is not great. However, recent extremely convincing data from studies in animals and humans show that strict diabetic control will ameliorate, prevent, or even reverse microangiopathic changes. For this reason, the goal of diabetic therapy should now be to return glucose concentrations to as near normal as possible without seriously disrupting a patient's daily pattern of living.

References

1. Davidson MB: The case for control in diabetes mellitus. West J Med 129:193-200, 1978

2. Engerman R, Bloodworth JMB, Nelson S: Relationship of microvascular disease in diabetics to metabolic control. Diabetes 26:760-769, 1977

3. Williamson JR, Kilo C: Current status of capillary basement-membrane disease in diabetes mellitus. Diabetes 26:65-73, 1977

4. Knowles HC: The problem of the relation of the control of diabetes to the development of vascular disease. Trans Am Clin Climatol Assoc 76:142-147, 1964

5. Strauss MB: Diabetic regimens—procrustean beds. N Engl J Med 281:1484-1486, 1969

6. Johnsson E: Retinopathy and nephropathy in diabetes mellitus. Comparison of the effects of two forms of treatment. Diabetes 9:1-8, 1960

7. Goodkin G: Mortality factors in diabetes—a 20-year mortality study. J Occup Med 17:716-721, 1975

8. Takazakura E, Nakamoto Y, Hayakawa H, et al: Onset and progression of diabetic glomerulosclerosis. A prospective study based on serial renal biopsies. Diabetes 24:1-9, 1975

9. Miki E, Fukuda M, Kuzuya T, et al: Relation of the course of retinopathy to control of diabetes, age, and therapeutic agents in diabetic Japanese patients. Diabetes 18:773-780, 1969

10. Miki E, Kuzuya T, Ide T, Nakao K: Frequency, degree, and progression with time of proteinuria in diabetic patients. Lancet 1:922-924, 1978

11. Job D, Eschwege E, Guyot-Argenton C, et al: Effect of multiple daily injections on the course of diabetic retinopathy. Diabetes 25:463-469, 1976

12. Eschwege E, Job D, Guyot-Argenton C, et al: Delayed progression of diabetic retinopathy by divided insulin administration: a further follow-up. Diabetologia 16:13-15, 1979

13. Ashikaga T, Borodic G, Sims EAH: Multiple daily insulin injections in the treatment of diabetic retinopathy. The Job study revisited. Diabetes 27:592-596, 1978

14. Pirart J: Diabetes mellitus and its degenerative complications: a prospective study of 4,400 patients observed between 1947 and 1973. Diabetes Care 1:168-188, 1978

Table 3-6. Total Plant-Fiber and Caloric Content of Selected Breads, Cereals, and Starchy Vegetables[a]

Food[b]	Portion Size	No. of Calories	Fiber (g)	Fiber (g)/100 Calories
Beans, white	½ cup	91	4.2 (1.5)[c]	4.7
Beans, kidney	½ cup	94	4.5 (1.8)	4.8
Beans, lima	½ cup	126	4.1 (1.5)	1.1
Bran (100%) cereal	½ cup	66	10.0 (2.3)	15.1
Bread, rye	1 slice	54	2.7	5.0
Bread, white	1 slice	74	0.8 (<0.1)	1.0
Bread, whole-grain wheat	1 slice	63	2.7 (0.4)	4.2
Corn, kernels	⅓ cup	41	2.1 (0.5)	5.2
Corn, grits	½ cup	59	1.9 (0.4)	3.2
Corn bread	1 square	151	2.7	1.8
Corn flakes	¾ cup	64	2.1 (0.2)	3.3
Crackers, graham	2 squares	53	1.4	2.7
Crackers, saltine	6	65	0.5	0.8
Oats, whole	½ cup	61	1.6	2.4
Pancakes	1	61	0.4	0.6
Parsnips	⅔ cup	72	5.9 (2.7)	8.2
Peas	½ cup	44	5.2 (1.5)	11.8
Potatoes, white	1 small	80	3.8 (0.6)	4.8
Rice, brown	½ cup	83	1.3 (0.2)	1.6
Rice, white	½ cup	79	0.5 (<0.1)	0.6
Roll, dinner	1	81	0.8	1.0
Rye flour, dark*	2½ Tbs	60	2.8	4.7
Rye wafers	3 squares	64	2.3	3.5
Spaghetti	½ cup	82	0.8	1.0
Squash, winter	½ cup	43	3.6 (1.8)	8.3
Sweet potatoes	¼ cup	72	2.9	4.0
Waffles	1 section	139	0.8	0.5
Wheat flour, whole-grain*	2½ Tbs	60	1.8	3.0
Wheat flour, white*	2½ Tbs	77	0.7	0.9
Wheat cereal, flakes	¾ cup	75	3.0	3.9
Wheat cereal, shredded	1 large	84	3.0 (0.5)	3.6

Abbreviation: Tbs, tablespoon(s).

[a]Adapted from Anderson JW, Ward K: Long-term effects of high-carbohydrate, high-fiber diets on glucose and lipid metabolism: a preliminary report on patients with diabetes. Diabetes Care 1:77–82, 1978.

[b]All values are for cooked or prepared foods unless the name of the food is followed by an asterisk.

[c]The crude-fiber content is shown in parentheses. The source for these values is Church C, Church H: *Food Values of Portions Commonly Used*, 12th ed. JB Lippincott, Philadelphia, 1975, pp 8–14, 77–85.

Calculating Diets

Dietary Goals

The important goals of dietary therapy for diabetic patients are as follows.

Calorie Control. Adjustment of the calorie level when necessary in order to attain a desirable body weight is the first step in dietary management of the diabetic patient.

Prevention or Delay of Cardiovascular Diseases. In the diabetic meal plan, foods that are relatively low in saturated fat and cholesterol must be deliberately selected. For example, nonfat or low-fat milk, low-fat cottage cheese, and well-trimmed meats are preferable to their high-fat counterparts. Chicken, fish, and turkey should be emphasized. No more than three whole eggs should be eaten per week. Animal fats (such as cream, lard, and bacon) and products made with coconut or palm oils, which are highly saturated, should be avoided (Table 3-7).

Increased Fiber Intake. As discussed under *Fiber Content*, the fiber content of the average American diet is low, and an increase through the inclusion of more

Table 3-7. Ratio of Polyunsaturated Fatty Acids (P) to Saturated Fatty Acids (S) in Various Dietary Oils and Fats[a]

Food	P:S
Oil (unhydrogenated)	
Walnut	7:1
Safflower	8:1
Sunflower	6:1
Corn	5:1
Soybean	4:1
Wheat germ	3.3:1
Cottonseed	2:1
Peanut	1.9:1
Olive	0.6:1
Other fat	
Butter	1:17
Coconut	1:48
Palm kernel oil	1:51
Palm oil	1:53

[a]Data adapted from US Department of Agriculture: *Composition of Foods. Fats and Oils: Raw, Processed and Prepared.* USDA Agricultural Handbook no. 8.4, 1979.

whole grains, legumes, fresh fruits, and fresh vegetables in allowed amounts is encouraged (Tables 3-4, 3-5, and 3-6).

Education of the Patient. Appropriate dietary instruction cannot be emphasized strongly enough and should be ongoing during the treatment of the diabetic patient, who needs reinforcement at each step of learning.

Dietary History

A thorough dietary history must be elicited at the outset of dietary therapy. This information familiarizes the physician with the eating habits of the patient and is invaluable in nutritional assessment and in the selection of foods for the diet. If carefully taken, the history will reveal (*a*) caloric intake, (*b*) quality of the normal diet, (*c*) food idiosyncrasies, (*d*) times, size, and content of meals, (*e*) frequency of eating at restaurants, (*f*) ethnic food preferences, (*g*) eating problems (dental, gastrointestinal, etc.), and (*h*) alcoholic beverage usage.

Dietary histories can be taken in three ways. First, in the 24-hour recall, the patient recalls exactly what and how much he or she ate during a 24-hour period and thus provides extremely specific, objective information. The disadvantage of this approach is that the food eaten on the day selected may not represent a typical day's intake. Second, in the general pattern, the patient describes his or her typical eating pattern. This approach provides information that is representative but not as specific or possibly as accurate as that provided in the 24-hour recall. Finally, the 24-hour recall and the general pattern may be combined.

Key questions in a dietary history include the following:

1. In what room do you eat most of your meals?
2. Do you watch television or read during meals?
3. What is your favorite food?
4. How many family members are there in your household?
5. If you are living alone, does it affect your appetite? [For example, an elderly person living alone may eat less because of loneliness or may eat more because of boredom.]
6. Who plans, shops for, and prepares meals?
7. Are you a fast or slow eater?
8. Do you "binge" on certain foods? Do you snack all day?
9. In one week, how many times do you eat ice cream, cake, cookies, or pie?
10. What do you think triggers your eating?

The practicing physician all too often does not have the time to go into great detail about the eating habits and schedules of the patient. However, a few moments devoted to obtaining this information pay off in determining the nutritional adequacy of the patient's normal diet. A dietary history form (Fig. 3-3) can be used as a part of the medical record.

Exchanges

The food exchange system used in the diabetic diet represents the combined efforts of the American Diabetic Association, the American Dietetic Association, and the US Public Health Service. It permits the widest possible selection of foods, thereby offering variety and versatility to the diet. In our experience,

---

Date _____

Name _____ Birthdate _____ Hospital No. _____

Diet Rx _____

Occupation _____

Ht _____ Wt _____ IBW _____ Goal wt _____

Recent wt gain or loss _____

Chol _____ TG _____ BP _____ Other _____

Insulin or oral agents _____ Rx meds _____ Self meds _____

Previous diets _____ What kind _____

Appetite _____

Eat out frequently _____ How often per week _____

Eating problems _____
 (dental, GI)

Rate of eating: Fast _____ Moderate _____ Slow _____

Where at home do you eat _____
 (e.g., front of TV, at table, room)

No. in household _____ Who plans meals _____ Shops _____

Who prepares meals _____ Salt usage _____ Alcohol usage _____

Favorite foods _____ Food dislikes _____

Do you ever binge _____ On what _____ How often _____

Exercise over and above day's routine _____
 (as walk, swim, bicycle, etc.)

Diet recall:

Meal pattern:

Comments and recommendations:

Figure 3-3. Diet history form for diabetic patients. IBW, ideal body weight; Chol, cholesterol; TG, triglyceride; BP, blood pressure; GI, gastrointestinal; Rx, treatment.

a slight modification of the standard exchange lists (the Meat Exchange List in particular) seems to meet the needs of our patients more fully.

The six exchange lists that we use are shown in Tables 3-8 through 3-13, along with the respective values of carbohydrate, protein, and fat. The word *exchange* refers to the fact that each item on a particular list, in the portion listed, may be interchanged with any other item on the same list. An exchange can be explained to the patient as a choice or substitution. The portion sizes must be strongly emphasized. Foods from all six lists, with the possible exception of the Milk Exchange List, should be represented in each diabetic diet to help ensure adequate nutrient intake.

An understanding of the purpose and contents of the exchange lists is important before calculation of the meal plan and instruction of the patient are begun. In addition, a group of foods to be avoided is listed in Table 3-14, and a group of foods that can be eaten in unlimited portions is listed in Table 3-15. The patient should be familiarized with all of these lists.

Milk Exchanges. The Milk Exchange List (Table 3-8) includes both fluid and dry milk and plain yogurt. Calculations are based on 1 cup of nonfat (skim) milk, which contains 12 g of carbohydrate, 8 g of protein, and no fat. Buttermilk is calculated based on the same figures. The use of regular whole milk (3.5% butterfat, 12 g of carbohydrate, 8 g of protein, and 10 g of fat) is strongly discouraged because of its saturated fat content. Low-fat milk (2% butterfat, 12 g of carbohydrate, 3 g of protein, and 5 g of fat) may be included in the meal plan as a compromise if nonfat milk is unacceptable. If a person dislikes milk or is unable to tolerate it, none is included in her or his pattern. However, in the absence of any of these problems, ½ to 2 cups per day of nonfat milk (or more) can and

Table 3-8. Milk Exchange List

---

1 milk exchange = 80 calories, 12 g of carbohydrate, 8 g of protein, and 0 g of fat

---

Skim or nonfat milk, 1 cup
Powdered milk (nonfat, dry), 1/3 cup
Evaporated skim milk, 1/2 cup
Buttermilk, 1 cup
Low-fat milk,[a] 1 cup
Yogurt (low-fat, plain),[a] 1 cup
Whole milk,[b] 1 cup
Evaporated whole milk,[b] 1/2 cup

---

[a]Each exchange counts as 1 milk exchange and 1 fat exchange.

[b]Each exchange counts as 1 milk exchange and 2 fat exchanges.

Table 3-9. Vegetable Exchange List[a]

*1 vegetable exchange = 28 calories, 5 g of carbohydrate,
2 g of protein, and 0 g of fat*

Artichoke (medium)	Endive	Onions
Asparagus	Escarole	Parsley
Bean sprouts	Greens	Radishes
Beets	Beet	Rhubarb
Broccoli	Chard	Sauerkraut
Brussels sprouts	Collard	String beans (green and wax)
Cabbage	Dandelion	Summer squash
Carrots	Kale	Tomatoes
Cauliflower	Mustard	Tomato juice
Celery	Spinach	Turnips
Chicory	Turnip	Vegetable juice
Chinese cabbage	Lettuce	Watercress
Cucumber	Mushrooms	Zucchini
Eggplant	Okra	

[a]One serving is equal to ½ cup of cooked vegetables or to any amount of raw vegetables.

should be included. Inclusion of more than 2 cups per day, however, further restricts the number of meat exchanges allowed the patient.

Vegetable Exchanges. A vegetable exchange (Table 3-9) consists of ½ cup of any cooked vegetable listed and contains 5 g of carbohydrate, 2 g of protein, and no fat. At least 1 vegetable exchange should be included in the meal pattern to provide fiber, vitamins, and minerals. Raw vegetables have a much higher water content than do cooked vegetables, and because more effort is required for chewing, most patients eat a smaller amount of raw vegetables. For these reasons, raw vegetables are included in the Unlimited Use List (Table 3-15); i.e., the quantity eaten is unrestricted. Vegetables may be steamed, boiled, or baked, and a variety of herbs and spices may be used to flavor them. Margarine or oil added to vegetables must be considered part of the fat exchange allowance.

Fruit Exchanges. The Fruit Exchange List (Table 3-10) includes both fruits and juices; each exchange contains 10 g of carbohydrate, no protein, and no fat. Fresh fruits are emphasized because of their fiber, vitamin, and mineral content. Canned fruits packed in water or their own unsweetened juices may be used as well. Economic circumstances may make it a hardship for some patients to purchase these water-packed fruits (or diet fruits, as they are often called). In

Table 3-10. Fruit Exchange List

1 fruit exchange = 40 calories, 10 g of carbohydrate, 0 g of protein, and 0 g of fat

Apple, 1 small	Loganberries, 1/2 cup
Apple juice 1/3 cup	Mango, 1/2 small
Applesauce, 1/2 cup	Nectarine, 1 small
Apricots (fresh), 2 medium	Orange, 1 small
Apricots (dried), 4 halves	Orange sections, 1/2 cup
Apricot nectar, 1/3 cup	Orange juice, 1/2 cup
Banana, 1/2 small	Papaya, 1/3 medium
Blackberries, 1 cup	Peach, 1 medium
Blueberries, 2/3 cup	Peach nectar, 1/3 cup
Boysenberries, 1 cup	Pear, 1 small
Cantaloupe, 1/4 small	Pear nectar, 1/3 cup
Cherries, 10 large	Persimmon, 1/2
Cranberry juice, 1/4 cup	Pineapple cubes, 1/2 cup
Dates, 2 small	Pineapple ring, 2
Fig (fresh), 1	Pineapple juice, 1/3 cup
Fig (dried), 1	Plums, 2 medium
Fruit cocktail, 1/2 cup	Pomegranate, 1/3 medium
Grapefruit, 1/2	Prunes, 2 medium
Grapefruit sections, 1/2 cup	Prune juice, 1/4 cup
Grapefruit juice, 1/2 cup	Raisins, 2 Tbs
Grapes, 12	Raspberries, 1/2 cup
Grapes (seedless), 12	Rhubarb (raw cubes), 1 cup
Grape juice, 1/4 cup	Strawberries, 1 cup
Guava, 1 small	Tangelo, 1 medium
Honeydew melon, 1/8 medium	Tangerines, 2 small
Kumquats, 4 medium	Watermelon cubes, 1 cup or 1/2 slice,
Lemon juice, 3/4 cup	10" x 3" thick
Lime juice, 3/4 cup	

Abbreviation: Tbs, tablespoons.

this case, regular canned fruit that has had the syrup washed off completely is an acceptable substitution.

Bread Exchanges. Included in the Bread Exchange List (Table 3-11) are various foods other than bread itself, each with approximately equal caloric and nutrient values. In addition to bread and bread products, the list includes cereals, tortillas, beans, and certain starchy vegetables such as corn and potatoes. Calculations are based on 15 g of carbohydrate, 2 g of protein, and no fat for each exchange. However, a few items on the list must also be counted as 1 fat exchange because of the method of preparation. In addition, legumes (dried peas and beans) must be counted as 1 meat exchange because of their protein content.

Table 3-11. Bread Exchange List

1 Bread exchange = 68 calories, 15 g of carbohydrate, 2 g protein, 0 g of fat

Breads
   White (including French and
      Italian), 1 slice
   Whole wheat, 1 slice
   Sourdough, 1/2 slice
   Rye or pumpernickel, 1 slice
   Raisin, 1 slice
   Bagel (small), 1/2
   Biscuit or muffin,[a] 1
   Corn bread (2-inch cube),[a] 1
   English muffin, 1/2
   Hamburger bun, 1/2
   Hot dog bun, 1/2
   Pancake,[a] 1
   Roll (plain), 1
   Tortilla (corn or flour), 1 small
   Waffle,[a] 1

Starchy vegetables
   Baked beans (no pork), 1/4 cup
   Dried beans (cooked),[b] 1/2 cup
   Dried peas (cooked),[b] 1/2 cup
   Chayote, 1/2 cup
   Corn, 1/3 cup
   Corn on cob, 1 small
   Jicama, 1/2 cup
   Mixed vegetables, 1/2 cup
   Green peas, 1/2 cup
   Parsnips, 2/3 cup
   Potato (white), 1 small
   Potato (mashed or boiled), 1/2 cup
   Potato (French fried),[a] 8
   Pumpkin, 3/4 cup
   Rice, 1/2 cup
   Rutabagas, 3/4 cup
   Winter squash, 1/2 cup
   Yam or sweet potato, 1/4 cup

Cereals
   Barley (cooked), 1/2 cup
   Bran flakes, 1/2 cup
   Unfrosted dry, cereal, 3/4 cup
   Cooked cereal, 1/2 cup
   Grits, 1/2 cup
   Wheat germ, 1/4 cup

Crackers
   Round butter type,[a] 5
   Graham (2 1/2-in square), 2
   Matzoh, 1/2
   Melba Toast, 4 slices
   Oyster, 20
   Pretzels (stick), 25
   Rye wafers, 3
   Saltines, 5
   Soda, 4
   Zwieback, 2

Flour Products
   Bread crumbs (dried), 3 Tbs
   Bread sticks (4 in long), 2
   Corn flake crumbs, 3 Tbs
   Corn meal (dry), 2 Tbs
   Cornstarch, 2 Tbs
   Flour, 2 Tbs
   Wheat germ, 1/4 cup
   Pasta, cooked (spaghetti, noodles,
      macaroni), 1/2 cup

Miscellaneous
   Angel food cake (baked in tube
      pan), 1 oz or 1 slice (2 in wide,
      4 in high)
   Gelatin (flavored), 1/2 cup
   Ice milk, 1/3 cup
   Sherbet, 1/4 cup
   Popcorn (popped, unbuttered),
      3 cups
   Soup, 3/4 cup
   Vanilla wafers, 4

Abbreviation: Tbs, tablespoons.
[a]Each exchange counts as 1 bread exchange *and* 1 fat exchange.
[b]Each exchange counts as 1 bread exchange *and* 1 meat exchange.

Table 3-12. Meat Exchange List

1 meat exchange = 55 calories, 0 g of carbohydrate, 7 g of protein, and 3 g of fat

Chicken, turkey (without skin), 1 oz	Egg,[a] 1
Fish, shellfish, 1 oz	Luncheon meat, cold cuts,[a] 1-oz slice
Tuna, salmon, mackerel (packed in water or rinsed well), 1/4 cup	Canadian bacon,[a] 1 oz
	Chesse (all kinds),[a] 1 oz
Anchovies, sardines (drained well), 1 oz	Frankfurter (10/lb),[b] 1
Liver, kidney, heart, sweetbreads, 1 oz	Peanut butter,[b] 2 Tbs
Cottage cheese (low-fat), 1/4 cup	Dried beans and peas,[c] 1/2 cup
Tofu, 3 oz	
Beef, veal, pork ham, lamb,[a] 1 oz	

[a]Each exchange counts as 1 meat exchange *and* 1 fat exchange.

[b]Each exchange counts as 1 meat exchange *and* 2 fat exchanges.

[c]Each exchange counts as 1 meat exchange *and* 1 bread exchange.

Many patients, in their desire to lose weight, feel that the foods on this list should be eliminated entirely. However, the importance of this group lies not only in its vitamin and mineral contribution (e.g., thiamine, niacin, pyridoxine), but also in its role as the prime source of complex carbohydrate and fiber in the diet.

Meat Exchanges. The Meat Exchange List (Table 3-12) requires careful and often repeated explanation to the patient. Each item is calculated as 1 meat exchange, which contains no carbohydrate, 7 g of protein, and 3 g of fat. However, some items (those footnoted in the list) count as more than 1 meat exchange. Most of these are higher in saturated fat and therefore contain more calories. For these reasons, they should be deemphasized in the diabetic diet. For persons who do not choose to eat meat, various foods on this list, such as cheese, cottage cheese, and tofu, can be substituted without a loss in protein. Perhaps this list would be better designated as a High-Protein Food Exchange List.

Fat Exchanges. Each item on the Fat Exchange List (Table 3-13) contains no carbohydrate, no protein, and 5 g of fat. The listed items are divided into two categories: those high in unsaturated fats and those high in saturated fats. The foods in the latter category should be deemphasized. For example, margarine made from a polyunsaturated oil, such as safflower oil, should be emphasized rather than butter.

Method for Calculating Diets

(1) Determine the appropriate calorie level for the patient, as outlined earlier in this chapter (*Total Number of Calories*). A 1,500-calorie diet will be used

Table 3-13. Fat Exchange List

---

1 fat exchange = 45 calories, 0 g of carbohydrate, 0 g of protein, and 5 g of fat

---

Unsaturated and Monosaturated Fats	*Saturated Fats*
Margarine (made from safflower, corn, cottonseed, and/or soy oil), 1 tsp	Bacon, 1 slice
Oil (safflower, corn, cottonseed, soy), 1 tsp	Bacon fat, 1 tsp
	Sausage, ½ oz or ½ link
Avocado (medium), ⅛	Butter, 1 tsp
Olives (small), 5	Half and half, 2 Tbs
Oil (olive or peanut), 1 tsp	Whipped cream, 2 Tbs
Mayonnaise, 1 tsp	Heavy cream, 1 Tbs
Nuts	Sour cream, 2 Tbs
Almonds (whole), 10	Cream cheese, 1 Tbs
Pecans (whole), 2	Lard, 1 tsp
Peanuts (Spanish, whole), 20	Salt pork (¾-in cube), 1
Peanuts (Virginia, whole), 10	Hollandaise sauce, 4 tsp
Walnuts (whole), 6	Coconut, 1 Tbs
Others (whole), 6	Chocolate, unsweetened (melted), 2 tsp
Pumpkin seeds, 1 Tbs	
Sunflower seeds (kernels), 2 Tbs	
Dressings	
French, 1 Tbs	
Italian, 1 Tbs	
Thousand Island, 1 Tbs	
Bleu cheese, 1 Tbs	
Mayonnaise-type, 1 tsp	
Tartar sauce, 1 Tbs	

Abbreviations: tsp, teaspoon(s); Tbs, tablespoon(s).

here for illustrative purposes. Refer throughout to the blank worksheet shown in Figure 3-4 and to the completed worksheet for the 1,500-calorie diet shown in Figure 3-5.

(2) Multiply the total number of calories by the following percentages: carbohydrate, 50%; protein, 17%; and fat, 33%. For the 1,500-calorie diet, the calculations would be as follows: 1,500 calories × 0.50 = 750 calories in carbohydrate; 1,500 calories × 0.17 = 255 calories in protein; and 1,500 calories × 0.33 = 495 calories in fat.

(3) Determine the number of grams of carbohydrate, protein, and fat by dividing the number of calories in each category by the appropriate number of calories per gram (i.e., carbohydrate, 4 calories/g; protein 4 calories/g; and fat,

Table 3-14. Foods to Avoid

Alcoholic beverages (unless approved by physician and worked into meal pattern)

Cakes

Candy

Chewing gum

Chocolate (except as listed in the Fat Exchange List, Table 3-13)

Condensed milk

Dietetic foods (unless allowed by dietitian)

Doughnuts

Fruited yogurt

Honey

Jam

Jelly

Nondairy creamers

Pastries

Pies

Soft drinks

Sugar (all kinds)

Sweetened beverages

Table 3-15. Unlimited Use List

Raw vegetables

Coffee, tea

Bouillon, broth, consommé

Cranberries (unsweetened)

Gelatin (unflavored)

Herbs, spices

Horseradish

Lemons (up to 2 per day)

Limes (up to 2 per day)

Pickles (dill)

Sugarless gum

Vinegar

Water (plain or carbonated)

Calories

Exchange Group	Value per Exchange (g)			No. of Exchanges	( ) CHO	( ) Pro	( ) Fat
	CHO	Pro	Fat				
Milk	12	8	—				
Vegetable	5	2	—				
Fruit	10	—	—				

1. Total CHO from sources other than bread and subtract total from g of CHO in prescription.
2. Divide resulting figure by 15 g of CHO per bread exchange. This calculation gives you the number of bread exchanges.

Bread	15	2	—				

3. Total Pro from sources other than meat and subtract total from g of Pro in prescription.
4. Divide resulting figure by 7 g of Pro per meat exchange. This calculation gives you the number of meat exchanges.

Meat	—	7	3				

5. Total fat from sources other than fat exchanges and subtract from g of fat in prescription.
6. Divide resulting figure by 5 g of fat per fat exchange. This calculation gives you the number of fat exchanges.

Fat	—	—	5				

   Totals:

Figure 3-4. Blank diet calculation sheet. CHO, carbohydrate; Pro, protein; HS, hour of sleep.

9 calories/g). For the 1,500 calorie diet, the calculations would be as follows: 750 carbohydrate calories ÷ 4 calories/g = 187.5 g of carbohydrate (188 g); 255 protein calories ÷ 4 calories/g = 63.75 g of protein (64 g); and 494 fat calories ÷ 9 calories/g = 55 g of fat. The results of this calculation for diets between 1,000 and 3,500 calories are listed in Table 3-2.

   (4) Determine the total number of exchanges from each exchange list. The exchange lists are placed on the worksheet so that the first four shown

$^1/_{10}$ of the total CHO _____
$^2/_{10}$ of the total CHO _____
$^3/_{10}$ of the total CHO _____
$^4/_{10}$ of the total CHO _____

Distributions

		Meals				*Snacks*		
		CHO	*Pro*	*Fat*		*CHO*	*Pro*	*Fat*
Breakfast:	Milk				AM			
	Fruit							
	Bread							
	Meat							
	Fat							
Total					Total			
Lunch:	Milk				PM			
	Vegetable							
	Fruit							
	Bread							
	Meat							
	Fat							
Total					Total			
Dinner:	Milk				HS			
	Vegetable							
	Fruit							
	Bread							
	Meat							
Total					Total			
		CHO	*Pro*	*Fat*				
Totals:	Breakfast							
	Lunch							
	Dinner							
	AM							
	PM							
	HS							

(milk, vegetable, fruit, and bread) are the carbohydrate sources (Tables 3-8 through 3-11).

(a) Write the appropriate number of grams of carbohydrate, protein, and fat in the parentheses above the headings CHO, Pro, and Fat on the worksheet. These are your target figures, and your final totals should be within 5 g of these numbers.

Calories: 1,500

Exchange Group	Value per Exchange (g)			No. of Exchanges	(188) CHO	(64) Pro	(55) Fat
	CHO	Pro	Fat				
Milk	12	8	—	2	24	16	0
Vegetable	5	2	—	2	10	4	0
Fruit	10	—	—	3	30	0	0
Subtotal					64		

1. Total CHO from sources other than bread and subtract total from g of CHO in prescription.
2. Divide resulting figure by 15 g of CHO per bread exchange. This calculation gives you the number of bread exchanges.

Bread	15	2	—	8	120	16	0
Subtotal					36		

3. Total Pro from sources other than meat and subtract total from g of Pro in prescription.
4. Divide resulting figure by 7 g of Pro per meat exchange. This calculation gives you the number of meat exchanges.

Meat	—	7	3	4	0	28	12

5. Total fat from sources other than fat exchanges and subtract from g of fat in prescription.
6. Divide resulting figure by 5 g of fat per fat exchange. This calculation gives you the number of fat exchanges.

Fat	—	—	5	9	0	0	45
Totals:					184	64	57

Figure 3-5. Completed diet calculation sheet for a diet containing 1,500 calories, 50% carbohydrate, 17% protein, and 33% fat. CHO, carbohydrate; Pro, protein; HS, hour of sleep.

    (b) Determine the amount of carbohydrate that should come from each relevant group of exchanges as follows.

        The number of *milk* exchanges may range from 0 to 2 cups in increments of ½ cup. The Milk Exchange List is the only one in which use of half an exchange is feasible and practical. Write the number of exchanges

$^1/_{10}$ of total CHO	18 g
$^2/_{10}$ of total CHO	36 g
$^3/_{10}$ of total CHO	54 g
$^4/_{10}$ of total CHO	72 g

Distributions

		Meals				Snacks		
		CHO	Pro	Fat		CHO	Pro	Fat
Breakfast:	Milk	12	8	—	AM			
$^2/_{10}$ = 36 g	Fruit	10	—	—				
	Bread	15	2	—				
	Meat	—	—	—				
	Fat	—	—	5				
Total		37	10	5				
Lunch:	Milk	6	4	—	PM			
$^3/_{10}$ = 54 g	Vegetable	5	2	—				
	Fruit	10	—	—				
	Bread	30	4	—				
	Meat	—	7	3				
	Fat	—	—	10				
Total		51	17	13				
					HS:	$^2/_{10}$ = 36 g		
Dinner:	Milk	—	—	—		6	4	—
$^3/_{10}$ = 54 g	Vegetable	5	2	—		—	—	—
	Fruit	10	—	—		—	—	—
	Bread	45	6	—		30	4	—
	Meat	—	21	9		—	—	—
	Fat	—	—	20		—	—	10
Total		60	29	29		36	8	10

		CHO	Pro	Fat
Totals:	Breakfast	37	10	5
	Lunch	51	17	13
	Dinner	60	29	29
	AM	—	—	—
	PM	—	—	—
	HS	36	8	10
		184	64	57

and the exchange values of carbohydrate, protein, and fat in the appropriate boxes on the worksheet.

One or 2 *vegetable* exchanges are planned per day. Write the exchange values of carbohydrate, protein, and fat in the appropriate boxes on the worksheet.

Generally, 3 or more *fruit* exchanges are planned per day, depending on preferences of the patient. *At least* 1 serving should be encouraged (and planned for in the pattern) for general good nutrition. A rule of thumb is that there should always be more bread exchanges than fruit exchanges in a pattern (i.e., an emphasis on complex rather than simple carbohydrates). The items on the Milk and Fruit Exchange Lists contain only simple carbohydrates, while, for all practical purposes, the items on the Vegetable and Bread Exchange Lists include only complex carbohydrates. Therefore, the total number of grams of carbohydrate from the former two groups must make up not more than 10% to 15% of the total number of calories. Table 3-2 lists the allowable amounts (in grams) of simple carbohydrates at each calorie level. For the 1,500-calorie diet, since 10% to 15% of the total number of calories is 38 to 56 g of carbohydrate, 2 milk exchanges (24 g of carbohydrate) and 3 fruit exchanges (30 g of carbohydrate) fall within the acceptable range.

At this point, total the carbohydrate column, and then subtract this total from the total amount of carbohydrate. For the 1,500 calorie diet, the calculation is 188 − 64 = 124 g (Fig. 3-5).

To determine the total number of *bread* exchanges, divide the difference between the total allowable amount of carbohydrate and the amount of carbohydrate obtained from the milk, vegetable, and fruit exchanges by 15 g of carbohydrate per bread exchange. For the 1,500-calorie diet, the calculation is 124 ÷ 15 = 8 (Fig. 3-5).

(c) Determine the number of *meat* exchanges by totaling the protein column and subtracting the sum from the total allowable amount of protein. Next, divide this difference by 7 g of protein per meat exchange. For the 1,500-calorie diet, the calculations are 64 − 36 = 28; 28 ÷ 7 = 4 meat exchanges.

(d) Determine the number of fat exchanges by totaling the fat column and subtracting the sum from the total allowable amount of fat. Next, divide this difference by 5 g of fat per fat exchange. For the 1,500-calorie diet, the calculations are 55 − 12 = 43; 43 ÷ 5 = 9 fat exchanges.

(e) When the figures are totaled, each column is within 5 g of the goal set.

(5) The next step is the division of the total number of exchanges into meals in a manner as compatible as possible with the patient's usual diet. The number of meals and snacks is dependent on both medication and current eating patterns.

(a) Patients who receive *oral agents or no medication* are ketosis-resistant and (as discussed in chapter 2) are often obese, needing caloric restriction as the primary goal of treatment. Three meals are generally planned, and snacks are prescribed if the patient desires. Since weight-reduction diets are most often prescribed for such patients, spreading food intake throughout the day is often necessary in order to prevent excessive hunger. In addition, patients who have a problem with continuous snack-ing often benefit from planned snacks.

As was mentioned earlier, patients who are taking *insulin* must eat not only at certain times but in amounts that will serve as an appropriate "buffer" against the effects of absorbed insulin. Usually three meals plus a bedtime snack are planned for patients taking insulin. Intermediate-acting insulin taken early in the morning may require an afternoon snack, especially if the evening meal is eaten late.

(b) If a person works unusual hours, such as an evening or night shift, division of meals must be adapted to this pattern, but long periods without food should be avoided. (See case study 3, Appendix I.) Most school-aged children will enjoy an afternoon snack and possibly one at midmorning as well. Remember that the insulin prescription is adjusted as much as possible to fit the patient's usual daily activity and eating patterns.

(6) Once the number of meals and snacks has been determined, the carbo-hydrate allotment must be divided among the meals. The allotment may be divided in many ways, such as one third at breakfast, one third at lunch, and one third at dinner; one fifth at breakfast, two fifths at lunch, and two fifths at dinner; or two sevenths at breakfast, two sevenths at lunch, two sevenths at dinner, and one seventh at bedtime. Division into tenths (two tenths at breakfast, three tenths at lunch, one tenth for an afternoon [PM] snack, three tenths at dinner, and one tenth for a bedtime snack) works well because breakfast is not as large as dinner and snacks are readily incorporated. The division of carbohydrate should mimic the patient's usual eating pattern as closely as possible, and we have found that a division by tenths, as shown in Table 3-16, gives the most flexibility.

First, divide the indicated fractions of the carbohydrate allotment into the total number of grams of carbohydrate in order to calculate the number of grams to be consumed at each meal. For the 1,500-calorie diet, the carbohydrate allot-ment could be divided into 3 meals plus a bedtime snack as follows: two tenths at breakfast, three tenths at lunch, three tenths at dinner, and two tenths at bedtime. Thus, the calculations would be 188 g × 0.2 = 37.6 = 38 g; 188 g × 0.3 = 56.4 = 56 g.

Second, divide the protein and fat allotments among the meals in a reasonable manner. A good rule of thumb is to include a form of high biological protein, such as a meat exchange or milk exchange, at each meal or snack.

Finally, convert the total number of exchanges from each list into meals. As can be seen in Figure 3-5, the final totals in the 1,500-calorie diet (184 g of carbohydrate, 64 g of protein, and 57 g of fat) are identical to those of the original calculation of exchanges. The carbohydrate content of each meal and snack is within 5 g of the target number for that meal (i.e., 38 g or 56 g). The pattern shown assumes that the patient does not require a meat exchange at breakfast but instead chooses cereal and milk, for example. If a meat exchange

Table 3-16. Convenient Distributions of Carbohydrate Intake Among Meals and Snacks

Eating Schedule	Breakfast	AM Snack	Lunch	PM Snack	Dinner	Bedtime Snack
			Fraction of Carbohydrate at Indicated Meal or Snack			
3 meals only	2/10		4/10		4/10	
3 meals plus bedtime snack	2/10		3/10		3/10	2/10
3 meals plus PM and bedtime snacks	2/10		3/10	1/10	3/10	1/10
3 meals plus AM, PM, and bedtime snacks	1/10	1/10	3/10	1/10	3/10	1/10

food is normally eaten at breakfast, one meat exchange can be taken from the evening meal and inserted at breakfast. If the largest meal is normally eaten at lunch, the number of exchanges at lunch and dinner can easily be reversed. Also, this particular pattern assumes that the patient can obtain milk at lunch. If milk is unavailable, the ½ cup of milk can be moved to dinner and a fruit exchange moved from dinner to lunch.

Nutritional Instruction for the Patient

Translation of the Meal Plan

The meal plan that has been calculated according to the physician's orders and the patient's prior dietary experience is copied onto the form shown in Appendix A and discussed with the patient. The person who actually does the meal planning, the shopping, and the preparation of foods should be present at the initial instructive session. The food exchanges are translated into actual amounts of food selected from the six exchange lists. The 1,500-calorie diet, calculated as shown in Figure 3-5, might be translated as shown in Table 3-17.

For many patients, the translation of food exchanges into actual amounts of food is the point of greatest difficulty in understanding their meal plans. However, facility in translating meal plans is most important because it leads to more variety in the diet, permits greater integration of the patient's meals with those eaten by the rest of the family, and allows the patient to eat in restaurants and at other social gatherings.

The information that is necessary for translation of the calculated meal pattern into actual foods is included in Appendices A through F in a form that

Table 3-17. Sample Selection of Foods in Accord with Food Exchanges
Calculated for the 1,500-Calorie Diet Described in Figure 3-5

Meal, Exchange(s)	Selected Food and Portion
Breakfast	
1 fruit	½ cup orange juice
1 bread	1 slice whole wheat toast
1 fat	1 teaspoon margarine
1 milk (nonfat)	1 cup nonfat milk
Free	Coffee
Lunch	Sandwich
1 meat	¼ cup water-packed tuna
2 bread	2 slices bread
2 fat	2 teaspoons mayonnaise
1 vegetable	Asparagus-tomato salad
1 fruit	1 small apple
½ milk (nonfat)	½ cup nonfat milk
Dinner	
3 meat	3 ounces baked chicken
3 bread	1 cup parsley potatoes; 1 small dinner roll
1 vegetable	½ cup carrots; lettuce-wedge salad
1 fruit	1 cup fresh strawberries
4 fat	1 tablespoon French dressing; 3 teaspoons margarine
Free	Tea with lemon
Bedtime snack	
2 bread	1 English muffin
2 fat	2 teaspoons margarine
½ milk (nonfat)	½ cup nonfat milk

should be understandable to most patients and their families. We usually give copies of this material to our patients for their personal use. Appendix B ("Introduction to the Diabetic Diet") provides the patient with general information. Appendix C explains what an exchange list is. In addition, copies of the actual exchange lists in Tables 3-8 through 3-13 must be given to the patient. A list of herbs, spices, and seasonings that can be used by diabetics is furnished in Appendix D. Once the rudiments of using exchange lists and fitting them into a general diet are mastered, many patients will be able to use the information provided in Appendix E ("Combination Foods") to enhance the variety of their diets. Finally, the enjoyment of dining out is possible for diabetics if the guidelines provided in Appendix F are followed. Patients who are allowed alochol in their meal plans should receive copies of Table 3-3.

The patient should write sample menus for one day under the supervision of the dietitian. This kind of practice session is time well spent since it helps the patient understand his or her diet more fully. Menu writing can also be practiced at home and samples brought to subsequent office visits. Emphasis should be placed on the patient's actually using these menus at home. This kind of planning by the patient may result in better dietary compliance than would a food diary kept by the patient, in which foods eaten are merely recorded, whether or not they are allowed.

Follow-up on Dietary Therapy

The diabetic patient's continuing care must include follow-up on dietary therapy. The sooner the patient can correctly interpret the dietary prescription, the better the potential compliance. Two ways to ascertain the level of the patient's understanding are a brief review of the food exchanges and a short discussion of practice menus filled out by the patient at home and brought to an appointment. After the basic dietary information is mastered, more complicated aspects of nutritional education that can be discussed are: (a) planning menus that will incorporate the diabetic diet into the family meal plan; (b) shopping, with emphasis on the fact that the foods a diabetic eats are ordinary groceries bought in a supermarket; and (c) eating away from home.

In addition to enabling the patient to master the dietary prescription, dietary follow-up has two other important functions. First, in order to ensure maximal compliance, some adjustments may have to be made after the patient's initial experience with the meal plan. The patient should be encouraged to speak freely about her or his reaction to the new diet. An extremely rigid attitude by the physician or dietitian will lead only to the patient's not following the diet plan and hiding that lack of compliance from those supervising her or his care.

Second, dietary follow-up should provide encouragement and ensure realistic expectations for the patient. A change in eating habits is not easy for most patients, and they become discouraged without appropriate recognition of their efforts. Many diabetics have commented to us that their physicians did not seem to appreciate the efforts involved in losing 1 or 2 pounds between office visits. Besides encouragement, patients need a realistic framework in which to judge their progress. One pound of fat is equal to 454 g. Since 1 g of fat yields 9 calories, a patient has to eat approximately 4,000 fewer calories (9 × 454) than he or she expends in energy in order to lose 1 pound of fat. The weight-reduction diets discussed earlier (10 calories/lb. of ideal body weight) provide approximately 500 fewer calories per day than the patient usually expends in energy. Therefore, a patient following such a diet should expect to lose approximately 1 pound per week. Although 50 pounds per year will be lost at a safe rate on this regimen, many patients understandably wish to see quicker results. However, since a permanent restructuring of eating habits is necessary for the long-term success of diabetic diets, severely unbalanced or hypocaloric diets are followed for only short periods. A slow, gradual weight loss has a much greater chance of being sustained.

Obese patients on hypocaloric diets must also be warned that most of the weight loss during the first 1 to 2 weeks is due to fluid losses, not loss of fat tissue. Whenever carbohydrate intake is decreased (regardless of total caloric intake), urinary sodium excretion increases and causes diuresis. This water loss begins within 1 to 3 days and may last as long as a week. The more obese the patient, the more pronounced will be the diuresis. If the patient expects this initial weight loss to be sustained, the resulting disappointment may lead to abandonment of the diet. Conversely, if a patient goes on eating binges, the increased carbohydrate intake over the usual level (whatever it may be) will cause decreased urinary sodium excretion. This situation will result in weight gain that is due to water retention and is out of proportion to the number of extra calories ingested, for just as a patient must eat ~4,000 fewer calories than he or she uses in order to lose 1 pound of fat, the patient must ingest 4,000 calories more than he or she expends in order to gain 1 pound of fat! When obese patients are viewed in that light, it becomes clear that their overeating has been an ingrained habit for a number of years. Therefore, it is not too surprising that weight reduction is extremely difficult for many of these patients in spite of its great therapeutic benefits.

Dietary Strategy during Illness

Patients taking insulin have a special problem when an illness affects their appetite or their ability to retain what they have eaten. Infection and stress are associated with insulin antagonism; therefore, most physicians recommend that patients take their usual dose of insulin during illness, since a reduction in dosage often leads to rapid deterioration of control. Thus, it is important for a patient to ingest an amount of carbohydrate that will prevent hypoglycemia. One course that may be followed in this situation is the replacement of the usual carbohydrate content of the diet with carbohydrate-containing foods that are the easiest to digest; dietary protein and fat are ignored until the patient can resume her or his usual diet. This approach can be utilized only if the gastrointestinal symptoms are mild enough to allow the patient to hold down some food. It also requires a thorough understanding of the exchange system.

The carbohydrate in a meal pattern may be replaced as follows: (*a*) Calculate the carbohydrate content of each meal using the following figures for the various exchange groups: milk, 12 g; vegetable, 5 g; fruit, 10 g; and bread, 15 g. For example, a meal containing 1 milk exchange, 1 fruit exchange, and 2 bread exchanges would contain 52 g of carbohydrate to be replaced. (*b*) Convert the carbohydrate content of each meal into the foods listed in Table 3-18. In the example just mentioned, the 52 g of carbohydrate could be replaced with 1 cup of grape juice and 5 saltine crackers, or with any other combination equaling

Table 3-18. Foods Commonly Used for Carbohydrate Replacement
During Illness

Food	Amount	Carbohydrate Content (g)
Fruit juices		
unsweetened orange, grapefruit	1/2 cup	10
apple, pineapple, cranberry	1/3 cup	10
grape, prune, nectars	1/4 cup	10
Applesauce	1/2 cup	11
Popsicle, twin bar	1/2	12
Regular soft drink (any kind)	4 oz	13
Plain yogurt	1 cup	13
Hot chocolate	1/2 cup	13
Chocolate milk	1/2 cup	14
Warm milk	1 cup	12
Chocolate pudding	1/4 cup	16
Cream soup (made with milk)	1 cup	15
Eggnog	1/2 cup	13
Ice cream	1/2 cup	14
Toast	1 slice	15
Crackers (saltine)	5	15
Hot cereal	1/2 cup	15
Dry cereal	3/4 cup	15
Gelatin (flavored)	1/2 cup	16
Graham crackers, squares	2	10
Custard	1/2 cup	15
Sherbet	1/4 cup	15
Mashed potatoes	1/2 cup	14
Baked potato	1 small	14

50 to 55 g of carbohydrate. The calculation for an entire day for a patient following the 1,500-calorie diet containing 188 g of carbohydrate, 64 g of protein, and 55 g of fat is shown in Table 3-19.

A less rigorous dietary approach during illness is presented in chapter 7 for the patient whose gastrointestinal symptoms prevent him or her from eating as much as is required in this approach or whose understanding of the exchange system is not sophisticated enough to permit these kinds of calculations.

Table 3-19. Sample Selection of Foods for Carbohydrate Replacement
During Illness

Meal, exchange(s)	Carbohydrate (g)	Replacement Food	Carbohydrate (g)
Breakfast			
1 fruit	10	5 saltine crackers	15
0 meat		1/2 cup grape juice	20
1 bread	15		
1 fat			
1 milk	12		
Total	37		35
AM snack: none			
Lunch			
1 meat			
2 bread	30	1 cup orange juice	20
1 vegetable	5	1 cup ice cream	28
2 fat			
1 fruit	10		
1/2 milk	6		
Total	51		48
PM snack: none			
Dinner			
3 meat			
3 bread	45	1/2 cup chocolate	
1 vegetable	5	pudding	32
4 fat		2 slices toast	30
1 fruit	10		
0 milk			
Total	60		62
Bedtime snack			
2 bread	30	1 cup grape juice	40
1/2 milk	6		
2 fat			
Total	36		40

Diet and Exercise

Although exercise is important in the treatment of diabetics, insulin-dependent
patients may require extra calories in order to avoid hypoglycemia. Exercise
tends to lower the blood sugar level by two mechanisms. First, injected insulin is

absorbed from subcutaneous tissue into the circulation faster when the patient exercises (4). Second, the insulin-sensitive tissues seem to respond more effectively to whatever insulin is present than in the absence of exercise (5). The insulin dose is usually dependent on the patient's normal caloric intake and exercise pattern. Therefore, unusual exercise (activities not performed on a daily, routine basis) should be accompanied by ingestion of extra calories in order to prevent hypoglycemia.

Table 3-20 lists caloric expenditures during a number of activities. We were unable to find any recommendations in the literature concerning the number of extra calories that should be consumed by diabetic patients in association with a given type of exercise. This lack of information no doubt reflects the number of variables involved—e.g., amount of insulin injected, site of injection, interval between injection and exercise, different kinds of activity, and biological variation among patients. Therefore, each patient must experiment. However, we would offer the following empirical advice as an initial approach to replacing calories just before the anticipated exercise.

No additional calories need to be ingested for light or moderate activity. Approximately half of the calories expended should be replaced in the form of the usual exchanges for marked and vigorous activity. If the period of exercise is limited, the milk and fruit exchanges, with their simple carbohydrate content, should be emphasized. Complex carbohydrates (bread and vegetable exchanges) are important in instances of more prolonged exercise (1 to 2 hours). If the period of exercise lasts longer than several hours, it may have to be interrupted for caloric intake. In addition, extra simple carbohydrate (fruit juices, candy bars, cookies, etc.) should be eaten in order to counteract vigorous activity. Patients may have to vary these recommendations based on their personal experiences. However, this initial approach should help both to prevent exercise-induced hypoglycemia and to limit unnecessary hyperglycemia due to the ingestion of too many calories (especially in the form of simple carbohydrates) for the amount of exercise performed.

Practical Summary

Ordering Diets

A diet for any diabetic patient is ordered as follows:

1. Determine the ideal body weight of the patient.
    (a) For females, allow 100 pounds for the first 5 feet of height. Allow 5 pounds for each inch over 5 feet.
    (b) For males, allow 106 pounds for the first 5 feet of height. Allow 6 pounds for each inch over 5 feet.

Table 3-20. Caloric Expenditure During Various Activities[a]

Level of Activity	No. of Calories Expended/hr[b]
Light	50-199
Lying down or sleeping	80
Sitting	100
Driving an automobile	120
Standing	140
Domestic work	180
Moderate	200-299
Walking (2½ mph)	210
Bicycling (5½ mph)	210
Gardening	220
Canoeing (2½ mph)	230
Golf	250
Lawn mowing (power mower)	250
Lawn mowing (hand mower)	270
Bowling	270
Marked	300-399
Fencing	300
Rowing (2½ mph)	300
Swimming (¼ mph)	300
Walking (3¾ mph)	300
Badminton	350
Horseback riding (trotting)	350
Square-dancing	350
Volleyball	350
Roller-skating	350
Table tennis	360
Vigorous	≥ 400
Ditch digging (hand shovel)	400
Ice-skating (10 mph)	400
Wood chopping or sawing	400
Tennis	420
Hill climbing (100 ft/hr)	480
Skiing (10 mph)	490
Squash	600
Handball	600
Bicycling (13 mph)	660
Scull rowing (racing)	840
Running (10 mph)	900

[a]Reprinted with permission from Bierman J, Toohey B: *The Diabetic's Sports and Exercise Book. How to Play Your Way to Better Health.* JB Lippincott, Philadelphia, 1977, pp 241-242.

[b]The number of calories expended by a 150-pound person is shown. Caloric expenditure will be slightly lower for lighter persons and somewhat higher for heavier subjects. A more detailed analysis of the metabolic costs of many more activities can be found in Consolazio CF: *Physiologic Measurements of Metabolic Function in Man.* McGraw-Hill, New York, 1963, pp 329-332.

(c) The resultant number of pounds is for a medium frame. Add 10% for a large frame size, and subtract 10% for a small frame size.

2. Determine the total caloric intake.
   (a) Allow 10 calories/pound of ideal body weight if the patient needs to lose weight.
   (b) Allow 15 calories/pound of ideal body weight for weight maintenance.
   (c) Allow 20 calories/pound of ideal body weight for patients who need to gain weight, for adolescent patients, or for patients whose usual physical activity is deemed excessive (i.e., heavy physical labor).
   (d) Lower the number of total calories by 10% for *each* decade after the age of 50 years because of the decreases in physical activity, lean body mass, and resting metabolic rates that are associated with aging.
   (e) Round off to the nearest 50 calories.

3. Distribute the calories among the categories of carbohydrate, protein, and fat.
   (a) Fifty per cent of the total number of calories should be carbohydrate, with approximately 35% to 40% in the form of complex carbohydrates (starches) and 10% to 15% in the form of simple carbohydrates.
   (b) Seventeen per cent of the total number of calories should be protein.
   (c) Thirty-three per cent of the total number of calories should be fat, with saturated (S) fat limited to one third of the total amount and cholesterol intake limited to approximately 300 mg per day. Of the remaining fat intake, one third is usually monounsaturated and one third is polyunsaturated (P). Table 3-7 lists the P:S ratio of a number of oils and other fats.

4. Translate the number of calories derived from carbohydrate, protein, and fat into the actual amount (in grams) of each food source by dividing the number of carbohydrate and protein calories by 4 and the number of fat calories by 9 (i.e., carbohydrate yields 4 calories/g, protein yields 4 calories/g, and fat yields 9 calories/g). Alternatively, consult Table 3-2, which contains the calculated amounts (in grams) of carbohydrate (both total and simple), protein, and fat for diets ranging between 1,000 and 3,500 calories.

5. If alcohol is allowed in the diet, the number of calories it contributes can be calculated by the following formula: 0.8 × proof × number of ounces = number of calories, where proof is twice the percentage of alcohol. Table 3-3 lists the exchange equivalents of some common alcoholic beverages.

6. The use of natural foods with a high fiber content should be encouraged. Tables 3-4 through 3-6 list the *total* plant-fiber content of selected foods. Most sources give only the crude-fiber content, a value that is much lower (see values in parentheses in the tables) and that should not be used to evaluate the fiber content of a diet. The average American (low-fiber) diet contains 6 to 12 g of total plant fiber/1,000 calories, while a typical high-fiber diet consists of 25 to 30 g/1,000 calories.

Calculating Diets

The basic units of diabetic diets are the food exchanges. The diet is selected from six different lists of foods (Tables 3-8 through 3-13) that are grouped according to their nutritional content. The term *exchange* refers to the fact that each item on a particular list (in the amount stated) may be interchanged with any other item on the *same* list. The amounts (in grams) of carbohydrate, protein, and fat in the food items on each list are as follows:

Exchange List	Table	Carbohydrate	Protein	Fat
Milk	3-8	12	8	0
Vegetable	3-9	5	2	0
Fruit	3-10	10	0	0
Bread	3-11	15	2	0
Meat	3-12	0	7	3
Fat	3-13	0	0	5

Some of the items on the Milk and Meat Exchange Lists also count as 1 or 2 fat exchanges. Dried peas and beans on the Bread Exchange List also count as a meat exchange. Other items on the Bread Exchange List may also count as a fat exchange, depending on their method of preparation. Certain foods can be eaten in unlimited quantities (Table 3-15), while others must be avoided altogether (Table 3-14).

The information obtained from a dietary history (Fig. 3-3) is extremely useful in translating the diet ordered by the physician into the actual meal plan for the patient. The steps involve: (*a*) determining the total number of exchanges from each exchange list; (*b*) dividing this total number of exchanges into meals; (*c*) distributing the allotment of carbohydrate among the meals; and (*d*) converting the total number of exchanges into a meal plan. The worksheet in Figure 3-4 facilitates this process, which is described in detail for a 1,500-calorie diet in this chapter; the completed worksheet for this diet is shown in Figure 3-5. The three case studies in Appendices G, H, and I relate some practical experiences in the calculation of actual diets.

Nutritional Instruction for the Patient

The information that is necessary for translation of a meal pattern into actual foods is included in Appendices A through F. Dietary follow-up should include: (*a*) opportunities for patients to write sample menus; (*b*) incorporation of meal patterns into the family meal plan; (*c*) information relevant to shopping for appropriate foods; (*d*) information relevant to eating away from home; (*e*) encouragement for patients on weight-reduction diets; and (*f*) information concerning realistic goals. For instance, expenditure of approximately 4,000 more calories than are consumed is required in order to lose 1 pound of fat. Therefore, patients should be told that a weight loss of 0.5 to 2.0 pounds per week (depending on the degree of obesity) is to be expected from the weight-reduction diets described in this chapter. The patient should be made aware that the greater weight loss during the first 2 weeks of a diet is due to diuresis associated with increased urinary sodium excretion, which in turn is secondary to lowered carbohydrate intake. Conversely, if a patient binges on carbohydrates, the resultant weight gain is due to water retention secondary to diminished urinary sodium excretion and is out of proportion to the number of extra calories actually ingested.

Dietary Strategy during Illness

Because insulin-requiring patients are usually advised (appropriately) by their physicians to continue taking the usual dose of insulin during an illness, marked impairment of food intake could cause hypoglycemia. One way of avoiding this problem is to replace the usual carbohydrate content of the diet with carbohydrate-containing foods that are easy to digest and to ignore protein and fat intake. (This approach is described in the section *Dietary Strategy during Illness*.) The foods to be used for carbohydrate replacement during an illness are listed in Table 3-18. This method requires a thorough knowledge of the exchange system and gastrointestinal symptoms that are mild enough to allow ingestion of a reasonable amount of food. A less rigorous dietary approach during illness is presented in Chapter 7 for patients whose gastrointestinal symptoms prevent ingestion of adequate amounts of food or whose understanding of the exchange system is not sophisticated enough to permit these kinds of calculations.

Diet and Exercise

Exercise in insulin-requiring diabetics may cause hypoglycemia because of both increased absorption of insulin from the injection site and enhanced effectiveness at the tissue level. The approximate caloric expenditures during a variety of activities are listed in Table 3-20. Although we could find no guidelines in the literature for caloric replacement during exercise, an initial (empirical) approach to the adjustment of caloric intake—in order both to prevent hypoglycemia and to avoid unnecessary hyperglycemia—is as follows: ingestion of no additional calories for light and moderate activity; ingestion (in the form of the usual exchanges) of approximately one half of the anticipated number of calories to be expended for marked or vigorous activity; ingestion of extra simple carbohydrates (fruit juices, cookies, candy bars, etc.) for vigorous activity; and ingestion of some calories after several hours of exercise if the activity is to continue. These recommendations may need modification based on the actual experience of individual patients.

Appendix A: Diabetic Meal Plan

_____ Calories   Total Exchanges: _____
_____ Carbohydrate (g)   Fruit _____
_____ Protein (g)   Milk _____
_____ Fat (g)   Vegetable _____
                                               Bread _____
                                               Meat _____
                                               Fat _____

MEAL PATTERN

BREAKFAST:
    Fruit Exchange _____
    Meat Exchange _____
    Bread Exchange _____
    Fat Exchange _____
    Milk Exchange _____

MIDMORNING:
_____

NOON:
    Meat Exchange _____
    Bread Exchange _____
    Vegetable Exchange _____
    Fat Exchange _____
    Fruit Exchange _____
    Milk Exchange _____

MIDAFTERNOON:
_____

EVENING:
    Meat Exchange _____
    Bread Exchange _____
    Vegetable Exchange _____
    Fat Exchange _____
    Fruit Exchange _____
    Milk Exchange _____

BEDTIME:
_____

    Dietitian: _____ , RD

    Phone: _____

Appendix B: Introduction to the Diabetic Diet

Your diet is a very important part of the treatment of diabetes. Along with medication and physical activity, the diet is used to keep your blood sugar level within a normal range. This is important because control of your blood sugar level can prevent or lessen the effects of complications in other organs of your body, such as the eyes, heart, and kidneys. Knowing *when, what,* and *how much* to eat is the key to following your diet.

It is important for you to eat three meals a day plus any snacks that have been planned for you. Try to eat at about the same time every day, and don't skip meals. Your body is not designed to go for long periods without food, and any medication you may be taking to control your blood sugar level will require regular eating habits.

Your foods and the amounts of each food will be selected from six different lists of foods. These *exchange lists* group foods according to their nutrient content. The foods on the lists are regular, nutritious foods; there is no reason to buy special "dietetic" foods. You may prepare the same foods for yourself that you prepare for your family and friends, although you may need to separate your portion before any sugar, fat, or thickening is added. A variety of seasonings may be used freely, but other foods must be measured and eaten in the amounts specified. After measuring foods carefully for a while, you should be able to estimate portion sizes accurately when you are eating away from home.

A meal plan designed to meet your needs will be given to you along with the food exchange lists. This plan will be based as much as possible on your present eating habits. The meal plan will show you how many choices to make from each list each day and will be the basis for planning your daily menus.

Certain foods are not on the exchange lists because they contain too many calories and too much sugar. High-sugar foods cause your blood sugar to rise very quickly to levels that are too high instead of remaining near the normal levels. These foods include sugar, honey, jams, jellies, pie, cake, cookies, candy, sweetened condensed milk, soft drinks, and chewing gum. Alcoholic beverages should not be consumed without permission from your doctor and, if consumed, should be worked into your diet by your dietitian.

If you need to lose weight, your prescribed calorie level will allow you to lose it gradually and to obtain proper nutrients at the same time. Losing weight will help to lower your blood sugar level and will help your heart, lungs, and other organs to work more efficiently.

You are encouraged to select plain foods and to combine them yourself instead of buying already-prepared foods that may have unknown or disallowed ingredients. Usually, the less processing a product has undergone, the less chance there is of hidden calories. There are many recipes for combining foods, and your dietitian can help you get started. Remember that you "eat" with your eyes as well as your mouth, so make your food look as attractive as possible. Herbs and spices may be used freely to add additional flavor.

When eating out, it is important for you to understand and follow your meal pattern. Choose meats that are not fried and do not have sauces or gravies; add your own dressing to salads in the amount you are allowed; and choose vegetables that are not creamed, fried, or in a sauce. Various breads are fine, and fresh fruit rather than sweets should be chosen for dessert. Coffee, tea, and milk (if milk is on your meal plan) are good beverages to choose.

Be sure to ask any questions you may have, and remember that if you understand and follow the plan for when, what, and how much to eat, you will be on the right track toward controlling your disease and living a normal life.

Appendix C: What is an Exchange List?

If variety is what you expect from your diet, exchange lists are just what you are looking for. To help you plan your meals and obtain the nutrients your body needs, foods have been divided into six different lists: the Milk Exchange List, the Vegetable Exchange List, the Fruit Exchange List, the Bread Exchange List, the Meat Exchange List, and the Fat Exchange List. Similar types of foods are grouped together, and the foods on each list contribute special nutrients to your diet. Foods from each list should be included in your diet each day since it takes all six groups working together to supply your nutritional needs for good health.

An *exchange* is a serving of food in a specific amount from a particular list. It can be substituted for any other food on the *same* list. Each exchange is approximately equal in number of calories and amounts of carbohydrate, protein, fat, vitamins, minerals, and fiber. The body needs all of these nutrients to function properly. The amount listed after each food is the portion that makes up 1 exchange. The portion sizes are very important and are different for each food, so pay close attention to the amounts listed.

For example, 1 slice of bread and 1/2 cup of mashed potatoes are each 1 bread exchange. If you are allowed 2 bread exchanges at a meal, you can have two different choices (such as the slice of bread *and* the mashed potatoes) or two times the listed amount of 1 exchange (such as 2 slices of bread *or* 1 cup of mashed potatoes). You may substitute the bread or potatoes for any other item on the Bread Exchange List but not for a food from any other list. You make choices from the other lists in the same manner.

The Meat Exchange List is divided into three parts: lean meat exchanges (all those not followed by a letter), medium-fat meat exchanges (those followed by the letter *a*, such as beef), and high-fat meat exchanges (those followed by the letter *b*, such as frankfurters and peanut butter). Each lean meat exchange counts as 1 meat exchange. Each medium-fat meat exchange counts as 1 meat exchange *and* 1 fat exchange. Each high-fat meat exchange counts as 1 meat exchange *and* 2 fat exchanges. For example, 3 ounces of chicken (a lean meat exchange) equals 3 meat exchanges; 3 ounces of lean beef (a medium-fat exchange) equals 3 meat exchanges *and* 3 fat exchanges; and 3 frankfurters (a high-fat meat exchange) equals 3 meat exchanges *and* 6 fat exchanges. You can see that when you choose your meat exchanges from the medium-fat and high-fat items, you will be able to make fewer selections from the Fat Exchange List.

Your dietitian will explain the lists to you and give you a meal pattern to follow; this pattern will be based on your appropriate calorie level and your eating habits. The dietitian will ask you what kind of work you do and where you usually eat your meals (at home, at work, in a restaurant, etc.). He or she will also need to know the foods you prefer, whether or not you cook for other family members, and your food shopping and spending patterns. In short, the meal pattern will be designed to meet *your* needs and will show you how many choices to make from each list at each meal. Sometimes compromises will have to be made between the kinds and amounts of food you prefer and what is best for your health.

Your meal pattern will not require a lot of special foods and special preparation. Basically, it will outline a healthy, nutritious pattern of eating, not only for you, but for other family members as well. You can cook the same foods for your family that you cook for yourself. As long as you follow your meal pattern, you can eat in restaurants and friends' homes as well as in your own home. The types of foods you eat are important, but many times the *amount* of food is more important.

You must be the person responsible for knowing how to plan your meals, so be sure to ask your dietitian any questions you have. You cannot be independent if you have to rely on someone else to understand your meal plan and prepare your food. Your dietitian will give you any help you need and will make changes in your meal pattern if necessary.

Appendix D: Herbs, Spices, and Seasonings

The following herbs, spices, and seasonings have few or no calories and may be used freely to add flavor to your foods. Those preceded by an asterisk (*) are very salty and should not be used if you must watch your salt intake.

Allspice
Angostura bitters
Anise
Basil
Bay leaf
Bell peppers (dried or fresh)
*Bouillon cube
Caraway seed
*Catsup
Celery
*Celery salt
Celery seed
Chervil
Chili peppers
Chili powder
Chives
Cinnamon
Cloves
Curry powder
Dill
Garlic (fresh)
Garlic powder
*Garlic salt
Ginger
Leeks
Lemon juice
Lemon rind

Lime juice
Mace
Marjoram
Mint
*Mustard (prepared)
Mustard (dry)
Nutmeg
Onion (fresh)
Onion juice
Onion powder
*Onion salt
Orange rind
Oregano
Parsley
Pepper (black or white)
Poppy seeds
Poultry seasoning
Rosemary
Saffron
Sage
*Soy sauce (bottled without sugar)
*Tabasco sauce
Tarragon
Thyme
*Worcestershire sauce
Vanilla extract
Vinegar

Appendix E: Combination Foods

After using the exchange lists and following your meal pattern for a while, you will probably want to add even more variety to your diet by combining foods occasionally. One way in which you are probably already combining foods is a tossed salad. By mixing choices from the Vegetable Exchange List, such as lettuce, tomato, cucumber, cauliflower, chopped onion, and bell pepper, you get an interesting variety of flavors and textures, few calories, and a lot of bulk. Since they are raw, these vegetables can be eaten in unlimited amounts. Salad dressing may be added as a fat exchange, or lemon juice can be used freely.

Another way to combine foods is in a small casserole. For example, combination of the following ingredients in the indicated amounts would make a one-serving casserole:

1/2 cup canned tomatoes	=	1 vegetable exchange
1/2 cup cooked rice	=	1 bread exchange
2 ounces cooked lean ground meat, drained	=	2 meat exchanges + 2 fat exchanges
1 teaspoon margarine	=	1 fat exchange
Chopped onion	=	free
Salt, pepper, spices to taste	=	free

One serving of this dish would count as 1 vegetable exchange, 1 bread exchange, 2 meat exchanges, and 3 fat exchanges. These exchanges would be subtracted from the total number of exchanges of each type allowed for that meal. In cooking for two persons, the amount could be doubled, with each person eating half.

Let us look at another combination in a quantity more like that you might find in a recipe book:

Chili (serves 4)

1 pound (16 oz.) lean ground meat, cooked, drained	=	12 meat exchanges (after cooking) + 12 fat exchanges
2 cups pinto beans, cooked	=	4 bread exchanges + 4 meat exchanges
1 16-oz can tomato sauce	=	4 vegetable exchanges
2 cloves garlic, crushed	=	free
3 or 4 green chilis or small amount chili powder	=	free
Chopped onion, small amount	=	free
Water to desired consistency	=	free
Spices as desired	=	free

Four servings would count as a total of 16 meat exchanges, 12 fat exchanges, 4 bread exchanges, and 4 vegetable exchanges. One serving would therefore count as 4 meat exchanges, 3 fat exchanges, 1 bread exchange, and 1 vegetable exchange.

There are recipe books in which the dishes are designed for calorie-controlled diets and the number of exchanges is given for each recipe. A list of such cookbooks is provided at the end of this section, and you may find others in a bookstore. Be sure, though, that the exchanges are given.

Don't forget about herbs and spices to season your foods and give added color and flavor. These foods have no calories and can be used freely. For example, lemon juice and garlic both add flavor to all kinds of foods.

Choosing food combinations when eating out can be very difficult, so stick to meats and vegetables without sauces, breading, and gravies. Avoid fried foods. You can see how chili prepared by someone else, for example, might have many ingredients that you would not be aware of (e.g., fat) so that figuring exchanges would be impossible.

There are many convenience foods in your market. Before using them, you must become familiar with the package labels and understand what they tell you about the products, their ingredients, and especially their nutrient content. Check with your dietitian before using a product about which you are not sure.

Also check with your dietitian if there is a particular food or recipe that you crave but that is not on your exchange lists. Chances are good that it can be worked into your meal pattern occasionally, either as is or modified slightly.

Remember, your dietitian wants you to be able to eat as many different foods as possible and does not want to take the pleasure of eating away from you. Check with her or him whenever you have any questions.

Cookbooks

A Cookbook for Diabetics by Maude Behrman.

Cookbook for Calorie Watchers by *Good Housekeeping.*

Cookbook for Diabetics by Gaynor Maddox.

Recipes for Diabetics by Billie Little.

The Art of Cooking for the Diabetic by Mary Hess and Katharine Middleton.

The Calculating Cook by Jeanne Jones.

Appendix F: Dining Out

When eating away from home, you must still follow your meal pattern and make appropriate choices. Remember to consider portion sizes, noting the amount listed after each exchange. Take your exchange lists along if necessary.

Measure foods at home so that you are able to judge the size of portions you are served when eating out. If a serving is too large, eat only the amount your diet allows, and ask for a doggy bag for the rest. A cafeteria is convenient because you can see the size of the serving before selecting it.

Choose foods that are not breaded, creamed, or in sauce or gravy. Avoid unfamiliar food combinations, because it is too easy for extra calories to be hidden in them. When foods are listed by special names on the menu, ask the waiter or waitress what is in the dish and how it is prepared.

The following are guidelines for making choices. Be sure to follow your meal pattern. Remember that not only what you eat but how much you eat is important.

DO ORDER	DO NOT ORDER
Appetizers	
Tomato or vegetable juice, unsweetened fruit juice, clear broth, bouillon, consommé, dill pickles, and raw vegetables are acceptable. Plain fish or meat is allowed if you eat less meat at the main course.	Canned fruit, fish or meat cocktails, alcoholic beverages (unless approved by your doctor and worked into your diet), creamed soups, crackers, chips, marinated vegetables, and nuts are not permissible.
Salads	
Fresh vegetable or fruit salads without dressing already added, chef's salads, cottage cheese, and fruit are allowed. Use a lemon wedge or vinegar in unlimited amounts. Other dressings must be counted as fat exchanges.	Salads with dressings added (including coleslaw and potato salad), molded salads, creamy mixtures, and cheese mixtures are not acceptable.
Meat, Fish, Poultry	
Anything that is roasted, baked, broiled, boiled, or charcoal grilled is a good choice. Trim off extra fat; remove skin from poultry. Bacon and sausage count as fat exchanges rather than meat exchanges.	Any choices that are fried, breaded, grilled, sautéed, stewed, braised, creamed, or in sauces or gravies are not allowed.
Eggs	
Soft, hard-cooked, or poached eggs are permissible.	Fried or scrambled eggs and omelets are not permissible.

Sandwiches

Single-item sandwiches and those made with meat, poultry, cold cuts, cheese, hot dogs, and hamburgers may be ordered. You must allow for the bread, fillings, and any condiments.

Hot-gravy sandwiches, club sandwiches, sandwiches grilled in fat, and those with cream cheese fillings, salad fillings (chicken, tuna), or avocado fillings are not acceptable.

Vegetables

Any stewed, steamed, boiled, or baked items are fine. If buttered, allow for the fat.

Items that are creamed, escalloped, au gratin, fried, sautéed, or in sauces are not acceptable.

Potatoes, Rice, Noodles

Baked, mashed, boiled, or steamed potatoes and boiled or steamed rice or noodles are good choices. If buttered, allow for the fat.

Do not choose potatoes that are French fried, home fried, browned, creamed, or escalloped; fried rice; or rice or noodles with gravy.

Breads and Cereals

Acceptable choices are any bread sliced to average thickness (as long as it is not sweetened or frosted), hard or soft rolls, bagels, English muffins, other muffins, biscuits, corn bread, crackers, unfrosted cold cereals, hot cereals without added sweetener, pancakes, waffles, French toast without syrup, and tortillas.

Sweet rolls, coffee cakes, Danish pastries, sweet breads, nut breads, fruit breads, doughnuts, fruit muffins, cakes, cookies, pies, and sweetened cereals are not allowed.

Fats

Butter, margarine, salad dressings, mayonnaise, cream cheese, tartar sauce, sour cream, bacon, or sausage may be selected. All choices should be made according to the number of fat exchanges allowed.

Gravy, fried foods, foods with cream sauces, and salads with dressing already added are not acceptable choices.

Desserts

Fresh fruit, sherbet, ice cream, angel food cake, or flavored gelatin is allowed.

Sweetened or canned fruits, custards, pies, puddings, cakes, pastries, candy, and chocolate are not permissible.

Beverages

Coffee and tea (black), milk (as allowed on your meal pattern), plain or carbonated water, and unsweetened juice may be chosen.

Chocolate milk, hot chocolate, milk shakes or malts, regular soft drinks, and sweetened fruit juices are unacceptable.

Appendix G: Case Study 1—Obese Female on Weight-Reduction Diet

L.W. is a 62-year-old Caucasian woman recently diagnosed to be diabetic with a fasting plasma glucose concentration of 278 mg/100 ml. She denies experiencing polyuria, polydipsia, or polyphagia. She is 5 feet 2 inches tall; her weight has been increasing gradually over the past 5 years and is currently at 180 pounds. She holds a full-time secretarial job and has little physical activity after work hours. A dietary history indicates that she eats one meal per day—dinner—with frequent afternoon and evening snacks. She names ice cream and strawberries as her favorite foods. She takes no medication for her diabetes.

An appropriate diet for L. W. can be calculated as follows:

1. Ideal body weight = 110 pounds

2. 10 calories/pound of ideal body weight (to lose weight) = 1,100 calories per day

3. Division of carbohydrate (CHO), protein (pro), and fat:
   50% CHO = 550 calories = 138 g
   17% pro = 187 calories = 47 g
   33% fat = 363 calories = 40 g

4. Breakdown of 1,100 calories by exchanges:

	CHO (g)	*Pro (g)*	*Fat (g)*
1 nonfat milk exchange	12	8	—
2 vegetable exchanges	10	4	—
2 fruit exchanges	20	—	—
6 bread exchanges	90	12	—
4 meat exchanges	—	28	12
5 fat exchanges	—	—	25
	132	52	37

= 1,069 calories

5. Distribution of CHO by meals:
   Target figures (CHO)
   $2/10$ at breakfast = 26 g
   $3/10$ at lunch = 39 g
   $3/10$ at dinner = 39 g
   $2/10$ at bedtime = 26 g

	Breakfast	*Lunch*	*Dinner*	*Bedtime*
1 nonfat milk exchange	1/2	—	—	1/2
2 vegetable exchanges	—	1	1	—
2 fruit exchanges	1	—	1	—
6 bread exchanges	1	2	2	1
4 meat exchanges	—	1	3	—
5 fat exchanges	1	1	3	—

	Breakfast	*Lunch*	*Dinner*	*Bedtime*
CHO (g)	31	35	45	21

32 g of simple CHO

100 g of complex CHO

6. Comments: L.W. was strongly advised to spread her intake over three meals and a bedtime snack, as shown on the above pattern, rather than concentrating it in one meal. Appropriate snacks from the Unlimited Use List were chosen by the patient when she made her practice menus. Because weight reduction was a high priority, the patient was urged to limit her ice cream intake to ½ cup once per week or less (½ cup of ice cream = 1 bread + 2 fat exchanges), and it was suggested that strawberries be included as a fruit exchange.

Appendix H: Case Study 2—Male on Weight-Gaining Diet

B.W. is a 38-year-old black man in whom diabetes mellitus was diagnosed 5 years ago. He states that since that time he has eliminated all "starches and sweets" from his diet to try to decrease his blood sugar level and has lost 30 pounds. He now weighs 130 pounds and is 5 feet 9 inches tall. A dietary history indicates that he prepares breakfast for himself at home, takes a lunch to his 8 AM-to-5 PM job, and eats dinner prepared by his wife. He takes intermediate-acting and regular insulin in the morning only.

An appropriate diet for B.W. can be calculated as follows:

1. Ideal body weight = 160 pounds
2. 20 calories/pound of ideal body weight (to gain weight) = 3,200 calories
3. Division of carbohydrate (CHO), protein (pro), and fat:
   50% CHO = 1,600 calories = 400 g
   17% pro =   544 calories = 136 g
   33% fat   = 1,056 calories = 117 g
4. Breakdown of 3,200 calories by exchanges:

	CHO (g)	Pro (g)	Fat (g)
3 nonfat milk exchanges	36	24	–
2 vegetable exchanges	10	4	–
6 fruit exchanges	60	–	–
20 bread exchanges	300	40	–
10 meat exchanges	–	70	30
17 fat exchanges	–	–	85
	406	138	115

= 3,211 calories

5. Distribution of CHO by meals:
   Target figures (CHO)
   $2/10$ at breakfast = 80 g
   $3/10$ at lunch = 120 g
   $3/10$ at dinner = 120 g
   $2/10$ at bedtime = 80 g

	Breakfast	Lunch	Dinner	Bedtime
3 nonfat milk exchanges	1	1	1	–
2 vegetable exchanges	–	1	1	–
6 fruit exchanges	1	1	2	2
20 bread exchanges	4	6	6	4
10 meat exchanges	1	4	4	1
17 fat exchanges	3	5	6	3
CHO (g)	82	117	127	80

96 g of simple CHO
310 g of complex CHO

6. Comments: The patient and his wife were instructed concerning the above pattern. It was suggested that the patient eat an afternoon snack to help spread out his carbohydrate intake through the day. However, this suggestion was not acceptable to the patient because of his work schedule. Both the patient and his wife were able to practice writing menus according to the above pattern for use at home. When the patient achieves his ideal body weight, the caloric intake will need to be reduced to a weight-maintaining diet (2,400 calories).

Appendix I: Case Study 3—Patient with Unusual Distribution of Meals

C.M. is a 47-year-old Mexican-American female homemaker who was recently discovered to be diabetic. She is 5 feet tall and weighs 130 pounds. Her husband works evenings from 4 PM to midnight. Therefore, her usual practice is to have her meal at 2 PM. She sometimes has a small meal at 9 AM and usually has a small evening snack at 7 PM. She takes intermediate-acting insulin in the morning.
   An appropriate diet for C.M. can be calculated as follows:

1. Ideal body weight = 100 pounds

2. 10 calories/pound of ideal body weight (to lose weight) = 1,000 calories

3. Division of carbohydrate (CHO), protein (pro), and fat:
   50% CHO = 500 calories = 125 g
   17% pro = 170 calories = 43 g
   33% fat = 330 calories = 37 g

4. Breakdown of 1,000 calories by exchanges:

	CHO (g)	Pro (g)	Fat (g)
0 nonfat milk exchanges*	—	—	—
2 vegetable exchanges	10	4	—
3 fruit exchanges	30	—	—
6 bread exchanges	90	12	—
4 meat exchanges	—	28	12
4 fat exchanges	—	—	20
	130	44	32

*Patient does not drink milk.

= 984 calories

5. Distribution of CHO by meals:
   Target figures (CHO)
   $2/10$ at breakfast = 26 g
   $4/10$ at lunch = 52 g
   $3/10$ at dinner = 39 g
   $1/10$ at bedtime = 13 g

	Breakfast	Lunch	Dinner	Bedtime
0 nonfat milk exchanges*	—	—	—	—
2 vegetable exchanges	—	1	1	—
3 fruit exchanges	1	2	—	—
6 bread exchanges	1	2	2	1
4 meat exchanges	1	1	1	1
4 fat exchanges	1	2	1	—

	Breakfast	*Lunch*	*Dinner*	*Bedtime*
CHO (g)	25	55	35	15

30 g of simple CHO

*Patient does not drink milk.   100 g of complex CHO

6. Comments: Because the patient takes intermediate-acting insulin, she was instructed to eat breakfast consistently and to eat dinner 1 hour earlier (at 6 PM) so that she could include a bedtime snack at about 9 PM to carry her through the night.

References

1. West KM: Diet therapy of diabetes: an analysis of failure. Ann Intern Med 79:425-434, 1973

2. Genuth SM: Insulin secretion in obesity and diabetes: an illustrative case. Ann Intern Med 87:714-716, 1977

3. Bagdade JD, Bierman EL, Porte D Jr: The significance of basal insulin levels in the evaluation of the insulin response to glucose in diabetic and non-diabetic subjects. J Clin Invest 46:1549-1557, 1967

4. Koivisto VA, Felig P: Effects of leg exercise on insulin absorption in diabetic patients. N Engl J Med 298:79-83, 1978

5. Kemmer FW, Berchtold P, Berger M, et al: Exercise-induced fall of blood glucose in insulin-treated diabetics unrelated to alteration of insulin mobilization. Diabetes 28:1131-1137, 1979

6. National Academy of Sciences: *Recommended Dietary Allowances*, 9th ed. National Academy of Sciences, Washington, D.C, 1980, p 46

7. Committee on Food and Nutrition of the American Diabetes Association: Principles of nutrition and dietary recommendations for individuals with diabetes mellitus: 1979. Diabetes Care 2:520-523, 1979

8. Chase HP, Glasgow AM: Juvenile diabetes mellitus and serum lipids and lipoprotein levels. Am J Dis Child 130:1113-1117, 1976

9. Mann GV: Diet–heart: end of an era. N Engl J Med 297:644-650, 1977

10. Glueck CJ, Mattson F, Bierman EL: Diet and coronary heart disease: another view. N Engl J Med 298:1471-1473, 1978

11. Stone DB, Connor WE: The prolonged effects of a low cholesterol, high carbohydrate diet upon the serum lipids in diabetic patients. Diabetes 12:127-132, 1963

12. Kaufmann RL, Assal JP, Soeldner JS, et al: Plasma lipid levels in diabetic children. Diabetes 24:672-679, 1975

13. Schlierf G, Reinheimer W, Stossberg V: Diurnal patterns of plasma triglycerides and free fatty acids in normal subjects and in patients with endogenous (type IV) hyperlipoproteinemia. Nutr Metab 13:80-91, 1971

14. Weinsier RL, Seeman A, Herrera MG, et al: High- and low-carbohydrate diets in diabetes mellitus. Ann Intern Med 80:332-341, 1974

15. Gastineau CF: Nutrition note: alcohol and calories. Mayo Clin Proc 51:86-87, 1976

16. Anderson JW, Chen W-JL: Plant fiber. Carbohydrate and lipid metabolism. Am J Clin Nutr 32:346-363, 1979

17. Anderson JW, Ward K: Long-term effects of high-carbohydrate, high-fiber diets on glucose and lipid metabolism: a preliminary report on patients with diabetes. Diabetes Care 1:77-82, 1978

18. Anderson JW, Midgley WR, Wedman B: Fiber and diabetes. Diabetes Care 2:369-379, 1979

19. Anderson JW, Ferguson SK, Karounos D, et al: Mineral and vitamin status on high-fiber diets: long-term studies of diabetic patients. Diabetes Care 3:38-43, 1980

20. Anderson JW, Sieling B: *HCF Diets: A Professional Guide to High-Carbohydrate, High-Fiber Diets*. University of Kentucky Diabetes Fund, Lexington, KY, 1979, pp 2-53

Chapter 4

Insulin Therapy

Insulin Preparations

Although the oral and intranasal administration of insulin is being studied, currently the only practical means of insulin administration is injection. Today insulin is marketed in 10-ml vials at three concentrations: 40, 80, and 100 U/ml (preparations U-40, U-80, and U-100, respectively). If a patient injects 0.5 ml, she or he receives 20 U of insulin with preparation U-40, 40 U with U-80, and 50 U with U-100. From another viewpoint, administration of 20 U of insulin requires injection of 0.5 ml of U-40, 0.25 ml of U-80 or 0.2 ml of U-100 insulin. Fortunately, calculations by the patient are obviated by the use of syringes with the number of units marked directly on the barrel. Of course, the particular syringe used must correspond to the appropriate concentration of insulin.

In 1973, U-100 insulin was introduced in the United States by both Eli Lilly & Company and E.R. Squibb & Sons, and a vigorous educational campaign was initiated to facilitate the transfer of patients from U-40 and U-80 insulins to U-100. The long-range goal was gradually to phase out U-40 and U-80 insulins so that medication errors would be eliminated. In 1976, approximately 10% of the total number of units of insulin sold by Lilly were sold as U-40, 25% as U-80, and 65% as U-100. The US Food and Drug Administration is now in the final phases of withdrawing U-80 insulin from the market. Thus, in the near future, only U-40 and U-100 insulins will be available in this country.[*]

In addition to differences in concentration, the other feature distinguishing the various insulin preparations from one another is their rate of absorption

---

[*]Since this chapter was written, U-80 insulin has been officially withdrawn and is no longer available. U-40 insulin still occupies 10% of the market.

after subcutaneous injection (Table 4-1). The values were obtained in studies with stable, well-controlled diabetic patients who had relatively low daily insulin requirements (1). After the patients were admitted to a metabolic ward, insulin therapy was discontinued, and the blood sugar level was allowed to rise above 200 mg/100 ml. At this time, a single large dose of insulin (usually about 80 U) was given, and the blood sugar level was determined every 4 hours. One sixth of a patient's total daily caloric intake was ingested after each blood sample was taken, and the study was continued for at least 36 hours. The relations summarized in Table 4-1 may not pertain exactly to the clinical situation, in which patients' physical activity and eating patterns differ from conditions imposed by the metabolic ward setting. These ranges are only approximations, and the response of an occasional patient may differ considerably from the values listed. However, these are probably the best data available on the time-activity relations of the various insulin preparations.

Regular insulin has no modifying agent and therefore is the only one that should be administered intravenously. In the Lente series, insulin is buffered by acetate, and the size of the crystal determines the rate of absorption. Lente insulin itself is a combination of 7 parts of Ultralente (large crystals) and 3 parts of Semilente (small crystals). This combination results in a time-course of action that is indistinguishable from that of neutral protamine Hagedorn (NPH) insulin. The protamine in the NPH preparation (originally formulated by Hagedorn) delays the absorption of insulin. The amount of protamine in NPH insulin is small enough (50 mg/100 U) that regular insulin added to the same syringe is still rapidly absorbed. In protamine zinc insulin (PZI), however, much more protamine

Table 4-1. Approximate Time-Activity Relation of Various Insulin Preparations

Kind of Insulin	Preparation	Onset of Action (hrs)	Maximal Action (hrs)	Total Duration of Action (hrs)
Short-acting	Regular[a]	0.5-1	2-4[b]	4-6
	Semilente	1-2	3-6	8-12
Intermediate-	NPH[c]	3-4	10-16	20-24
acting	Lente	3-4	10-16	20-24
Long-acting	PZI[d]	6-8	14-20	>32
	Ultralente	6-8	14-20	>32

[a]Also called crystalline zinc insulin (CZI).

[b]In some patients, the action of regular insulin may peak later than indicated here (between 4 and 8 hours) and last considerably longer. Therefore, addition of regular insulin to intermediate-acting insulin may cause afternoon hypoglycemia in these patients.

[c]Neutral protamine Hagedorn.

[d]Protamine zinc insulin.

(125 ml/100 U) is present. If regular insulin is added to a syringe containing PZI, the amount of long-acting insulin increases because the short-acting insulin is bound to the protamine. Only when the ratio of regular to PZI insulin exceeds approximately 1:1 does the patient receive any rapid-acting insulin. Regular insulin can be added to the Lente insulins, and, of course, the Lente series can be mixed in various proportions.

An intermediate-acting insulin preparation, either alone or in combination with regular insulin, is preferred for the following reasons. The action of the long-acting insulins peaks at times of little or no food intake. Therefore, the maintenance of acceptable glucose concentrations before breakfast and throughout the day often requires amounts of PZI or Ultralente insulin that pose a risk of hypoglycemia during the night. In addition, two separate injections would be required if short-acting insulin were considered necessary in a patient receiving PZI. Since the time-courses of action of Lente and NPH insulins are indistinguishable and since short-acting insulins can be added to the same syringe, either of these intermediate-acting insulins is suitable. If Lente insulin is used, Semilente can be added, but the greater delay in onset and the longer duration of its action as compared with regular insulin (Table 4-1) make the Semilente preparation less appropriate for use as a short-acting insulin.

Use of Insulins: General Considerations

The most effective way to use the available insulin preparations necessarily depends on the goals involved. It is obviously much easier to render an insulin-requiring diabetic asymptomatic (i.e., no nocturia, polyuria, or polydipsia; prevention of weight loss; and avoidance of increased susceptibility to infection) than to return the prevailing glucose concentrations to nearly normal levels. The evidence presented in chapter 2 relating good diabetic control to an amelioration of microangiopathic complications is a persuasive argument for dedicated efforts to achieve the best possible control in each patient. How can this goal be achieved? In theory, insulin should be used in a manner that maximizes the chances of maintaining nearly normal glucose levels at all times and minimizes disruption in the lives of diabetic patients.

Figure 4-1 shows the usual time-course of the activity of a single injection of insulin given before breakfast. Intermediate-acting insulin (NPH or Lente) is represented by the solid curve. There is usually a lag period of 3 to 4 hours before enough insulin is absorbed to have a measurable effect. Activity peaks around supper time (10 to 16 hours after injection), and the total duration of the effect is approximately 24 hours. Because of delayed absorption, hyperglycemia often occurs after breakfast. In order to avoid this problem, a small amount of short-acting insulin (regular; represented by the dotted line in the figure) can be added to the syringe with the intermediate-acting insulin. This short-acting insulin is absorbed rapidly and starts to work within 30 to 60 minutes; its activity peaks

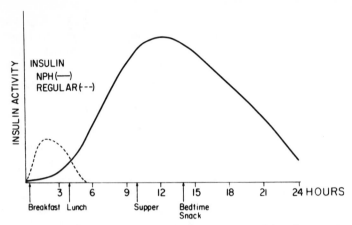

Figure 4-1. Time-course of action of one injection of insulin per day before breakfast. (Reprinted with permission from Davidson MB: The case for control in diabetes mellitus. West J Med 129:193–200, 1978.)

at 2 to 4 hours and may last as long as 4 to 6 hours. If it is to prevent hypergly-cemia, this single injection must cover the calories consumed at breakfast, lunch, dinner, and a bedtime snack and must also provide enough insulin to control hepatic glucose production throughout the night.

Three responses to a single injection in the morning are seen. In a small minority of patients, such an injection satisfactorily controls glucose concentrations during the following 24-hour period. Most commonly, however, the amount of intermediate-acting insulin that results in satisfactory control during the day is not adequate to prevent fasting hyperglycemia the following morning; the patient is also hyperglycemic during much of the night. Less often, the amount of intermediate-acting insulin appropriate for daytime needs is more than adequate for the night, and hypoglycemia occurs. If attempts are made to correct this situation, the patient is hyperglycemic throughout much of the day since the amount of intermediate-acting insulin is decreased in order to avoid night-time hypoglycemia.

Thus, since one injection per day usually does not result in optimal control, this approach is generally reserved for patients over 60 years of age. Their more limited life expectancy diminishes the long-term value of strict diabetic control, and hypoglycemia may be considered a greater threat than in younger patients because of the likely presence of cerebral and coronary vascular disease.

In my experience, a feasible way to achieve the dual goals of controlling glucose levels and minimizing disruptions of daily activity patterns is to inject insulin twice a day—before breakfast and before supper. The usual time-course of the activity of insulin given in this manner is depicted in Figure 4-2. The total insulin activity during a given period is the sum of all of the curves operating at that time. As indicated above, I prefer to administer an intermediate-acting

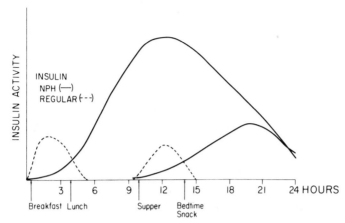

Figure 4-2. Time-course of action of two injections of insulin—one before breakfast and one before supper. (Reprinted with permission from Davidson MB: The case for control in diabetes mellitus. West J Med 129:193–200, 1978.)

insulin (NPH or Lente) supplemented as necessary with a short-acting insulin (regular) in the same syringe.*

In general, between two thirds and three fourths of the intermediate-acting insulin is given in the morning and the remainder before supper. If regular insulin is also required, 5 to 10 U at each time will usually suffice (in the nonobese patient). However, *only after the correct dose of intermediate-acting insulin has been established should short-acting insulin be added.* Regular insulin may be necessary in the morning to handle the breakfast calories because of the lag period before NPH insulin starts to work. Even though the intermediate-acting insulin administered in the morning exerts its maximal effect in the late afternoon and early evening, an amount appropriate to cover the interval before supper may be inadequate to cover the caloric intake of the largest meal of the day. In that case, regular insulin should be added to the second insulin injection. The advantage of this approach is that each component of the insulin prescription can be regulated independently (Table 4-2). Thus, as can be deduced from the intervals of maximal action of the various insulin preparations (Table 4-1), the urine or blood test that best reflects the patient's response to the morning NPH insulin injection is the one before supper; the following morning's test is the best indicator of the effect of NPH insulin given before supper; the test before lunch best reflects the action of regular insulin given before breakfast; and the test at bedtime is the most sensitive indicator of the action of regular insulin received before supper.

---

*Throughout this book, the terms *NPH* and *regular insulin* will be used interchangeably with the terms *intermediate-* and *short-acting insulin*, respectively.

Table 4–2. Timing of Most Appropriate Test of Effectiveness of
Insulin Injections

Type of Insulin, Time of Injection	Time of Test
Intermediate-acting, before breakfast	Before supper
Short-acting, before breakfast	Before lunch
Intermediate-acting, before supper	Before breakfast
Short-acting, before supper	Before bedtime

Initiation of Insulin Therapy in Hospitalized Patients

The initial dose of insulin given to a patient is to some extent empirically based. Lean individuals are given 15 U of NPH insulin: 10 U before breakfast and 5 U before supper. Obese patients (>125% of ideal body weight; see chapter 3) receive a total of 30 U of NPH insulin: 20 U in the morning and 10 U in the evening. A patient's response is monitored closely, and the amounts of intermediate-acting insulin are adjusted accordingly, usually by 4 or 5 U at a time. In extremely obese patients and in any others whose diabetes is poorly controlled (glucosuria of 1% or 2% and/or plasma glucose levels exceeding 300 mg/100 ml), increments of 8 to 10 U are advisable in order to achieve control faster. (An important point to remember is that these results are obtained at times of maximal action of NPH insulin and that glucose concentrations presumably are even higher at other times.) In the early stages of therapy with NPH insulin, amounts are adjusted daily. In contrast, when patients taking stable, established amounts of insulin inexplicably lose control, changes are made only after several days of poor test results. One exception is in cases of moderate to large ketonuria in the presence of glucosuria; these problems require more immediate action (see chapter 7).

For hospitalized patients, plasma glucose concentrations in specimens obtained before breakfast and before supper will determine what adjustments must be made in the amounts of NPH insulin administered. If a patient's hospital stay is to be minimized, these test results must be made available in time to change the appropriate NPH insulin dose if necessary. Since the amount of insulin given before breakfast depends on the result of the test before supper on the preceding day, this result must be communicated to the doctor during the evening. By the same token, the fasting glucose concentration must be made available to the physician during the day so that the evening NPH insulin dose can be altered if necessary.

The physician should write insulin orders on a continuing basis to ensure that the patient receives insulin at the proper times. Even if an appropriate change in dose is not made, at least the previous dose will automatically be given, and the orderly flow of gradually increasing amounts of insulin will not be interrupted. If the physician orders each insulin dose or each day's insulin prescription separately (with the intent of using the most recent appropriate glucose results to determine the amount of insulin given the next day), he or she may for some reason fail to write a particular order, and valuable time is lost. Even if the error is caught quickly and the patient receives insulin late, the response to that dose may not accurately reflect the efficacy of injected insulin because of the altered relation between the times of peak insulin action and meals. If the patient has been approaching reasonable control and his or her control deteriorates significantly because a dose is missed, the amount of insulin required to return to the control attained previously may exceed the requirement once control has been regained. (For reasons that are not entirely clear, diabetics are often less sensitive to insulin when their glucose levels are out of control than when these levels are in control.) In instances such as these, hospitalization is prolonged, and with current daily hospital rates, such errors can be expensive.

The final adjustments of insulin dosage are made after the patient has left the hospital. The patient's diet, activity, and emotional patterns will almost certainly be different when he or she returns to the usual environment, and these factors strongly influence the insulin requirement. For this reason, not only are decisions concerning the need for regular insulin usually delayed until the patient has left the hospital, but the amount of NPH insulin prescribed on discharge may be altered later. Several cases will serve to illustrate these points.

Patient 1

Case Study. This 48-year-old woman has had diabetes mellitus for 3 years. She is 5 feet 2 inches tall, has a medium frame, and currently weighs 165 pounds. Despite institution of an 1,100-calorie diet (which, she admits, is difficult for her to follow) and treatment with 750 mg of chlorpropamide (Diabinese) per day, her fasting plasma glucose levels consistently exceed 300 mg/100 ml. Fasting urine tests show 0.25% to 0.5% glucosuria, but these values increase to 1% to 2% during the day. The patient has only mild symptoms of polyuria and polydipsia, conditions that are due, no doubt, to her increased renal threshold (Tm) for glucose. Because of her failure to respond to maximal dosages of chlorpropamide, she enters the hospital for initiation of insulin therapy. She arrives in the morning before breakfast, and a blood specimen is taken so that a fasting plasma glucose level can be determined. Since the weight of the patient exceeds 125% of her ideal body weight (which is ∼110 pounds), a 20 U–10 U split NPH regimen is initially prescribed. The patient's response to insulin is summarized on the flow sheet in Table 4-3. She is discharged with a prescription for 45 U of NPH insulin before breakfast and 20 U of NPH insulin before supper.

Comment. A simple flow sheet like the one shown in Table 4-3 is extremely helpful in monitoring the progress of a patient in the hospital. Anyone reviewing the chart can quickly and easily determine the patient's degree of diabetic control and response to insulin. The flow sheet should be placed in the records in front

Table 4-3. Flow Sheet Showing Response of Patient 1 to Initiation of
Insulin Therapy

Date	Time	Plasma Glucose (mg/100 ml)	Insulin (U)	Remarks
9/19	0800	358		
	0920		20 (NPH)	
	1600	326	10 (NPH)	Urine 0.5%
9/20	0700	285	30 (NPH)	Urine 0.25%
	1600	278	15 (NPH)	Injected herself
9/21	0700	222	40 (NPH)	Urine negative
	1600	232	20 (NPH)	
9/22	0700	172	45 (NPH)	
	1600	163	20 (NPH)	
9/23	0700	178	45 (NPH)	

Abbreviation: NPH, neutral protamine Hagedorn.

of the patient's chart for easy access; its use will save time by making it unnecessary to go through the chart in order to locate the dose of insulin given (medication sheet and/or order sheet), the glucose response (laboratory results), and
the patient's subjective response (nurses' notes and physician's progress notes).
The flow sheet also saves time in constructing the temporal relations between
insulin administration, glucose concentrations, and the patient's reaction. Thus,
the flow sheet should be used for all insulin-requiring diabetics, regardless of the
reason for hospitalization. In many cases, twice-a-day glucose determinations
will not be ordered, and approximate urine test results can be recorded under
the column headed "Remarks."

With regard to the patient just described, the initial morning injection of
20 U of NPH insulin was clearly suboptimal since the 1600 glucose level (i.e.,
at 4 PM) was 326 mg/100 ml. As the morning dose of NPH insulin was increased,
the glucose concentration before supper gradually decreased to acceptable levels.
Similarly, the initial amount of NPH insulin (10 U) given before supper was
inadequate; the next morning's fasting glucose concentration was 285 mg/100 ml.
Increases over several days to a dose of 20 U in the evening finally brought the
fasting glucose level below 200 mg/100 ml. Note that the morning and evening
insulin doses were adjusted independently of each other. For example, on 9/22
the morning dose of NPH insulin was increased, whereas the evening dose
remained the same.

Although the patient's glucose concentrations after institution of insulin
therapy were much lower than her levels before insulin therapy, the recorded
values represent the minimal levels attained during the day, and the patient was
probably significantly hyperglycemic at most other times. Her fairly rapid

response to insulin was aided by her dietary compliance in the hospital and by the unexplained fact that once glucose levels begin to be brought under control, a patient's sensitivity to insulin (exogenous or endogenous) increases.

The final adjustments of the insulin dose after the patient's discharge from the hospital will have to take into account her probable increased level of activity (which will lower insulin requirements) and her probable increased caloric intake, as predicted on the basis of her previous lack of dietary compliance (which will raise insulin requirements). Although intermittent determinations of fasting and late-afternoon plasma glucose levels will be helpful in the choice of appropriate doses of NPH insulin, urine test results can also be used. Since the patient's Tm lies somewhere between 220 and 300 mg/100 ml (Table 4-3), results of all tests for glucosuria should be negative. Any spillage in the fasting or before-supper test will suggest that more NPH insulin is needed at the appropriate time. Once urine test results become negative, only plasma glucose concentrations will indicate the actual degree of control. When the appropriate amounts of NPH insulin have been decided upon, the need for regular insulin will be assessed by consideration of the results of urine tests before lunch and at bedtime. Consistent glucosuria at these times will indicate that small amounts of regular insulin should be added. Because of her obesity, the patient may require more than the 5 to 10 U of short-acting insulin that is usually adequate in the lean patient.

Patient 2

Case Study. A 32-year-old man (5 feet 11 inches, medium frame, 155 pounds) gives a 3-week history of polyuria, polydipsia, polyphagia, and weight loss (12 pounds). When he is seen during morning office hours, his urine shows 2% glucosuria and moderate ketonuria. His plasma glucose concentration is 425 mg/100 ml, and his undiluted plasma gives a mildly positive reaction for acetoacetate (ketone bodies) when mixed with nitroprusside powder. The patient is admitted to the hospital for initiation of insulin therapy (and of the general educational process). When he arrives at 3 PM, a stat glucose concentration is measured at 467 mg/100 ml. The patient's response to insulin during hospitalization is summarized on the flow sheet in Table 4-4. He is discharged on 25 U of NPH insulin before breakfast and 10 U of NPH before supper.

Comments. The mildly positive test for plasma ketone bodies indicated that the patient did not have ketoacidosis. If acidosis had been present, the test would have been strongly positive with undiluted serum and might have remained strongly positive through several dilutions.

On admission to the hospital, the patient was given 10 U of regular insulin in order to begin bringing his glucose levels under control faster than if only intermediate-acting insulin had been used. The 10 U of NPH insulin was administered for a more sustained effect overnight. (If only regular insulin had been

Table 4-4. Flow Sheet Showing Response of Patient 2 to Initiation of Insulin Therapy

Date	Time	Plasma Glucose (mg/100 ml)	Insulin (U)	Remarks
10/5	1500	467		Obtained on admission
	1600		10 (NPH) 10 (Regular)	
10/6	0700	323	10 (NPH)	Urine 1%
	1600	387	5 (NPH)	
10/7	0700	267	20 (NPH)	Injected himself
	1600	230	10 (NPH)	Urine 0.5%
10/8	0700	213	25 (NPH)	
	1600	185	10 (NPH)	Urine negative
10/9	0700	202	25 (NPH	
	1345			Patient hypo- glycemic because missed lunch; given orange juice stat followed by lunch
	1600	367	10 (NPH) 5 (Regular)	
10/10	0700	242	25 (NPH)	
	1600	178	10 (NPH)	
	0700	198	25 (NPH)	
	1600	183	10 (NPH)	
10/11	0700	173	25 (NPH)	

Abbreviation: NPH, neutral protamine Hagedorn.

used, the effect would have worn off by the next morning, and the patient would not have received any long-range benefit from his insulin therapy during the first day of hospitalization.) Since the patient was not overweight (ideal body weight, 172 pounds), the 10 U-5 U split NPH regimen was initially prescribed. As judged by results of urine tests for glucosuria, which became negative when the patient's plasma glucose level fell below 200 mg/100 ml, his Tm was appropriate. The administration of gradually increasing amounts of NPH insulin started to bring the glucose levels under control. However, on 10/9 the patient's lunch was delayed and he became hypoglycemic. The hormonal response to hypoglycemia (see chapter 10) raised his subsequent glucose level, and he was treated with a small amount of regular insulin to improve his control as quickly as possible. However, this episode temporarily obscured the usual responses to NPH insulin and necessitated a few additional days of hospitalization.

The usual caveats apply to the final adjustments of insulin dose after the patient's discharge from the hospital. In addition, this patient was initially placed on a hypercaloric diet (3,400 calories) so that he would gain weight. Once his ideal body weight was attained, his daily caloric intake was reduced to 2,600 calories, and a small downward adjustment of his insulin dose was deemed appropriate.

Initiation of Insulin Therapy in Nonhospitalized Patients

It is often unnecessary to hospitalize a diabetic for initiation of insulin therapy. An obvious exception is the patient who initially presents with diabetic keto-acidosis or with marked symptoms of uncontrolled diabetes. In such an instance, the patient should be hospitalized for intensive treatment with regular insulin and appropriate fluid replacement. The subsequent transition from regular to NPH insulin will be discussed in chapter 6.

Hospitalization does provide an opportunity to initiate the extensive and critically important educational process in which patients learn to take care of themselves (see chapter 8). However, in the absence of a metabolic need for hospitalization, many patients can begin insulin therapy in an office setting. This setting is particularly appropriate for diabetics who are switching from another mode of therapy to insulin and who presumably already have a basic knowledge of the pathophysiology of diabetes, diet, urine testing, etc. These patients need only to acquire information related to insulin therapy and its possible consequences (e.g., hypoglycemia).

In addition, many well-motivated and reasonably intelligent new diabetics requiring insulin can embark on their therapeutic and educational tasks in an office or outpatient setting. Obviously, a patient must have the opportunity to communicate frequently with the physician about insulin doses and with teaching personnel (if other than the physician) about other important points. As will be discussed in greater detail in chapter 9, the patient's reaction to the diagnosis of diabetes mellitus often involves a great deal of anger, depression, and denial. Not only are efforts at education poorly received under such circumstances, but patients often fail to call their physicians regularly for adjustment of insulin doses. In contrast to the situation in the hospital, where the patient is a captive audience and a formal system operates to ensure that insulin orders are reviewed, follow-up on adjustment of insulin doses outside the hospital can be inadequate if the patient does not take the initiative. Thus, when insulin therapy is begun for a nonhospitalized diabetic, the physician or office personnel should contact the patient on a prearranged schedule and should see the patient at frequent intervals. Although initiation of insulin therapy in the office or outpatient setting may be less efficient (and economical) from the physician's point of view, the greatly diminished disruption of the patient's life and the tremendous savings in health-care costs make this approach desirable when at all possible.

When insulin therapy is started outside the hospital, dose adjustments are necessarily based mainly on the results of urine tests. Therefore, the patient must thoroughly understand how to test for urinary glucose (and ketone bodies, if appropriate). Although recent evidence suggests that testing second-voided urine specimen gives results identical to those obtained with the first sample 66% of the time (2), it is probably wise to use results of double-voided urine specimens as the basis for initial insulin adjustments. This will minimize the possibility of hypoglycemia occurring as the insulin dose is increased. Before relying on urine test results, however, the physician must obtain a general idea of the patient's Tm for glucose. Simultaneous blood and second-voided urine tests for glucose must be performed under circumstances that will allow such a judgment to be made. For instance, if all tests are done when plasma glucose concentrations are greater than 300 mg/100 ml and urine tests show heavy glucosuria, it is impossible to determine the Tm. On the other hand, if the results of urine tests are negative or show minimal glucosuria while plasma glucose concentrations are high, the Tm is high. At plasma glucose levels below 200 mg/100 ml, negative urine test results are appropriate, and, again, no decision regarding the approximate Tm for glucose is possible. However, if glucosuria is present with glucose concentrations much below 200 mg/100 ml, the patient has a low Tm.

Therefore, simultaneous blood and double-voided urine tests must be done under both fasting and postprandial conditions until appropriate data for determining the Tm are in hand. Only then should the results of urine tests be relied upon exclusively as a basis for insulin dose adjustments. In practical terms, results of blood and urine tests must be matched frequently from the time the patient starts to take insulin until the fasting or late-afternoon plasma glucose concentrations fall to the point at which urine tests reveal no glucosuria. If the patient has either a high Tm (often associated with kidney disease or aging) or a low Tm (usually seen in pregnant women and in the few diabetics who also have independent renal tubular abnormalities), repeated determinations of plasma glucose concentrations at the appropriate times are necessary for proper adjustment of insulin doses.

Patient 3

Case Study. A 43-year-old man has had diabetes for 4 years. He is 5 feet 9 inches tall, with a stable weight of 158 pounds. He currently follows an appropriate diet and takes 750 mg of chlorpropamide per day. However, his fasting plasma glucose concentrations have consistently been measured at 220 to 265 mg/100 ml for the past 4 months. At present, the patient has 0.1% to 0.5% glucosuria before breakfast and excretes glucose in the urine throughout the day and evening. Office records indicate, however, that he did not have fasting glucosuria prior to 4 months ago, when his glucose concentrations before breakfast ranged between 130 and 187 mg/100 ml. Because of the patient's normal

Tm, his busy schedule, and his motivation and intelligence, insulin therapy is initiated in an office setting. The patient is obviously not overweight, so the 10 U-5 U split NPH regimen is initially prescribed. A nurse shows him how to inject insulin the first afternoon. He returns the following morning to inject it himself under her supervision. In addition to the technique of insulin injection, instruction is given on the care of insulin and syringes and on the signs, symptoms, and treatment of hypoglycemia. The patient's response to insulin therapy is summarized on the flow sheet in Table 4-5.

Comment. The patient, who kept faithful records, was contacted every second day. On 11/11 both the morning and evening doses of NPH insulin were increased because the urine tests before breakfast and before supper showed 0.5% glucosuria. (Since the conversation with the patient occurred in the late afternoon, the increase in the morning dose was not implemented until the following morning.) The fasting urine test gave negative results secondary to the increased amount of evening insulin, but the patient continued to excrete some glucose in the urine specimen tested before supper. Therefore, after consultation on 11/13, the morning dose of NPH insulin was raised further, with subsequent clearing of glucosuria in the late-afternoon urine test. However, the results of tests done before lunch remained positive, and on 11/16 the patient added a small amount of regular insulin to the morning injection. On this insulin regimen (20 U of NPH and 5 U of regular insulin before breakfast, 10 U of NPH insulin before supper), the patient's urine tests consistently yielded negative results except at times of dietary indiscretion.

This patient had a smooth transition from oral hypoglycemic agents to insulin therapy. The dose of insulin could be adjusted every second day because the pattern of results of urine tests was consistent. In many cases, however, these results are not consistent, and changes in the insulin dose must proceed more slowly until a definite pattern emerges.

Patient 4

Case Study. This 42-year-old woman has had diabetes for 8 years. She is 5 feet 7 inches tall, has a large frame, and currently weighs 202 pounds. In spite of a 1,500-calorie diet (which is poorly followed) and maximal amounts of oral hypoglycemic agents, her urine tests (when done) consistently reveal 1% to 2% glucosuria; this result corresponds to her recent plasma glucose concentrations of 320 to 415 mg/100 ml, as determined at office visits. Treatment with oral hypoglycemic agents is discontinued, and the 20 U-10 U split regimen of NPH insulin is prescribed because of the patient's obesity. Her response is summarized on the flow sheet in Table 4-6.

Comment. It was convenient for this patient to come to the office before breakfast for glucose determinations. She took her insulin, ate breakfast at a

Table 4-5. Flow Sheet Showing Response of Patient 3 to Initiation of Insulin Therapy

| | Insulin Dose (U) Before | | | | Urine Test Result (plasma glucose, mg/100 ml) Before | | | |
| | Breakfast | | Supper | | | | | |
Date	NPH	Regular	NPH	Regular	Breakfast	Lunch	Supper	Bedtime
11/8			5				2%	1%
11/9	10		5		0.5%	2%	1%	0.5%
11/10	10		5		0.5%	1%	0.5%	1%
11/11	10		10		0.5%	1%	0.5%	1%
11/12	15		10		0.1%	1%	0.25%	1%
11/13	15		10		Negative	1%	0.25%	0.5%
11/14	20		10		Negative	0.5%	Negative	0.25%
11/15	20		10		Negative	0.5%	0.1%	0.25%
11/16	20	5	10		Negative	0.1%	Negative	0.1%
11/17	20	5	10		Negative	Negative	Negative	Negative

Abbreviation: NPH, neutral protamine Hagedorn.

122

nearby coffee shop, and was contacted later that day about appropriate insulin dose adjustments, which she implemented that evening and the following morning. Initially, fasting glucose concentrations were determined in order to establish her Tm. On 4/5, both insulin doses were increased by 10 U because of persistent heavy glucosuria. On 4/7, the evening dose of NPH insulin was increased by 5 U only because the patient's fasting urine test results and glucose levels had shown some improvement. (This decision is in keeping with the policy of *gradually* increasing insulin doses in order to avoid hypoglycemia and its attendant disruption of metabolism for 12 to 24 hours.) The morning dose of NPH insulin was increased by 10 U since the tests done before supper gave consistently poor results. No change in either dose of insulin was made on 4/9 because the fasting tests showed definite improvement and the results of the late-afternoon urine tests suggested some improvement. (This decision is in keeping with the principle that changes in insulin therapy should be predicated on a consistent pattern of tests rather than on a group of tests that vary considerably.)

On 4/11 increases were made in both insulin doses because of unacceptable fasting and before-supper urine test results. On 4/13 the morning dose of NPH insulin was increased by only 5 U because late-afternoon tests, although showing definite improvement, still showed 0.25% glucosuria consistently. The evening dose of NPH insulin was not changed because the fasting glucose concentration and urine test results were continually improving. On 4/15 both doses of insulin were again increased; the evening injection was increased in an attempt to lower the fasting plasma glucose concentration below approximately 200 mg/100 ml, and the morning dose was increased because the tests before supper still showed some spillage.

On 4/17 the Tm was established as normal, and further determinations of plasma glucose levels could be made only at routine office visits (see chapter 7). The amounts of intermediate-acting insulin being administered were deemed appropriate; therefore, small amounts of regular insulin were added to each injection because of persistent glucosuria before lunch and before bed. Two days later (4/19), the urine tests showed some response to the addition of the short-acting component. Five more units of regular insulin were added to the morning dose because of persistent glucosuria before lunch. Arrangements were made to lengthen the period between consultations since the urine tests gave fairly consistent and almost acceptable results. On 4/23, the evening dose of NPH insulin was increased by 5 U in an attempt to eradicate intermittent fasting glucosuria. However, the patient experienced hypoglycemia in the early-morning hours of 4/25 and 4/27; she woke up perspiring and had feelings of tremulousness, hunger, and palpitations, all of which were relieved within 10 to 15 minutes by food. As expected, her urine test results deteriorated during that period, and the insulin prescription was returned to 60 U of NPH plus 10 U of regular insulin before breakfast and 35 U of NPH plus 5 U of regular insulin before supper. The fact that the morning and evening doses of insulin were changed independently of each other on 4/7, 4/13, 4/19, 4/23, and 4/27 attests to the efficacy of this approach.

Table 4-6. Flow Sheet Showing Response of Patient 4 to Initiation of Insulin Therapy

| | Insulin Dose (U) Before | | | | Urine Test Result (plasma glucose, mg/100 ml) Before | | | |
| | Breakfast | | Supper | | | | | |
Date	NPH	Regular	NPH	Regular	Breakfast	Lunch	Supper	Bedtime
4/3	20		10		2%	2%	2%	2%
4/4	20		10		2%	2%	2%	2%
4/5	20		20		1% (352)	2%	2%	2%
4/6	30		20		0.5%	2%	1%	1%
4/7	30		25		1% (301)	2%	1%	1%
4/8	40		25		0.5%	1%	0.5%	0.5%
4/9	40		25		0.25% (227)	1%	0.25%	0.5%
4/10	40		25		0.5%	1%	0.5%	1%
4/11	40		30		0.5% (253)	1%	0.5%	0.5%
4/12	50		30		0.25%	1%	0.25%	0.5%
4/13	50		30		0.1% (198)	1%	0.5%	0.5%

Date								
4/14	55	30			Negative	0.5%	0.1%	0.25%
4/15	55	35			0.1% (203)	1%	0.25%	0.5%
4/16	60	35			Negative	0.5%	0.1%	0.25%
4/17	60	35		5	Negative (178)	0.5%	Negative	0.1%
4/18	60	35	5	5	0.1%	0.5%	0.25%	0.1%
4/19	60	35	5	5	Negative	0.25%	Negative	Negative
4/20	60	35	10	5	0.25%	0.1%	0.1%	0.25%
4/21	60	35	10	5	0.1%	Negative	0.25%	0.25%
4/22	60	35	10	5	0.1%	0.1%	0.1%	Negative
4/23	60	40	10	5	0.25%	0.25%	Negative	0.1%
4/24	60	40	10	5	Negative	Negative	Negative	Negative
4/25	60	40	10	5	1% (reaction)	0.5%	0.25%	0.1%
4/26	60	40	10	5	Negative	0.25%	0.1%	Negative
4/27	60	35	10	5	0.5% (reaction)	0.5%	0.25%	0.1%
4/28	60	35	10	5	0.1%	0.1%	Negative	0.1%

Abbreviation: NPH, neutral protamine Hagedorn.

If this obese patient had been able to adhere to her hypocaloric diet, the resulting weight loss would no doubt have obviated her need for insulin and probably even sulfonylurea agents. Even though an appropriate diet would have been the most effective therapy for this patient, she was unable to benefit from this approach in spite of continued emphasis by persons involved in her medical care. In my view, the theoretical possibility of a simple, more effective treatment does not justify withholding other forms of therapy that will probably improve diabetic control. Without insulin, this patient's tissues would be exposed to chronic, moderate to marked hyperglycemia. Although insulin therapy is not fully effective because of the insulin antagonism associated with obesity, the lowering of the patient's glucose concentrations should prove helpful in retarding the development of microangiopathic lesions.

Furthermore, there is little, if any, valid evidence for the widely held belief that insulin therapy per se will lead to weight gain in obese patients who are not in a catabolic state. For weight gain to occur, intake and/or utilization of calories must increase. Let us consider the latter possibility first. Theoretically, the reversal of marked glucosuria could lead to weight gain since more carbohydrate calories would be deposited as fat. However, a careful consideration of the actual numbers involved reveals that this possibility is unlikely. Assume that the obese patient is ingesting 400 g of carbohydrate per day, 25% of which is lost as urinary glucose. This 100 g of glucose would furnish 400 calories if completely utilized by body tissues instead of excreted. Since approximately 4,000 excess calories are required for a 1-pound weight gain due to extra fat deposition, this patient would gain 1 pound every 10 days, or 3 pounds a month. These figures assume, of course, the complete reversal of marked glucosuria by insulin therapy. Thus, increased utilization of calories previously lost in the urine apparently would not cause much weight gain in obese patients taking insulin.

Increased intake of calories, then, is the only means by which these patients would gain weight. Although insulin may directly stimulate the appetite center in the hypothalamus in certain animal species under highly artificial laboratory conditions, we are aware of no evidence that, in the absence of hypoglycemia, insulin will directly lead to an increase in the caloric intake of humans. Since obese patients are notoriously resistant to the action of insulin and the overwhelming majority remain somewhat hyperglycemic even when taking large amounts of insulin, hypoglycemia-induced increases in caloric intake seem very unlikely. More likely, some of these patients voluntarily increase their caloric intake because they think that insulin will control their diabetes and that a strict dietary approach is not as important as in the past.

Initial Insulin Therapy Involving One Daily Injection

The principles delineated in the previous section on the initiation of insulin therapy with two daily injections also apply, for the most part, to therapy with a single daily injection. The appropriate dose of intermediate-acting insulin is established first. If short-acting insulin is necessary, only small amounts are used. If the patient is hospitalized, final adjustments, including the addition of regular insulin to the regimen, are made after discharge. The initial doses of 10 to 15 U of NPH insulin in lean patients and 25 to 30 U in obese patients are equivalent to the total amount used in the two-injection approach. The rates of increase of 5 U per day in lean patients and 10 U per day in obese and extremely hyperglycemic patients are also similar.

There are some differences, however. First, in the elderly patient—the most likely candidate for single-injection therapy—less stringent control may be acceptable because of decreased life expectancy and the greater risks of hypoglycemia. Second, results of the urine tests done on a given evening before supper *and* the following morning before breakfast help determine any changes in the dose of NPH insulin; that is, if either test yields an unacceptable result, the morning dose of NPH should be increased. As discussed previously, when the dose of intermediate-acting insulin is gradually increased, the test done before supper will usually show a quicker and more sensitive response than the next day's fasting test. Attempts are made to find a dose that will control both daytime and nighttime glucose levels. However, when the dose of NPH insulin is continually increased in an attempt to control the next morning's fasting glucose concentration or urine test result, hypoglycemia is often noted in the late afternoon. In such cases, switching some breakfast or lunch calories to a midafternoon snack may alleviate the problem and even allow further increases in the morning dose of NPH insulin. If this tactic should fail, two choices are left: either the patient can continue to take one daily injection of a dose that controls glucose levels during the day but allows significant fasting hyperglycemia, or the patient can switch to two injections per day.

Another pattern of response is (fortunately) infrequent. In this situation, NPH insulin acts much more slowly than usual (3), and nighttime or early-morning hypoglycemia occurs at insulin doses that fail to control the daytime hyperglycemia. Use of two daily injections of intermediate-acting insulin would not seem helpful in this instance. Since the dose that precipitated nighttime hypoglycemia was inadequate for daytime needs, addition of a second dose in the evening would only make matters worse unless the morning dose of NPH was reduced—a course that would cause further problems with daytime control. Several other approaches may be tried: (*a*) injecting the morning dose of NPH insulin earlier; (*b*) eating supper later; (*c*) delaying and/or increasing the bedtime snack; and (*d*) switching to shorter-acting insulin. If the first three options prove ineffectual or impractical, morning administration of Semilente insulin should be tried. If the effect of this morning dose does not last through the night, a second injection of a smaller amount of Semilente insulin before dinner should be tried. (Thus, Semilente insulin would be used in a split dose, in much the same manner as NPH insulin.) Alternatively (and much less likely), if the pattern of response to Semilente insulin resembles that to NPH insulin, regular insulin may have to be used. Again, if one injection fails to work throughout the night, a second smaller dose before supper should be added. (The delayed effect of insulin is sometimes associated with an increase in insulin-binding antibodies in the circulation. In this situation, greatly increased amounts of insulin are usually required, as will be discussed under *Insulin Resistance*.)

Most diabetics slated to receive one injection per day are elderly and are usually hospitalized for the initiation of insulin therapy for two reasons. First, the Tm for glucose in these patients is more likely to be high than in younger patients; if so, urine tests are an inadequate basis on which to judge the response to insulin and determinations of plasma glucose levels are required. Second, many of these patients need more instruction in the techniques of injecting insulin and properly handling syringes, needles, and insulin vials than can be given easily in an office setting.

While the patient is in the hospital, a second injection of a small amount of NPH insulin in the evening (especially early in the course of bringing the patient's glucose levels under control) is often helpful in expediting conversion to insulin therapy. The reasoning behind the second injection is simple. In the great majority of patients, the glucose concentration before supper represents the maximal effect of that morning's dose of NPH insulin. If this level is very high, the next day's fasting glucose concentration is almost certain to be markedly elevated also. Thus, the morning dose of NPH insulin has a high baseline glucose level upon which to work. Even though the dose of insulin has presumably been increased over the amount given the day before, glucose concentrations throughout the day are more likely to be lower when fasting hyperglycemia is diminished. Thus, administration of a small amount of NPH insulin in the early evening (if the patient's glucose concentration before supper is greatly increased) will usually shorten the hospital stay. If the glucose level is extremely high, small amounts of regular insulin may also be appropriate. For this approach, of course, the results of the late-afternoon glucose determination must be available to the

Table 4-7. Schedule of Evening Supplemental Insulin Doses in Patients Being Controlled by One Daily Injection

Glucose Level Before Supper (mg/100 ml)	Lean Patient (<125% IBW)		Obese Patient (>125% IBW)	
	NPH	Regular	NPH	Regular
250–299	5 U		10 U	
300–349	10 U		15 U	
350–399	10 U	5 U	15 U	10 U
>400	10 U	10 U	15 U	15 U

Abbreviation: IBW, ideal body weight. (For calculation, see chapter 3.)

Table 4-8. Flow Sheet Showing Response of Patient 5 to Initiation of Insulin Therapy

Date	Time	Plasma Glucose (mg/100 ml)	Insulin (U)	Remarks
6/5	1500	422		Obtained on admission
	1700		10 (NPH), 10 (Regular)	
6/6	0700	302	15 (NPH)	
	1600	317		
	1800		10 (NPH)	
6/7	0700	263	20 (NPH)	Urine negative
	1600	272		
	1830		5 (NPH)	
6/8	0700	243	25 (NPH)	
	1600	235		
6/9	0700	227	30 (NPH)	Injected himself
	1600	218		
6/10	0700	212	30 (NPH)	
	1600	206		
6/11	0700	219	30 (NPH)	

Abbreviation: NPH, neutral protamine Hagedorn.

physician within several hours. The schedule of supplemental evening insulin doses summarized in Table 4-7 has proved helpful.

Patient 5

Case Study. A 72-year-old man (medium frame, 5 feet 6 inches tall, 155 pounds) presents with the following history. He was told that he had "sugar in the urine" at a routine physical examination performed upon his retirement 4 years ago. Because he felt well, he ignored this finding and has not seen a physician since. The patient maintained his usual weight of 165 to 170 pounds until several months ago, when he noted increasing fatigue, nocturia ($\times$ 3), and mild increases in thirst and daytime urination. His appetite has remained good. A urinalysis in the office reveals 0.5% glucosuria but no ketonuria. The patient is admitted to the hospital that afternoon for initiation of insulin therapy. The glucose level on admission is 422 mg/100 ml, and a concomitant urine test again shows 0.5% glucosuria and no ketonuria. The patient's response to insulin is summarized on the flow sheet in Table 4-8. He is discharged from the hospital with a prescription for a morning dose of 30 U of NPH insulin.

Comment. This nonobese patient received small amounts of intermediate- and short-acting insulin shortly after admission; thus, his plasma glucose levels were lowered in anticipation of the initiation of therapy with gradually increasing amounts of NPH insulin the following morning. A supplemental evening dose of NPH insulin was given on 6/6 and 6/7 because of elevated glucose concentrations before supper on those days. An increased Tm was confirmed on 6/7, when the patient's urine was negative for glucose and the plasma concentration was 263 mg/100 ml. In contrast to Patients 1 and 2, younger individuals who were able to administer insulin to themselves after only 2 days of hospitalization, this 72-year-old man first gave himself insulin 4 days after admission. Note that the patient was discharged from the hospital with glucose levels consistently above 200 mg/100 ml. Tighter control was attempted after discharge. At a dose of 35 U of NPH insulin, fasting glucose concentrations hovered around 200 mg/100 ml; at 40 U of NPH insulin, fasting glucose levels ranged between 160 and 190 mg/100 ml, but the patient noted symptoms of hypoglycemia in the late afternoon. Because he lived by himself and either was away from his apartment during the middle of the day or was reluctant to prepare a midafternoon snack when at home, his morning dose of NPH insulin was decreased to 35 U, and mild fasting (and no doubt persistent) hyperglycemia was accepted.

Drawbacks of the Sliding-Scale Method

Two principles guide the physician in initiating insulin therapy. First, insulin should be administered in anticipation of subsequent events so that it is available to *prevent* inordinate hyperglycemia. To reiterate: a morning dose of NPH insulin exerts a gradual influence on plasma glucose levels throughout the day, with a maximal effect on the calories ingested during supper, which is usually the patient's largest meal. By the same token, morning and evening doses of regular insulin are given in anticipation of the acute influx of breakfast and dinner calories. Finally, the smaller dose of NPH insulin in the evening prevents significant fasting hyperglycemia by making gradually increasing amounts of insulin available throughout the night (as the effect of the larger morning dose of NPH insulin wanes) to restrain hepatic glucose production.

Second, the kind of insulin used (intermediate-acting) and the gradually increasing amounts initially prescribed should make for a relatively smooth transition from higher to lower plasma glucose levels. Large fluctuations in glucose concentrations, with the attendant disruption of carbohydrate homeostasis through secretion of contrainsulin hormones should be avoided.

These two principles are violated when the sliding-scale method of prescribing insulin is used. In this approach, different amounts of short-acting insulin are given (usually every 4 to 6 hours), depending on the outcome of urine tests for glucose and ketone bodies. First, treatment is given only after hyperglycemia is marked enough to result in glucosuria. Since the smallest amount of regular insulin is usually given for 0.5% glucosuria, treatment is withheld until relatively high plasma glucose concentrations ($\sim$220 to 250 mg/100 ml, or usually even higher) are attained. Thus, the principle of prescribing insulin to prevent significant hyperglycemia is certainly violated. Second, not only is the plasma glucose response to regular insulin fairly rapid, but the majority of the effectiveness of regular insulin is dissipated within 3 to 4 hours. In addition, the hormonal response to the rapid lowering of plasma glucose levels causes subsequently administered insulin to be less effective (see chapter 10). This effect leads to more hyperglycemia and thus larger amounts of insulin are required than if glucose concentrations had been lowered more gradually. The result is relatively large and rapid fluctuations of glucose levels treated with increasing amounts of short-acting insulin.

The sliding-scale method is critically dependent on the accuracy of urine testing, which involves at least three factors: the timing of collection, a consistent relation between the amount of urinary glucose actually present and that measured, and the Tm for glucose.

The collection and testing of the urine sample in the hospital is almost always the responsibility of the nursing staff. Unless the patient is on a diabetic ward where urine collection and testing are part of the daily nursing routine, this activity may be overlooked when other problems on the ward become pressing. Permanent insulin orders are much more dependable, even though they may need frequent modification. Dispensing of medication is such an integral part of the nursing routine that failure to give insulin that has already been ordered is most unusual.

Although both diabetics and the medical personnel caring for them rely heavily on the semiquantitative tests for urinary glucose, a number of factors (often beyond the patient's control) profoundly disrupt the relation between the amount of glucose present and the amount measured. Both falsely high and falsely low results are obtained frequently (see chapter 7). Thus, the dose of regular insulin administered may not correspond closely to the actual amount of urinary glucose.

Finally, if the Tm is abnormal, the patient can be seriously under- or overtreated. Two personal examples will illustrate this problem. An endocrinologic consultation was requested 5 days after prostate surgery for a 76-year-old diabetic man who was feeling lethargic, anorectic, and weak. The patient had been taking small amounts of NPH insulin before surgery. The sliding-scale method of insulin therapy had been ordered following surgery, but the patient had received no insulin in view of consistently negative results in urine tests for glucose. A determination of the plasma glucose concentration, as ordered by the endocrinology consultant, gave a result of 488 mg/100 ml. Obviously, the very high Tm in this elderly diabetic and the failure to measure plasma glucose levels conspired to deprive this patient of needed insulin.

The second patient was a pregnant diabetic woman who was admitted to the hospital several weeks before delivery. The sliding-scale method was prescribed to provide her with any additional insulin she might require during the last part of her third trimester. Her urine tests consistently revealed 2% glucosuria and gave moderate to large results for ketones. The patient received many extra units of regular insulin each day. The endocrinology consultant requested a random determination of the plasma glucose level, which was measured at 167 mg/100 ml. A 24-hour urine test for glucose revealed that this patient excreted 174 g per day. Since she was ingesting a 200-g carbohydrate diet, very little of her carbohydrate intake was being utilized. This loss resulted in starvation (or low-carbohydrate) ketosis (see chapter 7). Thus, neither the marked glucosuria nor the ketosis was due to uncontrolled diabetes. When the carbohydrate content of the patient's diet was increased to 250 g, the ketosis disappeared. Obviously, the lowered Tm associated with pregnancy was responsible for the administration of unnecessary insulin to this patient.

The sliding-scale method of prescribing insulin is usually used in two situations: either the initiation of insulin therapy in a patient or the treatment of a patient with insulin during a temporary situation in which the usual relations between eating and insulin therapy are disrupted (e.g., during and following surgery or in critically ill, hospitalized patients). In the first instance, the sliding-scale method is chosen in the hope that the amount of short-acting insulin required over several days will help determine the appropriate dose of inter-mediate-acting insulin. For the reasons just stated, this is a false hope, and the use of this approach simply lengthens the patient's hospital stay. Indeed, the proponents of this approach must recognize that it requires the use of dispro-portionately large amounts of regular insulin, because they recommend that the total dose of short-acting insulin given during the preceding 24 hours be reduced by one third to one half in calculating the dose of NPH insulin for the next day. In my experience, also, there is a large discrepancy between the amount of regular insulin initially given to a recently diagnosed diabetic and the amount of inter-mediate-acting insulin prescribed on discharge from the hospital.

The use of the sliding-scale method in the second situation should also be actively discouraged. It is easy to provide patients in these unusual circumstances with insulin in anticipation of their needs rather than after hyperglycemia has developed (see chapter 7). The other arguments against using this method (as just summarized) would certainly apply to the postoperative and/or critically ill patient.

Adverse Effects of Insulin Therapy

The adverse effects of insulin therapy include delayed local skin reactions to injected insulin, true insulin allergy, insulin resistance, insulin-induced lipo-atrophy, and insulin-induced lipohypertrophy. (Hypoglycemia is considered a therapeutic side effect of insulin administration, not an adverse effect.)

Some information regarding the structure, biosynthesis, and purification of insulin is necessary for an understanding of the pathogenesis of these complications of insulin therapy. Insulin is a polypeptide hormone with a molecular weight of approximately 6,000. As illustrated in the dark area of Figure 4-3, the insulin molecule consists of A and B chains joined by two disulfide bridges. In addition, a disulfide linkage connects amino acids 6 and 11 within the A chain. Based on the assumption that the A and B chains are synthesized separately and then joined in a final step to form the intact insulin molecule, scientists tried unsuccessfully for years to couple the A and B chains in test tubes. The reason for their failure was first discovered in the late 1960s by Dr. Donald Steiner at the University of Chicago. In a series of elegant experiments, he and his colleagues demonstrated that the steps by which insulin was synthesized in the pancreatic β-cell included: (*a*) the formation of a single long-chain polypeptide; (*b*) the curving of this string of amino acids back on itself in a configuration that aligns the future A and B chains of insulin opposite each other; (*c*) the closing of the two disulfide bridges to form a larger polypeptide (molecular weight, ~9,000) called proinsulin, which is illustrated by the entire structure in Figure 4-3, and

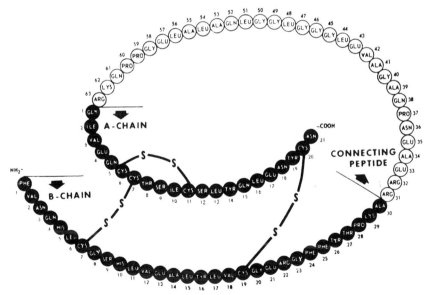

Figure 4-3. Structure of porcine proinsulin. Cleavage occurs at the points marked by straight lines, yielding equimolar amounts of connecting peptide and insulin. The letter S connected to the heavy bars represents disulfide linkages between the amino acids indicated. (Reprinted with permission from Chance RE: Amino acid sequences of proinsulins and intermediates. Diabetes 21 (Suppl 2):461-467, 1972.)

(d) the breaking of this curvilinear molecule at two points, yielding insulin (Fig. 4-3, solid circles) and the connecting peptide (Fig. 4-3, open circles).

Insulin and the connecting peptide (C peptide) are packaged in equimolar amounts in the granules of the β-cell and released into the circulation together. The C peptide has no known biological function but does serve as an important marker of insulin secretion in patients whose insulin levels cannot be measured directly (see chapter 10).

Insulin preparations used before the early 1970s contained significant amounts of protein impurities. When these preparations were examined by gel filtration, three components were seen (Fig. 4-4) and were labeled A, B, and C. The material isolated under peak A has been identified as several proteins with very large molecular weights, that under peak B as proinsulin and related compounds, and that under peak C as insulin itself or insulin that has been modified only slightly. Earlier insulin preparations were contaminated (~10%) with material that was not pure insulin. All of these larger-molecular-weight compounds are extremely antigenic and enhance the formation of IgG antibody directed not only against themselves but also against insulin. Before 1980, insulin preparations that were routinely available in the United States contained only the material collected under peak C. Such preparations are termed *single-peak* insulin and are contaminated with less than 1% of the larger-molecular-weight compounds (of which proinsulin is ~0.1%) and with 3% to 4% of slightly modified insulin. If this material is purified further by chromatography, the resulting preparation

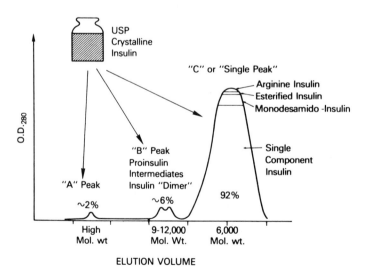

Figure 4-4. Schematic representation of the gel filtration pattern of USP beef or pork insulin on Sephadex G-50. (Reprinted with permission from Kahn CR, Rosenthal AS: Immunologic reactions to insulin: insulin allergy, insulin resistance, and the autoimmune insulin syndrome. Diabetes Care 2:283–295, 1979.)

contains only minuscule amounts (less than 10 ppm) of proinsulin, and a large amount of the slightly modified insulin is removed. This material is termed *single-component* (or *monocomponent*) insulin by European pharmaceutical companies and is more than 99% pure insulin.

In the spring of 1980, Eli Lilly & Company switched entirely from the production of single-peak insulin to a more purified preparation. Therefore, the purity of all insulin preparations produced by Lilly is comparable to that of single-component insulins. At the time of this writing, Squibb Pharmaceutical Company is still routinely producing single-peak insulin. The cost of the purer insulins is somewhat higher than that of single-peak insulin.

Both IgG and IgE antibodies to insulin are found in patients treated with insulin. Only rarely, however, do these antibodies cause clinical problems in diabetics. The IgE antibody seems to be directed specifically against insulin, and high titers are associated with systemic insulin allergy. The situation with regard to IgG antibodies is less clear. It was initially believed that insulin itself stimulated the formation of IgG antibodies. Later, this antigenic response was thought to be mainly (if not entirely) due to the impurities (proinsulin and other larger-molecular-weight compounds) in the preparation. Although single-peak and single-component insulins were once thought not to be antigenic, more recent studies clearly indicate that IgG antibodies are formed against these purer preparations (4, 5). Thus, although impurities may enhance the IgG antibody response to insulin, insulin itself is probably antigenic. However, the development of IgG antibodies to insulin may depend more on the species specificity of the insulin than on its purity or physical state of preparation (6).

Delayed Local Reaction at the Site of Injection

With earlier preparations of insulin, local skin reactions at the site of injection were common, occurring in up to 50% of patients receiving injections for the first time. In patients who have these reactions, symptoms start within 1 month of institution of insulin therapy. There is a 3- to 6-hour lag period before the appearance of the lesions, which are characterized by pruritic, erythematous, indurated areas from 1 to 5 cm in diameter. The lesions become maximal 18 to 24 hours later and last for several days. They are often heralded by a stinging or burning sensation at the time of injection. These reactions are self-limited, invariably disappearing within 1 to 3 months. Because the incidence and severity of these lesions have been markedly diminished by recrystallization of the older insulin preparations to rid them of contaminants, it is likely that the impurities cause these local reactions. The mechanism may involve a delayed hypersensitivity reaction (7). In any event, use of the new, purer preparations is expected to alleviate or eliminate this problem. To date, however, there is no information to substantiate this speculation.

Treatment of the local delayed reaction to insulin injections should be conservative. If the symptoms are not too troublesome to the patient, no therapy is indicated since the lesions will resolve spontaneously. Skin reactions to NPH insulin seem more common than those to the short-acting insulins. However, except in one instance (8), direct allergy to protamine has not been demonstrated. Still, a switch from NPH to Lente has been suggested, as well as a change from a beef or a mixed beef-pork source to a pure pork insulin. (The antigenicity of various insulins will be discussed under *True Insulin Allergy*.) Although these simple maneuvers may be tried, in my experience they seldom resolve the problem. A recent report (9) describes two patients in whom local reactions were caused by the zinc in the insulin preparation administered. Treatment with zinc-free insulin resolved the problem. The prevalence of zinc as the cause of delayed local reactions to insulin is unknown.

Other therapeutic approaches that have been suggested include systemic use of antihistamines or local injections of antihistamines or glucocorticoids. The adverse effects of these medications must be weighed against the possible benefits in this benign situation. If local injections of an antihistamine are tried, 1 mg of diphenhydramine (Benadryl) for each 10 U of insulin can be added to the same syringe. As long as small doses of steroids are used, adrenal suppression, insulin antagonism, and other adverse effects of glucocorticoid therapy should not be a problem. Two glucocorticoid preparations, hydrocortisone and dexamethasone, have been used in the same syringe with insulin. The initial doses of hydrocortisone and dexamethasone are 2 mg and 0.1 mg per injection, respectively. These amounts are gradually increased until the desired effect is achieved. The replacement doses of hydrocortisone and dexamethasone—i.e., the amounts that will suppress the hypothalamic-pituitary-adrenal axis—are 20 mg and 0.75 mg, respectively. It is important to use the smallest possible effective dose—one that preferably will be considerably smaller than a full replacement dose. Another important point is that the effect of dexamethasone lasts for more than 24 hours, while the effect of hydrocortisone lasts for about 8 hours. This shorter-lived effect of hydrocortisone is a theoretical argument for its use, since adrenal suppression may be less likely. On the other hand, if the local reaction flares up after the effect of the glucocorticoid wears off, dexamethasone may be the better agent.

True Insulin Allergy

Nature of Insulin Allergy. In contrast to the delayed local reaction, true allergy to insulin, also called systemic insulin allergy, is (fortunately) rare, occurring in approximately 0.1% of diabetics receiving insulin. It is much more common in patients with a history of interrupted insulin therapy than in those whose therapy has been continuous. The manifestations of insulin allergy are usually seen within 1 or 2 weeks of the resumption of interrupted insulin therapy. The hallmark of true insulin allergy is an *immediate* local reaction (within 30 to 60 minutes) that gradually increases until large areas surrounding the injection site are involved.

The reaction soon spreads into a generalized urticarial pattern and is occasionally associated with angioneurotic edema or even anaphylactic shock (10). These systemic reactions are often preceded by gradual increases in the severity of the immediate local reaction, which may serve as a warning that serious difficulties lie ahead unless appropriate therapy (desensitization) is instituted. Some patients, however, never progress to a generalized reaction.

These immediate reactions (both local and systemic) seem to be allergic responses to the insulin molecule itself. They are not alleviated by the use of extremely pure insulin preparations, either single-component preparations or (in earlier times) specially recrystallized insulin. The clinical similarity to penicillin allergy is striking, and, indeed, the immunologic characteristics of true insulin allergy are almost identical to those of penicillin allergy. Both types of allergy involve (a) exquisite sensitivity to minute amounts of the antigen on conjunctival or intradermal testing, (b) passive transfer of an antibody (recently identified as IgE) that is capable of sensitizing normal skin to a subsequent challenge by the antigen (positive Prausnitz-Küstner test), (c) high titers (as measured by direct assays) of IgE antibodies to the particular antigen in question, and (d) successful treatment by desensitization in almost all cases. Although true insulin allergy is mediated by the same antibody (IgE) that causes atopic disease (asthma, allergic rhinitis, urticaria), patients allergic to insulin apparently have no greater predisposition to atopy than do other patients. On the other hand, in a recent study (5), one third of patients with true insulin allergy had a history of penicillin allergy.

Patients with systemic insulin allergy have high titers of IgE antibodies; these levels decline rapidly (within days) after desensitization but only gradually (over months) after discontinuation of insulin (11, 12). These antibodies are thought also to characterize the immunologic response of patients who develop persistent, immediate local reactions without systemic symptoms, but this point has not yet been demonstrated directly. The IgE antibodies fix to mast cells, and when the IgE–mast cell combination is exposed to insulin, a complicated reaction causes the degranulation of the mast cells. The material released by the mast cells is composed of chemical inflammatory mediators, including large amounts of histamine, and is responsible for the urticaria and anaphylactic symptoms exhibited by patients with true insulin allergy.

Treatment of Insulin Allergy. Since pork and beef insulin differ slightly in their amino acid composition (as discussed later in this section), it is theoretically possible that IgE antibodies may be directed against insulin from only one of these species and that switching insulin preparations may be of value. However, such a switch is rarely, if ever, helpful; in fact, as stated previously, desensitization is the only effective treatment for systemic insulin allergy. To desensitize a patient, very small but gradually increasing amounts of insulin are injected after relatively short periods. These minute doses of the antigen bind to IgE, but the amount of histamine and other chemical mediators of inflammation released by the IgE–mast cell combination is too small to cause clinical symptoms. As the dose of injected insulin is gradually increased, the amount of IgE bound is thought to increase at a slow enough pace that the resultant mast cell degranulation causes no symptoms. Eventually, little or no free (unbound to insulin) IgE remains in the circulation, and the patient can tolerate the usual therapeutic dose of insulin.

Desensitization can be achieved by either of two methods. If the patient has received insulin within the preceding 24 hours, the dose is first decreased by 80% and then increased by 3 to 5 U per injection at daily or twice-daily intervals. In this manner, many patients can be adequately desensitized. If administration of 20% of the usual insulin dose still leads to symptoms of insulin allergy or if the patient has not received insulin within the preceding 24 hours, enough unbound IgE antibodies are probably present to cause difficulties. Under these conditions, injection of more than very small amounts of insulin will be extremely uncomfortable for the patient and possibly dangerous; therefore, a complete desensitization program is advisable.

Some authorities suggest skin testing with minute amounts of beef and pork insulin and desensitization to the insulin from the species that elicits the less marked reaction. We prefer to desensitize routinely to a mixed beef-pork preparation for several reasons. First, and most important, successful desensitization to both beef and pork insulins might prevent a catastrophic reaction should the wrong kind of insulin inadvertently be administered in the future. Second, although most patients are less allergic to pork insulin, uninterrupted supplies of insulin from this source may be jeopardized relatively soon. Third, whether monospecies insulin can always be obtained even at the present time depends on a patient's locale, travel habits, and level of understanding of the problem (which must be communicated to and correctly perceived by physicians and other personnel who may assume the patient's care). Finally, monospecies insulin is slightly more expensive than the mixed preparation. All of these potential problems can be circumvented if successful desensitization (which is the rule) to a mixed beef-pork insulin preparation is achieved. If desensitization proves difficult, then separate testing of beef and pork insulins can be performed, and desensitization to the less antigenic form can be undertaken.

A reasonable schedule for complete desensitization is presented in Table 4-9. The footnote to the table describes the four diluted insulin solutions used, and the table gives details of administration. All injections may be given subcutaneously. If rapid desensitization is required (i.e., if the patient's glucose levels are out of control and substantial amounts of insulin are needed soon), insulin is given every 30 minutes. If subtherapeutic amounts of insulin can be tolerated for a day or two, insulin is administered every 2 hours. Regular insulin is given for the first 12 injections (until a dose of 5 U is reached). After that, the required therapeutic dose of either intermediate-acting or fast-acting insulin (depending on the circumstances) may be tried. Since continued exposure to insulin is necessary in order to maintain the desensitized state, two injections per day should be given, at least during the period immediately following successful desensitization.

Table 4-9. Desensitization Schedule for Patients with True (Systemic) Insulin Allergy

Order of Doses	Solution[a]	Volume Injected (ml)	Amount of Insulin Injected (U)
1	D	0.1	0.001
2	D	0.2	0.002
3	D	0.4	0.004
4	C	0.1	0.01
5	C	0.2	0.02
6	C	0.4	0.04
7	B	0.1	0.1
8	B	0.2	0.2
9	B	0.5	0.5
10	A	0.1	1
11	A	0.2	2
12	A	0.5	5[b]

[a]Solutions are designed as follows: A, 1 ml of U-100 (regular insulin) + 9 ml of normal saline (final concentration, 10.0 U/ml); B, 1 ml of solution A + 9 ml of normal saline (final concentration, 1.0 U/ml); C, 1 ml of solutions B + 9 ml of normal saline (final concentration, 0.1 U/ml); and D, 1 ml of solution C + 9 ml of normal saline (final concentration, 0.01 U/ml).
[b]Required therapeutic dose may be tried after this point.

If a severe local or systemic reaction occurs during the gradual increase of the amount of insulin administered, the dose should be reduced by one dilution and the schedule resumed. If it proves impossible to progress because of severe reactions to the mixed beef-pork preparation, *intradermal* testing with pure preparations of each type of insulin should be done, and the patient should be desensitized to the less antigenic type. If the weakest dilution (0.001 U) listed in Table 4-9 elicits a positive reaction to both types, then even weaker dilutions must be tried. If a dilution containing 0.001 U causes no reaction to either beef or pork insulin, tests with gradually increasing amounts of each, as outlined in Table 4-9, should be continued until one preparation elicits a positive reaction. Desensitization to the other preparation should then be completed.

In practice, 90% of patients can be desensitized to pork insulin, and only 10% require desensitization to beef insulin (5). However, since these data were obtained in studies in which desensitization to pork insulin was attempted first, it is quite possible that a similar proportion of patients could also be desensitized to beef insulin. If desensitization to pork insulin is desired (either initially or after failure of desensitization to a mixed beef-pork preparation), an insulin allergy desensitization kit can be obtained from Eli Lilly & Company. This kit contains 10 vials of single-peak pork insulin in concentrations such that 0.1-ml injections will deliver the amounts of insulin listed for the first 10 doses in Table 4-9.

During the course of desensitization, adequate anaphylactic precautions must be taken. Epinephrine, diphenhydramine (Benadryl), and intubation equipment must be immediately available. A physician should be present for at least 30 minutes after the administration of each increasing amount of insulin. If this restriction should prove difficult (during the night, for example), the continued administration of the last dilution that was well tolerated by the patient should be performed by an experienced nurse. In this case, injections should be given at 2-hour intervals. The presence of the physician and anaphylactic precautions are mandatory when insulin-allergic patients are receiving increasing amounts of insulin since anaphylactoid reactions can occur suddenly, even when previous smaller doses of insulin administered at 30-minute intervals have not elicited any local reactions (13).

Desensitization is successful in approximately 95% of patients manifesting systemic insulin allergy (5). Approximately 50% of patients with persistent local reactions of the immediate type also seem to be helped by desensitization (5). Once desensitized, these patients should not have their insulin therapy interrupted. Since a schedule calling for two injections a day has the theoretical advantage of supplying insulin more constantly to the circulation (as well as usually improving diabetic control), such a regimen should probably be used for all patients who have been successfully densensitized. However, some patients require repeated desensitization in spite of continuous insulin administration.

Treatment of true insulin allergy with glucocorticoids should be avoided if possible because of the effectiveness of desensitization and the long-term adverse effects of steroid therapy. However, if repeated desensitizations are ineffective, prednisone may bring relief, probably by blocking IgE production. An initial dose of 30 to 40 mg per day should be tapered as rapidly as possible to the lowest amounts feasible, with the patient's allergic manifestations serving as the endpoint. If discontinuation of prednisone is not possible within several weeks, alternate-day therapy may be tried in order to minimize the adverse effects of the glucocorticoid. Since so little experience with glucocorticoid therapy for patients with true insulin allergy has been reported, it is difficult to offer firm recommendations. Fortunately, the need for glucocorticoid therapy in this situation is unusual.

Insulin Resistance

Insulin resistance is defined clinically as a situation in which a patient requires more than 200 U of insulin daily for more than 2 days. This definition was coined more than 35 years ago, when it was erroneously believed that the human pancreas secreted approximately 200 U of insulin per day. Although it is now known that the normal pancreas secretes only 20 to 40 U of insulin per day, this clinical definition is helpful because it delineates a very small group of patients with a number of unusual underlying problems.

Use of the term *insulin resistance* in this context must be clearly differentiated from its more general use (usually in research areas) to describe situations in which any impairment of insulin action is noted. The broad spectrum of insulin antagonism includes (*a*) situations in which the pancreas hypersecretes a quantity of insulin that maintains carbohydrate metabolism within normal limits; (*b*) mild glucose intolerance; (*c*) definite diabetes controlled by diet alone, by oral hypoglycemic agents, or by the usual amounts of insulin; and (*d*) cases in which the insulin requirement of a patient clearly falls outside the doses required by the great majority of diabetics. The situations to be discussed under the clinical definition of the term *insulin resistance* represent the far end of this spectrum, at which the action of insulin is markedly inhibited. For instance, although every acromegalic patient with or without diabetes mellitus manifests insulin resistance in the general sense, only those requiring the large amounts of insulin specified in the clinical definition of this term need special therapeutic consideration.

Conditions Associated with Insulin Resistance. The conditions associated with the clinical definition of insulin resistance are listed in Table 4-10. Infection, regardless of the causative organism, clearly is a state in which insulin antagonism exists, but the mechanism(s) involved are unknown. The insulin requirements of most diabetics with infections rise, but the requirement reaches 200 U per day in only a small minority of patients. Since the host's defenses against infections caused by bacteria and certain fungi are impaired in the setting of uncontrolled diabetes, it is important to increase the insulin dose appropriately in a vigorous attempt to lower glucose concentrations.

Although obese diabetics require significantly more insulin than their non-obese counterparts, relatively few obese patients could be termed insulin-resistant in the clinical sense of the term. In my experience, there seems to be a rough correlation between the patient's degree of obesity and the insulin requirement. Obese diabetics who are truly insulin-resistant are usually more than 100% above

Table 4-10. Conditions Associated with Insulin Resistance

Infection

Gross obesity

Cushing's syndrome

Acromegaly

Hemochromatosis

Lipodystrophic diabetes

Acanthosis nigricans

Werner's syndrome (adult form of progeria)

Insulin degradation at injection site

Idiopathic or immune-mediated (mediated by IgG antibody)

---

their ideal body weight. The clinical approach to obese diabetics will be considered in chapter 7.

Glucocorticoids are potent insulin antagonists that increase hepatic gluconeogenesis (see chapter 2) and also interfere with the ability of insulin to enhance glucose utilization by the peripheral tissues. Most cases of insulin resistance secondary to Cushing's syndrome are iatrogenic, i.e., glucocorticoid therapy is prescribed for treatment of other severe problems (asthma, lupus erythematosus disseminata, myasthenia gravis, rejection of transplanted organs, etc.). In general, the increase in the insulin requirement is proportional to the amount of glucocorticoids given. Thus, most patients classified as clinically insulin-resistant are taking at least 50 mg of prednisone or its equivalent. (That is not to say that most patients taking 50 mg or more of prednisone will be clinically insulin-resistant.) Non-iatrogenic cases of insulin resistance caused by excessive doses of glucocorticoids are unusual.

Acromegaly is the clinical syndrome caused by excessive secretion of growth hormone from a pituitary tumor. One metabolic aspect of this syndrome is insulin antagonism induced by growth hormone, the mechanism of which is unknown at present. Like obese patients and those affected by excessive doses of glucocorticoids, acromegalic patients may manifest a spectrum of conditions ranging from normal carbohydrate metabolism to diabetes of varying severity. Effective therapy exists for most patients with acromegaly, and those whose condition falls under the clinical definition of insulin resistance are few.

Although the great majority of patients whose diabetes is secondary to hemochromatosis do not develop insulin resistance, the number of patients with insulin resistance who have hemochromatosis is certainly higher than would be expected. Insulin resistance has also been reported in isolated cases of acute and chronic hepatic degeneration, hepatic infarcts, common-duct stones, fatty liver, Laennec's cirrhosis, and hepatic failure. The mechanism involved in insulin resistance associated with hemochromatosis and other liver diseases is unknown. Although most reports of such cases originated before IgG antibodies were routinely measured, the production of such antibodies clearly cannot explain many of these cases.

Patients with lipodystrophic diabetes (14) are often unresponsive to large amounts of insulin. Total lipodystrophy, often called lipoatrophy, is a syndrome characterized by a complete loss of adipose tissue associated with some or all of the following: ketosis-resistant diabetes, hyperlipoproteinemia, hepatomegaly, increased basal metabolic rates (but normal thyroid test results), and acanthosis nigricans. Partial lipodystrophy, in which loss of adipose tissue occurs only in parts of the body, is more common and is also associated with some or all of the features just listed. Partial lipodystrophy takes two general forms. In the cephalothoracic form, the loss of fat occurs in the upper part of the body, with normal or even excessive amounts of adipose tissue remaining in the lower half. In the second form, the loss of fat occurs in the lower half of the body and sometimes in the upper extremities, but adipose tissue remains over the face and trunk (15). The reason for the ineffectiveness of insulin in patients with any form of lipodystrophy is unknown. These rare lipoatrophic syndromes with marked systemic effects should not be confused with insulin-induced (local) lipoatrophy, one of the adverse effects of insulin (described in a later section of this chapter).

Insulin resistance is occasionally seen in patients who have acanthosis nigricans without lipoatrophy. All but one of such individuals studied have been females in whom obesity, hirsutism, amenorrhea, and/or polycystic ovaries were also noted. These individuals may tolerate thousands of units of insulin. (In one patient, 177,500 U was ineffective.) Recent evidence indicates that insulin resistance in these patients is caused by a marked defect in the binding of insulin to its receptor (16). There are two clinical subtypes. In younger females (type A), the number of insulin receptors available for binding is markedly decreased. This seems to be a primary abnormality. Type A patients manifest no immunologic features. In contrast, older patients with this syndrome (type B) have antibodies to the insulin receptor itself. These antibodies do not affect the number of receptors available but interfere with the affinity of insulin for its receptor. Some type B patients have intermittent hypoglycemia, which is occasionally life-threatening. The hypoglycemia is thought to be due to an insulin-like effect caused by the binding of the antireceptor antibody to the receptor. Why binding of the antireceptor antibody to the receptor only intermittently triggers post-receptor events mimicking the action of insulin is unclear. These older, type B patients also manifest other immunologic features, such as very high erythrocyte sedimentation rates, elevated levels of antinuclear and anti-DNA antibodies, decreased complement levels, and proteinuria.

Werner's syndrome, the adult form of progeria (17), is a rare familial condition that appears in adults and is characterized by diabetes, short stature, slender extremities but stocky trunk, premature graying of the hair, baldness, cataracts, skin ulcers, early appearance of atherosclerosis, and premature death. Although diabetes is usually mild, these patients are often unresponsive to large amounts of insulin for unknown reasons.

Destruction of subcutaneously injected insulin in a 16-year-old diabetic girl has been reported (18). This patient's condition could not be controlled by even as much as 3,000 U injected insulin per day. Control was achieved by continuous intravenous infusion of approximately 50 to 60 U over a 24-hour period. Fortunately, this kind of insulin resistance seems rare indeed.

Usually, all of the conditions listed in Table 4-10 and discussed so far can be easily excluded in the differential diagnosis. Most often, a patient's insulin resistance falls into the category described by the term *idiopathic*. In actuality, this designation is not entirely accurate since the basis for the high insulin requirements is known. Every person receiving insulin injections develops IgG insulin-binding antibodies during the ensuing weeks or months. These antibodies are produced whether or not the patient is diabetic. (For example, they were found to be present in mentally ill patients undergoing insulin-shock treatment 30 to 40 years ago.) Their production is unaffected by the source or purity of the insulin preparation used. In the vast majority of diabetics, modest titers of IgG antibodies to insulin (< 10 mU of insulin bound/ml) cause no difficulty. In approximately 0.1% of insulin-requiring patients, the titers increase to very high levels (ranging from 50 to many thousands of milliunits of insulin bound per milliliter). The reason for this markedly enhanced response and the subsequent decline to normal levels is completely unknown. As with true insulin allergy, intermittent insulin therapy seems to predispose the patient to insulin resistance. Indeed, both insulin allergy (IgE-mediated) and insulin resistance (IgG-mediated) are not infrequently seen in the same patient. Although this cause of insulin resistance is an immunogenic one, nitrogen mustard, 6-mercaptopurine, and azathioprine have all been ineffective in alleviating the condition. Other unsuccessful modes of therapy include tolbutamide, phenformin, starvation, hypophysectomy, and dimercaprol or British antilewisite (BAL).

Treatment of Insulin Resistance. Several approaches can be effective in patients with IgG-mediated (idiopathic) insulin resistance. Theoretically, it may be possible for the patient to switch to another insulin preparation that the IgG antibodies either will not recognize or will bind to much more weakly. Mammalian insulins differ in their primary amino acid structure only in positions 8, 9, and 10 on the A chain and position 30 on the B chain (Table 4-11). However, more is involved in the formation of antibody to insulin than the primary structure of the molecule. Since species as disparate as humans and guinea pigs will form antibodies to their own insulins, it is thought that the insulin molecule is somehow altered during the extraction process and that its secondary and/or tertiary structures (i.e., the spatial orientation of the amino acids in two and

Table 4-11. Species Differences in Amino Acid Sequence of Mammalian Insulins

| | Position | | | |
| | A Chain | | | |
Type of Insulin	8	9	10	*B Chain: 30*
Beef	Alanine	Serine	Valine	Alanine
Pork	Threonine	Serine	Isoleucine	Alanine
Human	Threonine	Serine	Isoleucine	Threonine
Other				
Dog	Threonine	Serine	Isoleucine	Alanine
Sperm whale	Threonine	Serine	Isoleucine	Alanine
Rabbit	Threonine	Serine	Isoleucine	Serine
Horse	Threonine	Glycine	Isoleucine	Alanine
Sheep	Alanine	Glycine	Valine	Alanine
Sei whale	Alanine	Serine	Threonine	Alanine

three dimensions, respectively) may therefore be important in eliciting IgG antibody formation. Furthermore, as discussed earlier in this chapter, the less pure the insulin preparation, the greater is the potential for antibody production; that is, contamination with larger-molecular-weight proteins and proinsulin seems to stimulate an immune response to insulin. On the other hand, the primary amino acid structure must also play a role since, with preparations of comparable purity, beef insulin is more antigenic than pork insulin (6). Thus, multiple factors (primary, secondary, and possibly tertiary structure; the amount of contaminating larger-molecular-weight proteins; and the species source) influence the IgG response to insulin.

From a clinical point of view, switching insulin preparations is not usually an effective way to treat insulin resistance. First, although the IgG antibodies in the non-insulin-resistant patient usually bind more avidly to beef insulin than to pork insulin, there is cross-reactivity. Thus, although the patient's IgG may be directed primarily against beef insulin, the titers are so high that the antibodies also neutralize virtually all of the pork insulin. Second, since impure preparations enhance the immune response to insulin, it was hoped that single-component insulin (an extremely pure preparation) would be effective in treating insulin resistance. However, this has not been the case (4, 5).

Finally, although two insulin preparations have been extremely effective in treating insulin resistance, neither is readily available to physicians in this country at present. If insulin is treated with sulfuric acid under the appropriate chemical conditions, the modified insulin molecule that emerges retains some biologic activity but shows a markedly reduced affinity for binding to IgG antibodies to insulin and very little antigenicity in patients never before treated with insulin. It is not surprising, then, that sulfated beef insulin has been used effectively in therapy of insulin resistance (19). However, although sulfated insulin was first prepared and tested by a Canadian laboratory approximately 15 years ago, it is still not available in the United States.

The (nonmammalian) fish insulins differ markedly from mammalian insulins in structure. For instance, cod and beef insulins differ in 14 positions on the A chain and 9 positions on the B chain. As might be anticipated, antibodies directed against beef insulin do not bind cod insulin. However, cod insulin retains its biologic activity in mammals and therefore is effective in treating insulin resistance (20). Unfortunately, nonmammalian insulins are not available in this country. On a practical basis, then, switching to pork insulin is the only option available, and although such a change may be tried, other avenues of therapy are usually necessary.

Some physicians treat insulin resistance with high doses of glucocorticoids. Although the mechanism by which these agents decrease insulin requirements is not known with certainty, inhibition of IgG antibody production has been postulated. Even if antibody formation were immediately curtailed, however (and this is probably not the case), high insulin requirements would persist for a while since the half-life of IgG is approximately 3 to 4 weeks. Thus, the clinical response to glucocorticoids is often delayed for 1 or 2 weeks, with initial responses occasionally occurring as late as a month after commencement of therapy. During the initial period of treatment, a deterioration in diabetic control and even higher insulin requirements are common, secondary to the insulin antagonism caused by high doses of glucocorticoids. If this therapeutic approach is tried, doses equivalent to approximately 60 mg of prednisone should be used initially and maintained for at least several weeks or until insulin requirements are definitely lowered. The amount of steroid administered is then decreased rapidly, either until the patient can be taken off of the medication entirely or until a level is reached below which insulin requirements definitely increase again. Patients frequently require 5 to 10 mg of prednisone for maintenance therapy. Some individuals who are in remission and either are taking low doses of steroids or have discontinued therapy completely may relapse and need subsequent courses. In view of the adverse effects of long-term glucocorticoid administration, complete discontinuation of therapy should be attempted repeatedly. If it is not possible to discontinue treatment, alternate-day therapy should be tried, although there are no published results concerning its efficacy.

Insulin resistance is self-limited, with antibody titers and insulin requirements returning to the usual levels within several months to a year. Because of the potential hazards of long-term glucocorticoid administration, the relatively long lag period before this type of therapy becomes effective (during which time the patient may be critically ill), the frequent deterioration in diabetic control after initiation of steroid therapy, and the temporary nature of the clinical course of insulin resistance, I avoid administering glucocorticoid therapy altogether and simply use enough insulin to keep the patient (relatively) asymptomatic and to prevent the development of ketosis.

A special preparation of highly concentrated regular pork insulin (U-500) is available for this purpose. The high concentration of insulin in this preparation (500 U/cc) is very convenient for these patients, since the usual U-100 insulin would have to be injected in large volumes. Even though the U-500 preparation contains regular insulin, the action is prolonged because of the extremely high antibody titers. After absorption from the subcutaneous injection site, the insulin is quickly bound by the enlarged pool of circulating IgG antibodies before it acts on the insulin-sensitive tissues. Free insulin is subsequently released at a rate that clinically approximates a time-course of action lying between those of Semilente and the intermediate-acting insulins. Thus, two injections per day of U-500 regular pork insulin in appropriate amounts will usually "control" an insulin-resistant diabetic. Obviously, in this temporary situation, good control is difficult to achieve and should probably not be sought. The goals should be to keep the patient from developing ketosis and to lower glucose concentrations to a degree such that the symptoms of hyperglycemia (polyuria, polydipsia, nocturia, and increased susceptibility to infection) are avoided.

Several important considerations must be kept in mind during the treatment of IgG-mediated insulin resistance with U-500 regular pork insulin. Small increments in insulin dosage are usually ineffective if more insulin is needed. The increase per dose should be at least 10 U and probably close to 20 U, depending on the clinical picture. That is, if the patient's glucose levels are clearly out of control and have shown little or no response to the current insulin regimen, increases of 20 to 25 units should be prescribed. If the patient has begun to respond to increased amounts of insulin, the additional increases in dose should be smaller—i.e., 10 to 15 units each time. However, it must be emphasized again that responses to these large amounts of insulin are usually not consistent and predictable in patients with insulin resistance. The dose of insulin may be varied considerably with little change in glucose levels, or conversely, glucose concentrations may vary considerably despite administration of a fixed amount of insulin. Thus, simply keeping the patient free of ketosis and symptomatic hyperglycemia is a realistic goal but can often be quite a therapeutic challenge.

Return of Insulin Sensitivity. Insulin sensitivity can return relatively quickly. The reason for a marked decrease in IgG production is unknown. At this point in the clinical course, hypoglycemia can become a serious problem as the large amounts of already-bound insulin are released and act on the tissues. Furthermore, the number of available binding sites for the recently injected insulin on the circulating antiinsulin IgG pool is not large. For this reason, the dose of insulin must be decreased in large decrements (20 to 40 U) once symptoms of hypoglycemia are detected. The reversal of insulin resistance is one of the few situations in which I will lower the insulin dose in *anticipation* of hypoglycemia. If the fasting and/or before-supper glucose concentrations are below 200 mg/100 ml or if a patient with an appropriate Tm for glucose has negative results in tests for glucosuria at these times, the dose of insulin should be decreased. If the degree of diabetic control remains the same, further decreases in the dose of insulin should be tried until control deteriorates. If the insulin-resistant state has finally been reversed, the cutoff will be at the usual therapeutic dose of insulin. If not, continued administration of larger amounts of insulin and continued close follow-up will be required.

A smooth transition from insulin resistance to insulin sensitivity is usually not apparent, and insulin requirements may have to be juggled from day to day, depending on the patient's responses. However, at some point in the clinical course, excessive production of IgG antibodies to insulin ceases, and the return of insulin sensitivity becomes obvious. This change usually takes place over several weeks, an interval consistent with the half-life of IgG antibodies. Although the timing of the decision to return to therapy with intermediate-acting insulins will vary from patient to patient, once less than 100 U of regular insulin is being given at each injection, NPH or Lente insulin generally may be tried again. A short interval (2 to 4 hours) between the injection of U-500 regular pork insulin and a clear metabolic (marked lowering of glucose concentrations) and/or clinical (symptoms of hypoglycemia) response suggests that the high titers of IgG antibodies have diminished; thus, a short interval may serve as a clue about when to resume therapy with intermediate-acting insulins.

Insulin-Induced Lipoatrophy

Insulin-induced lipoatrophy (Fig. 4-5) is a loss of subcutaneous fat at the sites of insulin injection. Although this condition seems to be more common in young females than in other patients, it certainly is not limited to this group of insulin-requiring diabetics. Even though this form of local lipoatrophy is a benign condition, the cosmetic effect can be disturbing, especially to adolescent girls and young women. Although the cause of this reaction is not known for certain, an immune response to contaminants in the administered insulin preparation may be involved. In one retrospective study (21), lipoatrophy was found to be more common in patients who had received preparations containing the more immunogenic beef insulin (16%) than in those given only pork insulin (5%). Patients with lipoatrophy often describe a local, delayed dermal reaction at the site of injection (5); such a response might be associated with delayed hypersensitivity to impurities in the insulin preparation (7). Finally, the condition of some patients improves in response to local injections of dexamethasone (22).

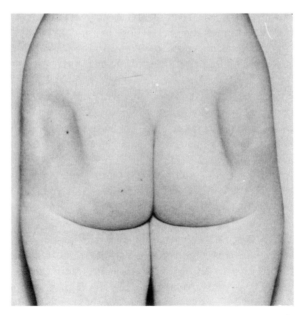

Figure 4-5. Insulin-induced lipoatrophy in a young woman. (Reprinted with permission from Mazzaferi EL: *Endocrinology Case Studies.* Medical Examination Publishing Co, Flushing, NY, 1975, p 161.)

An effective treatment is now available for insulin-induced local lipoatrophy. This treatment simply (and perhaps paradoxically) involves the injection of recently manufactured, purer insulin preparations directly into the involved areas. The response is probably due to a local lipogenic effect of insulin; this effect is possible because the previous (immunologically induced?) lipolytic response to the impurities in the older preparation is now absent. The technique for injection in these atrophic areas is shown in Figure 4-6, and the results 6 months later are shown in Figure 4-7. In a series of more than 300 patients (5), more than 80% were successfully treated by injection of single-peak, mixed beef-pork insulin. Approximately one quarter of those in whom this approach was not helpful responded to injection of a single-peak, pure pork preparation. The remainder were successfully treated when an even purer preparation (single-component) of pork insulin was used (5).

Several other considerations need to be kept in mind. First, patients who may still be experiencing local dermal reactions to insulin are often refractory to treatment for lipoatrophy until the skin reaction abates. Second, local injections must be given for 2 to 4 weeks before normal subcutaneous fat tissue begins to reaccumulate. Third, areas that have filled in may lose their fatty tissue again unless they are reinjected periodically (every 2 to 4 weeks). Fourth, although lipoatrophy was common with the much earlier insulin preparations, occurring

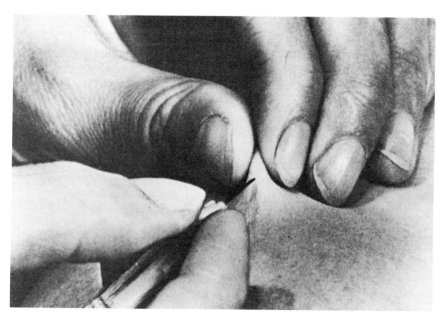

Figure 4-6. Injection of insulin into the affected area of a patient with lipoatrophy. Note the thin skin fold. (Reprinted with permission from Hulst SGTh: Treatment of insulin-induced lipoatrophy. Diabetes 25:1052–1054, 1976.)

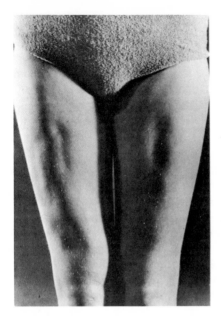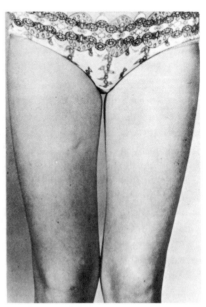

Figure 4-7. Insulin-induced lipoatrophy before (*left*) and after (*right*) 6 months of treatment with a purified insulin preparation. (Reprinted with permission from Hulst SGTh: Treatment of insulin-induced lipoatrophy. Diabetes 25:1052–1054, 1976.)

in 44% of patients less than 20 years of age and 15% of those over the age of 20 (23), it might be anticipated that this syndrome would become rare or even disappear altogether since single-peak insulin is now routinely used. However, in my experience and the experience of others (5), an occasional patient develops lipoatrophy when taking single-peak insulin. In those cases, single-component pork insulin is reported to be "virtually 100% effective" (5). Finally, once insulin lipoatrophy is successfully treated, use of the insulin preparation that was effective should be continued. Return to a less pure preparation can be associated with recurrence of lipoatrophy both at new injection sites and in areas previously afflicted but no longer being injected after reaccumulation of fat (5, 24).

Insulin-Induced Lipohypertrophy

Some diabetics receiving insulin manifest lipohypertrophy of subcutaneous fat tissue at the site of injection (Fig. 4-8). This condition is no doubt due to a local lipogenic effect of insulin. Although patients are less likely to comment on lipohypertrophy than on atrophy, a careful study of almost 600 patients (23) revealed some increase in subcutaneous fat at the sites of insulin injection in approximately 40% of males and 18% of females less than 20 years old and in 20% of males and 12% of females over the age of 20 years. One factor that probably predisposes to this reaction is repeated injections in the same place.

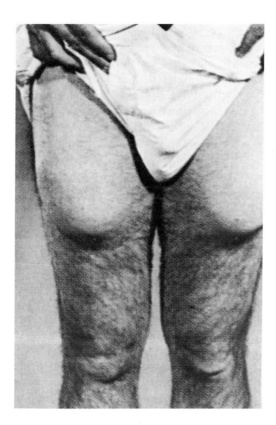

Figure 4-8. Insulin-induced lipohypertrophy. (Reprinted with permission from Krall LP, Zorilla E: Disorders of the skin in diabetes. In *Joslin's Diabetes Mellitus.* Edited by Marble A, White P, Bradley RF, Krall LP. Lea and Febiger, Philadelphia, 1971, p 654A.)

Once lipohypertrophy develops, patients may tend to continue injecting at this site since many report less pain than at other sites. In addition to cosmetic considerations, continued injection into these areas is probably not wise since absorption of insulin from such sites is thought to be erratic. (However, I have been unable to find any documentation of this widely held belief.) There is no good evidence that switching either to purer preparations or to insulin from another species is helpful. Avoidance of these lipohypertrophic areas for future insulin injection sometimes results in a gradual disappearance of this extra tissue.

Practical Summary

Insulin is packaged in 10-cc vials at concentrations of 40 or 100 U/ml (U-40, or U-100). Insulin preparations differ in their time of onset, peak, and duration of action after injection (Table 4-1). I use two injections of intermediate-acting

(NPH or Lente) insulin per day (before breakfast and before supper), supplemented with small amounts of short-acting (regular) insulin in the same syringe if necessary. The use of two injections allows the patient more flexibility and almost always affords tighter control. (See chapter 2 for a discussion of the importance of strict control.) The proper amount of intermediate-acting insulin is first determined, and only then is short-acting insulin added. The urine or plasma glucose test that best reflects the effectiveness of each component of the insulin prescription is shown in Table 4-2.

The initial dose of NPH insulin for lean patients is 10 U in the morning and 5 U before supper. In obese individuals whose weight is more than 125% of their ideal body weight (see chapter 3 for calculation of ideal body weight), the doses are 20 U and 10 U, respectively. Each dose can be adjusted independently of the other, depending on results of the appropriate test (i.e., the before-supper test for the morning dose of NPH insulin, and the fasting test for the before-supper dose of NPH insulin). The doses are increased gradually (4 to 5 U each time) until both the fasting and before-supper glucose concentrations are less than 200 mg/100 ml. In very obese subjects and those whose glucose levels are greater than 300 mg/100 ml, increments of 8 to 10 U are sometimes advisable. In hospitalized patients, plasma glucose levels are determined twice a day and used as guidelines for daily adjustments in doses of NPH insulin. When appropriate glucose levels have been attained, the patient is discharged from the hospital; final adjustments of the dose of NPH insulin and the addition of regular insulin (when necessary) are dealt with outside the hospital. In an office setting, results of urine tests (after the approximate renal threshold, or Tm, for glucose has been determined) serve as the primary guidelines for insulin adjustments every 2 to 3 days. The appropriate urine test for determining the need for adding regular insulin to the morning insulin dose is made before lunch; the need for regular insulin before supper is determined by the results of the before-bedtime urine test.

For patients over the age of 60 years and for those who refuse to take two injections per day, a single injection before breakfast is indicated. Again, the appropriate dose of NPH insulin is determined before any regular insulin is added to the regimen. In this situation, the total daily dose used at the initiation of therapy for patients taking more than one injection per day is given in a single dose before breakfast. A patient's response is reflected both in the before-supper test on the same day and in the following morning's fasting test. The dose of NPH insulin is gradually increased until (ideally) plasma glucose concentrations measured by both tests are less than 200 mg/100 ml. In order to expedite this process while the patient is in the hospital, small amounts of NPH insulin and sometimes regular insulin are given in the evening if the before-supper glucose level is very high (Table 4-7).

Three patterns of response are seen after a single morning injection of NPH insulin. Ideally, the glucose level is controlled throughout the subsequent 24-hour period, but this result is unusual. More commonly, daytime glucose concentrations can be kept at reasonable levels, but the effect of insulin wears off overnight and moderate to marked fasting hyperglycemia ensues. Increasing the dose of intermediate-acting insulin in order to control the fasting glucose concentration often results in afternoon hypoglycemia. If intake of some calories as a midafternoon snack does not alleviate this circumstance, either significant fasting hyperglycemia must be accepted or two injections of insulin per day must be given. A delayed peak in the action of NPH insulin, with nighttime hypoglycemia, occurs infrequently. In this situation, the patient should be given short-acting insulin (usually Semilente), and two injections are often necessary.

The sliding-scale method (determination of each dose of regular insulin based on results of the preceding urine test for glucose) should not be used for the following reasons. First, this method does not anticipate increases in glucose concentrations but delays treatment until hyperglycemia exceeding the Tm for glucose occurs. Second, regular insulin lowers the glucose level fairly rapidly, thereby stimulating the release of contrainsulin hormones. Subsequent doses will not be as effective because of the resulting insulin antagonism, and much larger amounts of regular insulin will be required than the amount of NPH that the patient eventually receives on a routine basis. Third, the relation between the results of urinary glucose tests and plasma glucose concentrations is inexact, in part because of such factors as varying renal thresholds among patients, interference by drugs and other substances with urine tests for glucose, and incomplete emptying of the bladder. Fourth, urine samples are not always collected and analyzed appropriately on busy hospital wards.

There are five adverse effects of insulin therapy. The first is a *local delayed reaction* to insulin at the injection site. Such common dermal reactions are thought to be related to cell-mediated hypersensitivity to impurities in insulin preparations. Pruritic, erythematous, indurated papules (1 to 5 cm) appear 3 to 6 hours after injection and may last for 24 to 48 hours. They invariably disappear after several months. No treatment is usually indicated, although switching to a different insulin preparation, systemic administration of antihistamines, and administration of either antihistamines or glucocorticoids in the same syringe as insulin have all been advocated.

The second adverse effect is *true insulin allergy*, also termed *systemic insulin allergy*. This rare complication (in 0.1% of patients taking insulin) begins as an immediate reaction (within 30 minutes) at the injection site that quickly spreads over large parts of the body as an urticarial rash. Angioneurotic edema and anaphylactic shock can also occur. The pathogenesis and clinical picture of this allergic reaction to the insulin molecule itself are very similar to those of penicillin allergy: the allergy is more common in patients whose insulin therapy has been interrupted; it is mediated by IgE antibodies; skin tests are positive; and desensitization, the treatment of choice (see Table 4-9 for schedule), is effective in approximately 95% of cases.

The third adverse effect is immune-mediated *insulin resistance*. Insulin resistance is defined as a clinical situation in which a patient requires more than

200 U of insulin per day. The conditions considered in the differential diagnosis are shown in Table 4-10. Most of the conditions listed are easily ruled out, and the diagnosis of IgG antibody-mediated insulin resistance is made by exclusion. Every subject (whether or not a diabetic) who receives insulin for approximately a month develops IgG antibodies to insulin. In a very few of these patients (~0.1%), the antibody titer increases considerably for unknown reasons, and large amounts of insulin are required. An intermittent history of insulin therapy is also common in these patients. Switching from beef or beef-pork mixtures to pure pork insulin is occasionally helpful. Although glucocorticoid therapy has been recommended, we avoid it because of the adverse effects of the drug and the self-limited nature of insulin resistance. (The condition usually resolves spontaneously within several months to a year.) I recommend simply to administer the amount of insulin that the patient requires. A U-500 insulin preparation from Eli Lilly & Company reduces the volume that must be injected in order to achieve this goal. Although this preparation is regular insulin, its time-course of action in insulin-resistant patients approximates that of intermediate-acting insulin because of the high titers of IgG antibody present. Therefore, it is usually given twice a day. Caution must be exercised when insulin resistance wanes (usually over a period of several weeks) in order to avoid profound hypoglycemia secondary to administration of these large amounts of insulin.

The fourth adverse effect is *insulin-induced lipoatrophy* (Fig. 4-5). This loss of subcutaneous fat at injection sites is most common in young females and is thought to be due to a lipolytic reaction to impurities in insulin preparations. Use of varied injection sites will minimize this effect. In addition, injection of the recently available, purer insulin preparations directly into the atrophic areas (Fig. 4-6) reverses this process in the great majority of cases (Fig. 4-7). Although one would expect that the use of these purer insulin preparations would prevent the appearance of lipoatrophy, we have seen several patients who have recently started insulin therapy and have developed this condition.

The fifth adverse effect is *insulin-induced lipohypertrophy* at the injection site (Fig. 4-8). This hypertrophy is due to a local lipogenic effect of insulin. Use of varied injection sites will obviously minimize this effect. However, because of decreased sensation at the affected sites during injection, patients tend to use those sites repeatedly, and accumulation of subcutaneous fat ensues. Although I could find no documentation in the literature, it is commonly believed that absorption of insulin from lipohypertrophic sites is erratic. Therefore, injection into these areas should be avoided.

References

1. Waife SE (ed): *Diabetes Mellitus*, 8th ed. Eli Lilly and Co, Indianapolis, 1979, pp 29-49

2. Guthrie DW, Guthrie RA, Hinnen D: Single vs. double voided techniques for urine testing. Diabetes Care 2:269-271, 1979

3. Hallas-Moller K: The lente insulins. Diabetes 5:7-14, 1956

4. Yue DK, Turtle JR: New forms of insulin and their use in the treatment of diabetes. Diabetes 26:341-345, 1977

5. Galloway JA, Bressler R: Insulin treatment in diabetes. Med Clin North Am 62:663-680, 1978

6. Neubauer HP, Schöne H: The immunogenicity of different insulins in several animal species. Diabetes 27:8-15, 1978

7. Federlin K: *Immunopathology of Insulin. Clinical and Experimental Studies.* Springer-Verlag, New York, 1971, pp 31-88

8. Shore RN, Shelley WB, Kyle GC: Chronic urticaria from isophane insulin therapy. Arch Dermatol 111:94-97, 1975

9. Feinglos MN, Jegasothy BV: 'Insulin' allergy due to zinc. Lancet 1:122-124, 1979

10. Hanauer L, Batson JM: Anaphylactic shock following insulin injection: case report and review of the literature. Diabetes 10:105-109, 1961

11. Patterson R, Mellies CJ, Roberts M: Immunologic reactions against insulin. II. IgE anti-insulin, insulin allergy and combined IgE and IgG immunologic insulin resistance. J Immunol 110:1135-1145, 1973

12. Mattson JR, Patterson R, Roberts M: Insulin therapy in patients with systemic insulin allergy. Arch Intern Med 135:818-821, 1975

13. Goldman RA, Lewis AE, Rose LI: Anaphylactoid reaction to single-component pork insulin. JAMA 236:1148-1149, 1976

14. Senior B, Gellis SS: The syndromes of total lipodystrophy and of partial lipodystrophy. Pediatrics 33:593-612, 1964

15. Davidson MB, Young RT: Metabolic studies in familial partial lipodystrophy of the lower trunk and extremities. Diabetologia 11:561-568, 1975

16. Kahn CR, Flier JS, Bar RS, et al: The syndromes of insulin resistance and acanthosis nigricans. Insulin-receptor disorders in man. N Engl J Med 294:739-745, 1976

17. Epstein CJ, Martini GM, Schultz AL, Motulsky AG: Werner's syndrome: a review of its symptomatology, natural history, pathological features, genetics, and relationship to the natural aging process. Medicine 45:177-221, 1966

18. Paulsen EP, Courtney JW III, Duckworth WC: Insulin resistance caused by massive degradation of subcutaneous insulin. Diabetes 28:640-645, 1979

19. Davidson JK, DeBra DW: Immunologic insulin resistance. Diabetes 27:307-318, 1978

20. Yalow RS, Berson SA: Reaction of fish insulins with human insulin antiserums. Potential value in the treatment of insulin resistance. N Engl J Med 270:1171-1178, 1964

21. Deckert T, Andersen OO, Poulsen JE: The clinical significance of highly purified pig-insulin preparations. Diabetologia 10:703-708, 1974

22. Kumar D, Miller LV, Mehtalia SD: Use of dexamethasone in treatment of insulin lipoatrophy. Diabetes 26:296-299, 1977

23. Marble A, Renold AE: Atrophy of subcutaneous fat following injections of insulin. Proc Am Diabetes Assoc 2:171-186, 1942

24. Teuscher A: Treatment of insulin lipoatrophy with monocomponent insulin. Diabetologia 10:211-214, 1974

25. Bhaskar R, Chou MCY, Field JB: Time-action characteristics of regular and NPH insulin in insulin-treated diabetics. J Clin Endocrinol Metab 50:475-479, 1980

Chapter 5

Oral Hypoglycemic Sulfonylurea Agents

Introduction of the Sulfonylurea Agents

During World War II, French scientists studying the antibiotic potential of modified sulfonamides noted that the mice used in their experiments were unexpectedly dying. Further investigations revealed that hypoglycemia was the cause of death. Because of the overwhelming need for and interest in the antibiotic properties of the sulfonamides, this serendipitous discovery was not considered further until after the war. The first sulfonylurea agent, carbutamide, was introduced into clinical practice for the treatment of diabetes mellitus in 1955 in Germany. (Its use was subsequently discontinued in the United States because of adverse reactions.) Tolbutamide (Orinase) was introduced in the United States the following year, and chlorpropamide (Diabinese) became available a year later. In the 1960s two more sulfonylurea agents, acetohexamide (Dymelor) and tolazamide (Tolinase) were introduced into clinical practice in the United States. Thus, four sulfonylurea compounds, whose chemical structures are shown in Figure 5-1, are available in the United States for the treatment of diabetes mellitus. The sulfonylurea component of these compounds, which is responsible for their hypoglycemic effects, is enclosed by dashed lines in the figure. The different groups attached to the common sulfonylurea structure give each compound unique pharmacologic properties.

In recent years, this first generation of oral hypoglycemic agents has been followed by a second generation of sulfonylurea compounds (Table 5-1). Although these agents are not currently available in the United States several may soon be. The range of doses for the first-generation compounds is from 100 to 3,000 mg; thus, it is apparent from the table that the second-generation agents are more effective on a milligram/milligram basis. Only one published study has directly compared the efficacy of first- and second-generation sulfonylurea

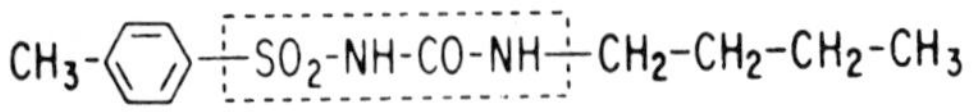

$$CH_3-\langle\ \rangle-SO_2\text{-}NH\text{-}CO\text{-}NH-CH_2\text{-}CH_2\text{-}CH_2\text{-}CH_3$$

Tolbutamide
(1-butyl-3-p-tolylsulfonylurea)

$$CH_3-\langle\ \rangle-SO_2\text{-}NH\text{-}CO\text{-}NH-N\begin{matrix}CH_2\text{-}CH_2\text{-}CH_2\\CH_2\text{-}CH_2\text{-}CH_2\end{matrix}$$

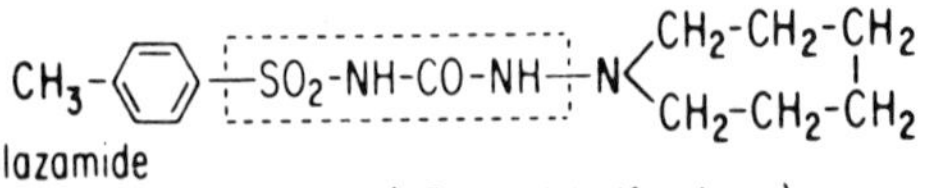

Tolazamide
(1-(hexahydro-1-azepinyl)-3-p-tolylsulfonylurea)

$$CH_3\text{-}CO-\langle\ \rangle-SO_2\text{-}NH\text{-}CO\text{-}NH-\langle\ \rangle$$

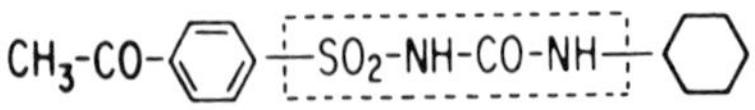

Acetohexamide
(N-(p-acetylbenzenesulfonyl)-N'-cyclohexylurea)

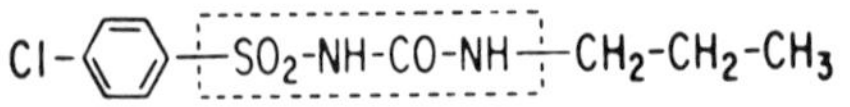

$$Cl-\langle\ \rangle-SO_2\text{-}NH\text{-}CO\text{-}NH-CH_2\text{-}CH_2\text{-}CH_3$$

Chlorpropamide
(1-propyl-3-p-chlorobenzenesulfonylurea)

Figure 5-1. Chemical structure of the four sulfonylurea agents currently available in the United States. The common sulfonylurea structure, enclosed by dotted lines, is the active component of each molecule. The attached groups are responsible for the various metabolic fates of each drug. (Adapted with permission from Williams RH, Porte D Jr: The pancreas. In *Textbook of Endocrinology,* 5th ed. WB Saunders, Philadelphia, 1974, pp 502–626.)

Table 5-1. Second-Generation Sulfonylurea Agents

Generic Name(s)	Trade Name(s)	Dosage Range (mg)
Glibenclamide or glyburide	Euglucon, Daonil, Micronase, Diabeta	1.25–20
Glipizide	Glibenese	2.5–45
Glibornuride	Glutril	12.5–100
Glisoxepide	Pro-Diaban	2–16
Gliquidone	Glurenorm	15–120
Glycodiazine[a]	Redul, Glymidine, Lycanol, Gondafon	500–1,500

[a]This compound is actually a modified sulfonamide rather than a sulfonylurea.

agents (1). Newly diagnosed, lean, type 2 diabetic patients in whom dietary therapy alone was ineffective were treated with either glibenclamide or chlorpropamide and observed for 2 years. With 2- to 2.5-hour post-breakfast glucose concentrations as a measure of the patients' response to the drug, the second-generation sulfonylurea agent was not found to be more effective than the first-generation agent.

Since only the compounds shown in Figure 5-1 are available in the United States today, the second-generation sulfonylurea agents will not be considered further here. They are listed in Table 5-1 so that the physician will recognize them when they are introduced in this country.

Mechanism of Action

Sulfonylurea agents are ineffective in animals whose β-cells have been removed by pancreatectomy or destroyed by chemicals. These compounds do not work in diabetics who are ketosis-prone—the biochemical manifestation of marked insulin deficiency (see chapter 2). With the advent of a radioimmunoassay that could measure insulin concentrations in the physiologic range, these levels were found to be increased in both peripheral and portal veins after the *acute* administration of these compounds. These data strongly suggested that the hypoglycemic effect of the sulfonylurea agents is due to a stimulation of insulin secretion. However, the *chronic* administration of these agents is associated with continued improvement in diabetic control but a return of insulin concentrations to pretreatment or even lower levels.

This sequence of events (2) is illustrated in Figure 5-2. Eleven obese (>120% of ideal body weight), ketosis-resistant (type 2) diabetics who had fasting blood sugar levels of more than 150 mg/100 ml and were currently being treated by means of diet alone were admitted to a clinical research center. For the first 3 days, they continued to adhere to their diets; then they were studied for 48 hours. The subjects continued to follow their diets on the fourth day but fasted from after supper on that day until breakfast on the sixth day. Multiple blood samples were obtained for measurements of plasma glucose and serum insulin concentrations throughout this 48-hour period. Chlorpropamide (500 mg daily) was then added to the dietary regimens of the patients, and the study was repeated 5 days later. The average fasting values of glucose and insulin on the mornings of the second, third, and fourth days were selected as basal levels. Each patient served as her or his own control, and all concentrations measured subsequently were expressed as a percentage change compared with the basal value. After 5 days of treatment with chlorpropamide, glucose concentrations were lower and insulin levels were higher than when dietary therapy alone was used (Fig. 5-2, left).

Four patients were studied again after 5 weeks of treatment. When the results of this additional study are compared with the data obtained after 5 days of drug

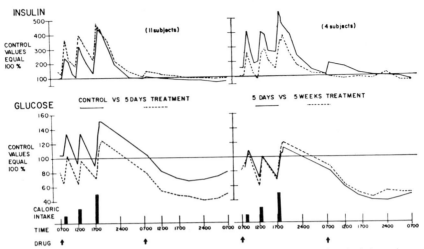

Figure 5-2. Effect of acute (5 days) and chronic (5 weeks) administration of chlorpropamide on plasma glucose and insulin concentrations throughout a 48-hour period in ketosis-resistant diabetics. (Reprinted with permission from Chu P-C, Conway MJ, Krouse HA, Goodner CJ: The pattern of response of plasma insulin and glucose to meals and fasting during chlorpropamide therapy. Ann Intern Med 68:757–769, 1968.)

therapy (Fig. 5-2, right), it is clear that glucose concentrations remained lower but insulin levels returned to the levels measured before drug treatment. Other workers have reported similar findings.

How do sulfonylurea agents help lower blood glucose concentrations? There are two possibilities. After the initial enhancement of insulin secretion by sulfonylurea agents, continued exposure leads to greater sensitivity of the pancreatic β-cell to glucose. Thus, the early increase in insulin secretion lowers glucose concentrations, and the pancreatic β-cell can respond to these decreased concentrations; in contrast, prior to drug treatment, a much greater hyperglycemic stimulus is necessary to stimulate the same amount of insulin secretion. This scenario will be extremely difficult to prove.

The second possibility is that the hypoglycemic actions of sulfonylurea agents are unrelated to their effects on the β-cell. Data showing decreased insulin synthesis and lower insulin levels after administration of sulfonylurea agents to diabetics in whom control has improved are consistent with an extrapancreatic effect of these drugs (3, 4).

Although a number of extrapancreatic effects of sulfonylurea agents have been reported (3, 4), most evidence favors the potentiation of insulin activity as the primary mechanism of action. This mechanism is illustrated in Figure 5-3. Type 2 diabetics with fasting hyperglycemia were brought under good control by means of diet alone ($n = 5$) or with the addition of a second-generation sulfonylurea agent to their dietary regimen ($n = 8$). Insulin tolerance tests were

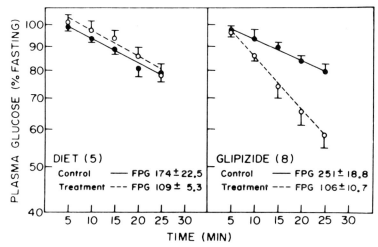

Figure 5-3. Insulin (0.1 U/kg) tolerance tests before and after achievement of control in ketosis-resistant diabetics. FPG, fasting plasma glucose. See text for description. (Reprinted with permission from Lebovitz HE, Feinglos MN, Bucholtz HK, Lebovitz FK: Potentiation of insulin action: a probable mechanism for the anti-diabetic action of sulfonylurea drugs. J Clin Endocrinol Metab 45:601–604, 1977.)

performed before and after control was achieved. The fasting glucose concentration was considered 100%, and the glucose levels after injection of insulin were expressed as a percentage of the fasting value. The slope of the resulting straight line shows the rate of fall of glucose concentrations and is a measure of the effectiveness of the injected insulin. Insulin sensitivity remained constant in patients controlled by means of diet alone. In contrast, insulin sensitivity was markedly increased in the patients treated with the sulfonylurea agent, although the degree of control attained, as assessed by fasting glucose concentrations, was similar in the two groups.

The point at which sulfonylurea agents potentiate insulin action may be the initial step of hormonal binding. Insulin exerts a number of transport and intracellular effects. Many of the latter effects are independent of transport. Recent evidence, however, provides rather convincing support for the theory that *all* aspects of the action of insulin are causally related to a signal generated by the interaction between insulin and its receptor in the plasma membrane of the cell (Fig. 5-4). Decreased insulin binding has been found in many (but not all) ketosis-resistant diabetics. Treatment of these patients for several months with a first-generation drug returns the depressed level of binding toward normal (Fig. 5-5). Data from studies in animals also support this mode of action for the oral hypoglycemic agents. After mice were treated for 10 days with a second-generation sulfonylurea agent, they responded to a dose of intraperitoneal (ip) insulin that had no hypoglycemic effect in control animals (Fig. 5-6, A). Thus,

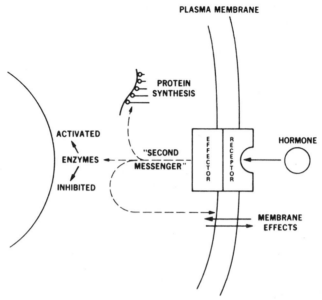

Figure 5-4. Schematic representation of hormonal action on cellular metabolism. Insulin (in this case) binds to a receptor that transmits a signal through an effector system. This unknown signal then affects membrane function (transport of glucose, amino acids, and potassium) as well as intracellular pathways (enzyme activation, protein, and RNA and DNA synthesis); these effects are independent of the effects of the signal on transport. (Reprinted with permission from Receptors for Peptide Hormones: new insights into the pathophysiology of disease states in man. Ann Intern Med 86:205–219, 1977.)

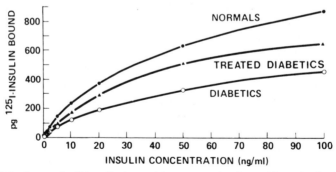

Figure 5-5. Amount of insulin bound to monocytes from 40 control subjects and 16 ketosis-resistant diabetics before and after treatment with chlorpropamide. (Reprinted with permission from Olefsky JM, Reaven GM: Effects of sulfonylurea therapy on insulin binding to mononuclear leukocytes of diabetic patients. Am J Med 60:89–95, 1976.)

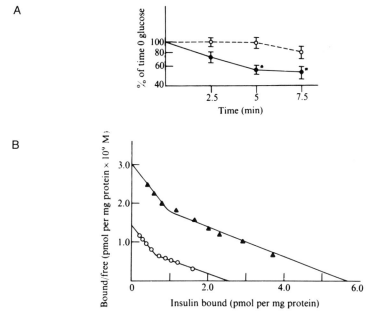

Figure 5-6. (A) Response of glucose concentrations to intraperitoneal injection of 2.5 mU of insulin in control mice (*open circles*) and in mice treated with glipizide for 10 days (*closed circles*). The data are expressed as a percentage of the glucose level before injection, which is considered 100%. Brackets enclose SE. Asterisks denote significant statistical differences ($P < 0.05$). **(B)** Insulin binding by hepatic plasma membranes from control mice (*open circles*) and from mice treated with glipizide for 10 days (*closed triangles*). (Reprinted with permission from Feinglos MN, Lebovitz HE: Sulphonylureas increase the number of insulin receptors. Nature 276:184–185, 1978. Copyright © 1978, Macmillan Journals Limited.)

the sulfonylurea agent potentiated the effect of insulin. Associated with this increased sensitivity to insulin was a marked enhancement of insulin binding to hepatic plasma membranes from these mice (Fig. 5-6, B). Sophisticated analysis of the binding data indicates that sulfonylurea agents affect insulin binding by increasing the number of receptors rather than by affecting the affinity between the hormone and its receptors.

In summary, sulfonylurea agents initially stimulate insulin release but, when given chronically, seem to inhibit both the synthesis and the secretion of insulin. The long-term effect of these oral hypoglycemic agents is a potentiation of insulin action, perhaps because of an increase in the number of receptors located on the plasma membrane. However, the relation between insulin binding and insulin action is complex (5). Further evidence is certainly needed on whether the primary mechanism by which sulfonylurea agents potentiate insulin action is mediated by an increase in the number of insulin receptors.

Pharmacology

Sulfonylurea agents are rapidly absorbed from the gastrointestinal tract. Appreciable concentrations in plasma can be measured by 1 hour after ingestion. The compounds are transported in the blood bound to serum proteins. Plasma levels of drug vary widely for reasons that are not entirely clear. In the case of tolbutamide, rates of disappearance vary over a 10-fold range among individuals. This variation is due to genetic differences in the enzyme of the rate-limiting degradative step (6). Thus, although generalizations will be made concerning the pharmacology of these drugs, the data cited may not strictly apply to individual patients.

Tolbutamide is oxidized in the liver, and its metabolites, which are inactive, are excreted by the kidney. The approximate half-life of the parent compound is 4 to 5 hours, and the duration of action is from 6 to 12 hours. Therefore, this drug should be taken 2 or 3 times a day.

Early investigators concluded that chlorpropamide was not metabolized in humans but rather was simply bound to serum proteins and excreted in the urine. This metabolic fate would account for its long half-life of about 36 hours and its prolonged duration of action of up to 60 hours. However, in more recent experiments, most of the amount of the drug administered was recovered in the form of urinary metabolites (7). Again, wide variability was noted. Although the discrepancies concerning the metabolic fate of chlorpropamide have not been resolved, from a clinical viewpoint the prolonged duration of action allows administration of the drug only once a day. Because of its long half-life, however, steady-state levels are not reached for 7 to 10 days.

Acetohexamide is degraded by the liver and kidneys. Its metabolites, however, have hypoglycemic activity, and one of them, hydroxyhexamide, is 2.5 times as potent as the parent compound. The metabolites are excreted by the kidneys. The fact that hydroxyhexamide is actively secreted by the renal tubules probably accounts for its uricosuric effect, mediated via inhibition of tubular reabsorption of uric acid. (In type 2 diabetics with hyperuricemia, an additional benefit of acetohexamide is a mild decrease in serum concentrations of uric acid [8].) Therefore, although the half-life of acetohexamide is 1 to 2 hours, its duration of action ranges from 12 to 24 hours mainly because of the activity of hydrohexamide, whose half-life is 4 to 5 hours.

Tolazamide is metabolized to six major by-products, three of which have some hypoglycemic activity. However, the effect of the metabolites is weaker than that of the parent compound. The degradative products are excreted by the kidney. The serum half-life of tolazamide and its active metabolites is about 7 hours. The duration of action ranges from 12 to 24 hours and the drug can usually be given once daily.

Adverse Effects

Sulfonylurea agents have been taken by millions of diabetics for a number of years and are well tolerated by most patients. The incidence of adverse effects is approximately 5%; use of the drugs must be discontinued in only 2%. Many years of experience with these drugs has fostered the clinical impression that tolbutamide may have slightly fewer adverse effects than the other three first-generation agents. Hypoglycemia, although considered to be an adverse effect, is actually an extension of the pharmacologic effect of the sulfonylurea agents.

The most common adverse effects of the sulvonylurea agents are gastrointestinal and cutaneous. The gastrointestinal effects are dose related and may disappear when the dose is reduced. Often these reactions will abate within several weeks even if the dose is not reduced. The gastrointestinal symptoms include anorexia, heartburn, nausea with occasional vomiting, feelings of abdominal fullness, and flatulence. The common adverse cutaneous effects are morbilliform, maculopapular, or urticarial rashes, which are often characterized by erythema and pruritus. There may be some cross-reactivity among the sulfonylurea agents.

A disulfiram-like reaction can be caused by sulfonylurea agents. Disulfiram (Antabuse) is a drug used in the treatment of alcoholism. After administration of disulfiram, ingestion of alcohol will cause some or all of the following reactions within 5 to 10 minutes: feelings of warmth, flushing, headache, nausea, vomiting, sweating, and thirst. More severe reactions occur occasionally, including respiratory difficulty, chest pain, hypotension, orthostatic syncope, confusion, and vertigo. Reactions can last from 30 minutes to several hours. Usually, only relatively mild symptoms develop in the disulfiram-like reactions precipitated by sulfonylurea agents. The prevalence of these reactions is unclear; various reports have cited prevalences from less than 1% to 33% among patients taking chlorpropamide. This discrepancy is obviously related to the amount of alcohol consumed by patients and the perseverance of the physician in questioning patients. Disulfiram-like reactions have most often been reported to occur with chlorpropamide therapy.

The other adverse effects of the sulfonylurea agents are uncommon ($< 1\%$) or rare (isolated case reports). Other skin reactions include photosensitivity, erythema multiforme, and exfoliative dermatitis. Adverse hematologic effects may include leukopenia, agranulocytosis, thrombocytopenia, hemolytic or aplastic anemia, and pancytopenia. Intrahepatic cholestatic jaundice has been reported; this condition can be reversed by discontinuation of the drugs. Fevers, eosinophilia, nonspecific proctocolitis, hepatic porphyria, and porphyria cutanea tarda have also been reported. Sulfonylurea agents may decrease the thyroidal uptake of radioactive iodine to some extent, but they have not been shown to cause goiters or hypothyroidism.

Chlorpropamide and tolbutamide may cause inappropriate antidiuretic hormone secretion. This problem has been reported most often with chlorpropamide therapy (9). The drugs cause this condition not only by stimulating the release of the hormone by the hypothalamus, but also by potentiating its inhibitory effect on free water excretion by the distal renal tubule. Therefore, serum sodium concentrations fall to abnormally low levels, and patients present with headache and lethargy that may progress to stupor, coma, and seizures. Elderly patients are much more susceptible to this effect, especially if they are also taking a diuretic. Tolazamide and acetohexamide do not cause inappropriate antidiuretic hormone secretion. Both of these drugs appear to have a mild diuretic effect.

A possible deleterious effect of the sulfonylurea agents on the cardiovascular system will be considered in much greater detail later in this chapter.

Drug Interactions

Other drugs can affect the hypoglycemic action of sulfonylurea agents in two general ways. First, drugs that either impair glucose tolerance (chapter 1) or cause hypoglycemia (chapter 10) would be expected to influence the effect of sulfonylurea agents in diabetic patients. This interaction would be *indirect,* since the interfering drugs would act by the same mechanisms as in nondiabetic subjects. Potassium-losing diuretics, glucocorticoids, estrogen compounds, and diphenylhydantoin (Dilantin) can impair the action of sulfonylurea agents. Conversely, salicylates, propranolol, monoamine oxidase inhibitors, oxytetracycline and ethanol (although not a prescribed drug) can potentiate the hypoglycemic effect of sulfonylurea agents.

Second, drugs may have a *direct* effect on the action of the sulfonylurea agents. That is, an interaction occurs in which the interfering drug affects the absorption, distribution, metabolism, or excretion of the sulfonylurea agents themselves. For instance, phenylbutazone enhances the hypoglycemic effect of acetohexamide by interfering with the renal excretion of hydroxyhexamide, its major degradative product, which is more potent than the parent compound. A moderate number of drugs displace the sulfonylurea agents from their protein binding sites, interfere with the enzymes responsible for their degradation, and/or alter their half-lives in the circulation (10). However, some of these effects are contradictory; e.g., although displacement of sulfonylurea agents from protein binding sites should decrease their half-lives, a number of drugs have been found to displace these agents and to increase their half-lives. Furthermore, most of these interfering drugs have not been shown to have a clinical effect on the action of the oral hypoglycemic agents. Therefore, only the relatively few drugs that have actually caused hypoglycemia by potentiating the effects of the sulfonylurea agents will be considered here.

Most instances of hypoglycemia caused by the drugs listed in Table 5-2 occurred in patients taking tolbutamide or chlorpropamide. This result probably reflects the much longer period of clinical experience with these two sulfonylurea agents than with acetohexamide and tolazamide. Since the metabolism and excretion of all four agents are generally similar, it seems prudent to consider a patient taking any sulfonylurea agent to be at increased risk when a drug listed in Table 5-2 is added to his or her regimen. In addition to the sulfonamides listed, sulfamethoxazole (Gantanol, Bactrim, Septra) prolongs the half-life of tolbutamide; thus, patients who are taking sulfamethoxazole plus a sulfonylurea agent should be monitored closely. Many of the drugs listed in Table 5-2 are likely to be used frequently in a diabetic population. Sulfonamides are excellent first-line antibiotics for the treatment of uncomplicated infections of the lower urinary tract. Although chloramphenicol is not widely prescribed, it is excellent for treatment of certain opportunistic infections that are more prone to occur in diabetics (e.g., infections with *Bacteroides*). Bishydroxycoumarin is used to treat certain forms of vascular disease—e.g., transient ischemic attacks, which are certainly more common in diabetics. Clofibrate is often used for the treatment of certain types of hyperlipidemia that are resistant to dietary therapy; therefore, this drug is likely to be prescribed for diabetics.

The University Group Diabetes Program Study

The results of a study by the University Group Diabetes Program (UGDP) (11, 12) seemed to show that mortality from cardiovascular causes was significantly

Table 5-2. Drugs that Potentiate the Hypoglycemic Effects of the Sulfonylurea Agents

Generic Name	Trade Name(s)
Sulfonamides	
Sulfisoxazole	Gantrisin, Sodiozole, Sosol, Unisulf
Sulfaphenazole	Orisul, Sulfabid
Sulfadiazine[a]	Coco-Diazine, Microsulfon
Sulfamethizole[a]	Thiosulfil, Utrasul, Microsul, Azotrex
Sulfadimethoxine	Madribon
Sulfadimidine	
Sulfafurazole	
Chloramphenicol	Chloromycetin
Bishydroxycoumarin	Dicumarol
Phenylbutazone	Butazolidin
Oxyphenbutazone	Tandearil
Clofibrate	Atromid-S

[a]Combination of these two sulfonamides is marketed as Suladyne.

higher among patients treated with tolbutamide than among their counterparts given a placebo. This finding obviously has important implications for decisions about therapy for type 2 diabetics. Since the UGDP results were published, however, a controversy in the scientific community has become so heated as to engender (unsuccessful) attempts through legal action to gain access to the original raw data. Therefore, before the clinical use of the sulfonylurea agents is considered, it is necessary to discuss in some detail the UGDP study, its possible flaws, and independent data that may bear on it.

Design of the Study

The UGDP study was initiated in 1959. Its purpose was to examine the effects of control of glucose levels in ketosis-resistant diabetics on the complications of diabetes and to assess the natural history of the diabetic syndrome. Recruitment of patients began in 1961 and was completed 5 years later. To be eligible for the study, a patient had to meet the following criteria: (a) The diagnosis of diabetes had to have been made within 1 year of selection. (b) The patient had to tolerate a month of dietary treatment alone. (c) The patient had to have an anticipated survival time of at least 5 years. The diagnosis of diabetes was confirmed by a 3-hour oral glucose tolerance test, whose results were defined as abnormal if the sum of the fasting and postchallenge whole-blood glucose concentrations exceeded 500 mg/100 ml. Patients who met these criteria and agreed to participate were recruited from 12 university-affiliated clinics (some of which were cardiology clinics!).

The patients were randomized into one of four treatment groups: tolbutamide (1.0 g before breakfast and 0.5 g before supper); lactose placebo (2 pills before breakfast and 1 pill before supper); insulin variable, abbreviated IVAR (intermediate-acting insulin given in a conventional manner in order to lower glucose concentrations to as near normal as possible); and insulin standard, abbreviated ISTD (10 to 16 U of intermediate-acting insulin per day, depending on the patient's body size). ISTD was included as a control in order to ascertain whether insulin had any effects independent of its glucose-lowering capabilities. This low dose of insulin should have had a minimal hypoglycemic effect in these patients, many of whom were obese. There were a few more than 200 patients in each group. All patients were given a baseline examination and monitored every 4 months.

The use of tolbutamide was discontinued in the UGDP study in October 1969, and an announcement to that effect appeared in the *Wall Street Journal* in March 1970. The data upon which this decision was based were published 9 months later (11, 12). The UGDP investigators concluded that tolbutamide therapy was associated with a significant increase in mortality from cardiovascular causes over that among patients given placebo (Table 5-3). The overall mortality figures of the placebo and tolbutamide groups did not differ, however. Many renowned scientists argued that the flaws of the UGDP study invalidated this conclusion.

Defects in the Study

In my view, four major defects in the design, execution, and analysis of the UGDP study support the position of its detractors.

Discrepancies in Baseline Cardiovascular Risk Factors. The existence of similar baseline cardiovascular risk factors in the placebo and tolbutamide groups is critical to the validity of the conclusion about tolbutamide. Although the patients were randomized into the four groups, the tolbutamide-treated patients may very well have been at greater risk of cardiovascular catastrophes than their counterparts receiving the placebo. Eight of the nine risk factors listed in Table 5-4 were found in a higher percentage of the tolbutamide group than of the placebo group. The percentage of patients with cholesterol concentrations above 300 mg/100 ml (a rather important cardiovascular risk factor) was significantly higher in the tolbutamide group than in the placebo group (12). As might be expected, both the total number of risk factors and the percentage of subjects who had more than two risk factors were also significantly higher in the tolbutamide group (13). Although statistical approaches can be used to isolate and evaluate the effect of each risk factor separately, the synergistic effect of multiple risk factors in a single patient cannot be assessed. Thus, patients receiving tolbutamide in the UGDP study were probably at greater risk of death from cardiovascular causes before they were given tolbutamide than were those destined to receive the placebo. This unfortunate difference in baseline characteristics may have been due to a low prevalence of risk factors in the placebo group. In fact, the percentage of patients with 7 of the 9 risk factors listed in Table 5-4 was lowest in the placebo group. This observation may help to explain the spuriously low mortality from cardiovascular causes noted during the first part of the UGDP study in this group (a point that will be discussed later).

Two other observations that have not been widely publicized support the argument that patients in the tolbutamide group were at greater risk of subsequent cardiovascular events than those in the placebo group. In 1966, the UGDP investigators submitted a 6-year progress report to the National Institute of Arthritis and Metabolic Diseases. This report contained information concerning the initial criteria used to diagnose electrocardiogram (ECG) abnormalities and the method used to assess the cardiac status of each patient by assignment of a cardiac score (13). Neither the ECG criteria nor the data on cardiac scores were included in the published results of the study (11, 12). On the basis of these initially agreed upon (but later discarded) criteria, 24% of the tolbutamide group,

Table 5-3. Cause of Death in UGDP Study Patients[a]

	Number (%) Dead, by Treatment Group				
Cause of Death	PLBO (n = 205)	TOLB (n = 204)	ISTD (n = 210)	IVAR (n = 204)	
Cardiovascular					
Myocardial infarction	0	10	3	2	
Sudden death	4	4	4	5	
Other heart disease	1	5	1	2	
Extracardiac vascular disease	5	7	5	3	
All cardiovascular causes	10 (4.9)	26 (12.7)	13 (6.2)	12 (5.9)	
Noncardiovascular					
Cancer	7	2	4	2	
Cause other than above	3	2	2	3	
Unknown cause	1	0	1	1	
All causes	21 (10.2)	30 (14.7)	20 (9.5)	18 (8.8)	

Abbreviations: PLBO, lactose placebo, TOLB, tolbutamide; ISTD, insulin standard; IVAR, insulin variable.

[a]Reprinted with permission from University Group Diabetes Program: A study of the effects of hypoglycemic agents on vascular complications in patients with adult-onset diabetes. II. Mortality results. Diabetes 19(Suppl 2):789–830, 1970.

Table 5-4. Percentage of Patients with Selected Baseline Cardiovascular Risk Factors in the Placebo and Tolbutamide Groups of the UGDP Study[a]

Risk Factor	Percentage of Indicated Group	
	PLBO	TOLB
Age (>55 yrs)	41.5	48.0
Hypertension	36.8	30.2
Digitalis use	4.5	7.6
Angina pectoris	5.0	7.0
Abnormal ECG	3.0	4.0
Cholesterol, $\geqslant$ 300 mg/100 ml	8.6	15.1
FBS, $\geqslant$ 110 mg/100 ml	63.5	72.1
Percentage of IBW, $\geqslant$ 125	52.7	58.8
Arterial calcifications[b]	14.3	19.7

Abbreviations: PLBO, lactose placebo; TOLB, tolbutamide; ECG, electrocardiogram; FBS, fasting whole-blood glucose concentration; IBW, ideal body weight.

[a]Adapted with permission from University Group Diabetes Program: A study of the effects of hypoglycemia agents on vascular complications in patients with adult-onset diabetes. II. Mortality results. Diabetes 19(Suppl 2):789–830, 1970.

[b]Noted on x-ray of right thigh.

but only 15.2% of the placebo group, had one or more major ECG abnormalities. This difference, like that in cholesterol levels, was statistically significant.

Although the cardiac score had some limitations, it was the only method available to the UGDP investigators for reporting the severity of cardiovascular impairment (13). Patients were assigned cardiac scores based on the baseline presence of ECG abnormalities, angina pectoris, and laboratory evidence suggestive of a previous myocardial infarction. If none of these factors was present, the cardiac score was 0. Electrocardiographic abnormalities, consisting of changes in ST and T waves, intraventricular conduction defects, and/or significant arrhythmias, rated 1 point. Angina pectoris was assigned 1 point. Either the presence of large Q waves on the ECG or a history of elevated levels of cardiac enzymes (both findings that would presumably document a previous myocardial infarction) rated 1 point.

Apparently, the cardiac score served as an excellent predictor of a fatal cardiovascular event, since in 1969 only 6.2% of the 661 patients with a baseline cardiac score of 0 had died from cardiovascular causes, as compared with 25.7% of the 148 patients with cardiac scores greater than 0. The mean baseline cardiac score was 56% higher in the tolbutamide group than in the placebo group (0.42 versus 0.27). In addition, the percentage of patients with a cardiac score greater than 0 was also higher in those receiving the active drug (28% versus 17%). Both of these differences between the two groups were statistically significant. Therefore, the original ECG findings and the baseline cardiac scores (neither of which were formally published) further suggest that the placebo and tolbutamide groups were not at equal risk of subsequent cardiovascular death.

Faulty Analysis of Data. The second drawback to the UGDP study was the manner in which data for patients who dropped out of the study or whose medication was changed were handled statistically. The usual procedure in therapeutic trials is to exclude data for such patients from statistical analysis and not to ascribe subsequent events to the patients' original treatment (13). The UGDP investigators chose to ascribe all subsequent events to the original treatment, regardless of whether the patient had discontinued the treatment or been switched to another form of therapy. Approximately 25% of patients in both the tolbutamide group and the placebo group had either dropped out (i.e., were unavailable for follow-up for $\geqslant 1$ year) or changed medications by the time the use of tolbutamide was discontinued in 1969 (14). Thus, the deaths of some patients were attributed to a form of treatment to which they had not been exposed for a number of years before their demise.

Spurious Cardiovascular Mortality. The third factor that may invalidate the conclusions of the UGDP study regarding tolbutamide is the spuriously low cardiovascular death rate reported for the placebo group during the first part of the study. If this low rate had been the result of random fluctuations, the rate of death from cardiovascular causes should have increased among the placebo group during the subsequent period. In fact, it did. After the use of tolbutamide was discontinued in 1969, the patients who had received this agent, as well as the subjects in the remaining three groups, continued to be monitored. The percentage of patients in each group who died from cardiovascular causes is summarized in Table 5-5. The early phase of the study is defined as the period between the patient's entry and December 1969. (Tolbutamide was discontinued in October 1969.) The late phase covered the years 1970 through 1974. The number of subjects at risk during the late phase of the study represents the number at risk during the early phase minus the number who died (from noncardiovascular as well as cardiovascular causes) before 1970. The percentage of cardiovascular deaths in the placebo group more than doubled during the late phase, while it remained constant in the two groups receiving insulin. The similarity in the overall rates of cardiovascular death by the end of 1974 for the placebo, ISTD, and IVAR groups supports the theory that the cardiovascular death rate among placebo-treated patients prior to 1970 was spuriously low because of random fluctuations.

Further evidence for an unusually low cardiovascular death rate in the placebo group emerges when the deaths rates among men and women are examined separately. It is recognized that the lower risk of cardiovascular disease in the general female population disappears in the female diabetic population; the

Table 5-5. Cardiovascular Deaths in the Early (before 1970) and Late (1970–1974) Phases of the UGDP Study[a]

Group	Number Dead/Number at Risk (% dead)		
	Early Phase	Late Phase	Total
PLBO	10/205 (4.9)	19/182 (10.4)	29/205 (14.1)
TOLB[b]	26/204 (12.7)		
ISTD	13/210 (6.2)	14/190 (7.4)	27/210 (12.9)
IVAR	15/204 (7.4)	14/183 (7.7)	29/204 (14.2)

Abbreviations: PLBO, lactose placebo; TOLB, tolbutamide; ISTD, insulin standard; IVAR, insulin variable.

[a]Adapted with permission from Kilo C, Miller JP, Williamson JR: The Achilles heel of the University Group Diabetes Program. JAMA 243:450–457, 1980. Copyright © 1980, the American Medical Association.

[b]Tolbutamide was not used in the late phase of the study.

risk is approximately equal in diabetic men and diabetic women (15). However, among women receiving a placebo, the percentage of cardiovascular deaths was less than 20% of that among their male counterparts (Table 5-6). The male-to-female ratio of cardiovascular deaths was 5.3, a value that contrasts markedly with those for the other three groups (all <2.0). Thus, the spuriously low cardiovascular death rate during the early part of the UGDP study seems to have been restricted to women receiving the placebo. Since approximately 70% of the UGDP patients were women, this unexpected finding would obviously bear on a comparison of the cardiovascular death rates for the tolbutamide and placebo groups.

Impact of Diabetic Control on Cardiovascular Mortality. Our fourth major reservation about the conclusions of the UGDP study concerns the impact of diabetic control on possible tolbutamide-induced cardiovascular mortality. If tolbutamide did indeed cause an increase in the rate of cardiovascular deaths, this effect seemed to be restricted to patients whose glucose levels remained out of control despite treatment with this agent (Table 5-7). The percentage of cardiovascular deaths was much higher in patients who were receiving tolbutamide and whose fasting whole-blood glucose concentrations remained higher than 200 mg/100 ml than in any other group. This apparent deleterious effect of tolbutamide in uncontrolled diabetics remains to be confirmed. However, the clinical applicability of this result may not be broad, since sound medical practice would dictate a change in therapy for diabetic patients with persistent fasting hyperglycemia of this magnitude.

Thus, serious questions can be raised about the validity of the conclusion by the UGDP investigators that tolbutamide therapy is associated with a significant increase in mortality from cardiovascular causes. These and related arguments

Table 5-6. Cardiovascular Deaths in the Early Phase (before 1970) of the UGDP Study, by Sex of Patient[a]

	Number Dead/Number at Risk (% dead)		Ratio of Men
Group	Men	Women	to Women
PLBO	7/63 (11.1)	3/142 (2.1)	5.3
TOLB	11/63 (17.5)	15/141 (10.6)	1.6
ISTD	5/57 (8.8)	8/153 (5.2)	1.2
IVAR	4/46 (8.7)	11/158 (7.0)	1.7

Abbreviations: PLBO, lactose placebo; TOLB, tolbutamide; ISTD, insulin standard; IVAR, insulin variable.

[a]Adapted with permission from Kilo C, Miller JP, Williamson JR: The Achilles heel of the University Group Diabetes Program. JAMA 243:450–457, 1980. Copyright © 1980, the American Medical Association.

Table 5-7. Cardiovascular Deaths Related to Fasting Whole-Blood Glucose Concentrations in UGDP Study Patients[a]

	Number Dead/Number at Risk (% dead) with Indicated FBS[b]	
Group	<200 mg/100 ml	>200 mg/100 ml
PLBO	5/98 (5.1)	2/53 (3.8)
TOLB	11/117 (9.4)	11/44 (25.0)
ISTD	12/111 (10.8)	5/42 (11.9)
IVAR	10/140 (7.1)	2/23 (8.7)

Abbreviations: PLBO, lactose placebo; TOLB, tolbutamide; ISTD, insulin standard; IVAR, insulin variable; FBS, fasting whole-blood glucose concentrations.

[a]Adapted with permission from Kilo C, Miller JP, Williamson JR: The Achilles heel of the University Group Diabetes Program. JAMA 243:450–457, 1980. Copyright © 1980, the American Medical Association.

[b]Patients were categorized according to the mean of the last 3 fasting whole-blood glucose concentrations during the early phase of the study or the last value before death.

have caused the American Diabetes Association, which initially supported the UGDP study, to reassess its position and withdraw its endorsement (16).

Other Prospective Studies of Tolbutamide

Several other prospective studies of tolbutamide did not demonstrate higher rates of cardiovascular death. In one study, a diagnostic survey for diabetes mellitus was done in 1962 among the population of Bedford, England. Blood samples were taken 2 hours after ingestion of a 50-g glucose load, and three groups of subjects were identified: those with whole-blood glucose concentrations of less than 120 mg/100 ml, those with values exceeding 200 mg/100 ml, and those with intermediate levels (120 to 199 mg/100 ml). The patients in the first group were considered normal, those in the second group were referred to their physicians with a diagnosis of diabetes, and those in the third group were termed "borderline diabetics" and enrolled in a prospective, double-blind study (17). The 248 subjects recruited for the study were given either placebo tablets or 0.5 g of tolbutamide twice a day. They were seen at intervals of approximately 6 months. Mortality among these subjects during an 8-year follow-up period is depicted in Figure 5-7. Initially, tolbutamide seemed to afford some protection against death from vascular causes. However, as the study progressed, the difference between the two groups diminished. There was certainly no hint of increased mortality from cardiovascular causes in the tolbutamide group.

The second prospective study included patients who had recently had a documented myocardial infarction (18). Subjects with overt diabetes and those taking medications known to interfere with glucose tolerance were excluded. The remaining 158 patients were randomized into two groups; one received placebo tablets ($n = 83$) and the other received 0.5 g of tolbutamide twice a day ($n = 95$). The survival rate among these patients during a 5-year period is depicted in Figure 5-8. All deaths were of probable cardiac origin. Although treatment with tolbutamide significantly increased the rate of survival during

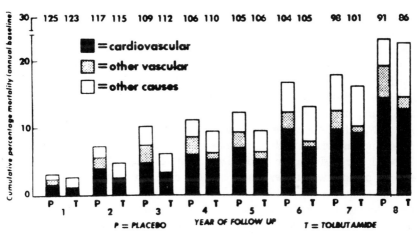

Figure 5-7. Deaths (expressed as cumulative percentages) among subjects in the Bedford study, who were monitored for up to 8 years. The number of patients at risk in each group each year is indicated at the top of the graph. (Adapted from Keen H, Jarrett RJ, Fuller JH: Tolbutamide and arterial disease in borderline diabetics. In *Proceedings of the Ninth Congress of the International Diabetes Federation.* Edited by Malaisse WJ, Pirart J. Excerpta Medica, Amsterdam, 1974, pp 588-602.)

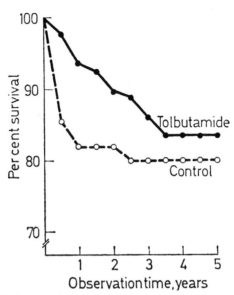

Figure 5-8. Cumulative survival rates among patients recovering from a myocardial infarction and receiving either placebo tablets or tolbutamide. (Reprinted with permission from Paasikivi J, Wahlberg F: Preventive tolbutamide treatment and arterial disease in mild hyperglycaemia. Diabetologia 7:323-327, 1971.)

the first 2 years, this protection disappeared over a longer follow-up period. Tolbutamide therapy was certainly not associated with increased mortality from cardiovascular causes.

Subjects in the third prospective study were recruited from a multiphasic screening program (19). Those who were suspected of having diabetes were given an oral glucose tolerance test. Patients with abnormal results were given either placebo ($n = 85$) or 0.5 g of tolbutamide twice a day ($n = 174$). During the next 8 years, only 4 persons died—1 with a myocardial infarction in the placebo group and 3 of carcinoma in the tolbutamide group. Thus, once again, tolbutamide was not associated with an increase in mortality from cardiovascular causes.

Several points should be emphasized. First, although the design of each of the three prospective studies was somewhat different from that of the UGDP study, these studies did follow a total of 392 subjects treated with tolbutamide (almost double the number in the UGDP study) for similar periods. Second, in none of the studies (including the UGDP study) was the incidence of nonfatal cardiovascular events increased in patients taking tolbutamide. This fact speaks against a generalized toxic effect of tolbutamide on the vasculature since, if such an effect were exerted, more morbidity (in addition to higher mortality) would be expected. If the conclusions of the UGDP study are valid at all, tolbutamide must affect a patient's ability to survive such an event instead of causing conditions that are more likely to precipitate the event. Third, the possibility that tolbutamide does indeed increase mortality from cardiovascular causes in poorly controlled diabetics could not be tested in the three prospective studies just described since most of the patients were only mildly diabetic (or, as defined in chapter 1, had impaired glucose tolerance). Some of the subjects in the post-myocardial infarction study even had normal results in an intravenous glucose tolerance test (18).

Finally, the results of the well-known Framingham study also bear on this question. Over 5,000 men and women living in Framingham, Massachusetts, were given cardiovascular examinations every 2 years. Of this cohort, 239 had diabetes when initially examined. After 16 years, mortality from cardiovascular causes was highest among patients given insulin, intermediate among those treated by means of diet alone, and lowest among those receiving oral hypoglycemic agents; most of the last group were taking tolbutamide (15). Among patients with the most severe diabetes, who would be likely to receive insulin, high cardiovascular mortality would be expected. The metabolic abnormality in patients taking oral hypoglycemic agents, however, would presumably be greater than in those using dietary therapy alone. Thus, the lower cardiovascular mortality in the group being treated with oral hypoglycemic agents was somewhat unexpected and certainly argues against an association between tolbutamide administration and increased cardiovascular mortality.

In light of all these data, I do not hesitate to prescribe sulfonylurea agents to type 2 diabetics under the appropriate conditions. This conclusion is based on what I perceive to be serious flaws in the UGDP study and the lack of supporting data in four other studies. One of the ironies of the UGDP study is that the original question of whether improved diabetic control has a beneficial effect on chronic complications cannot be answered by the data that were obtained, since the degree of control attained in the placebo group was similar to that attained in the tolbutamide group (12). Administration of the tolbutamide in a fixed dose may have precluded achievement of better control.

Clinical Use of the Sulfonylurea Agents

General Guidelines

General guidelines for use of the sulfonylurea agents are shown in Figure 5-9. The goal of therapy is to maintain the postprandial glucose concentrations (PPG) measured 1 to 2 hours after the patient's usual meal below 200 mg/100 ml. First, I will give a general description of how this goal may be realized. Then I will make specific recommendations about which drug and what dosage should be used under various circumstances.

As discussed in chapter 2, the use of oral hypoglycemic agents is contraindicated in ketosis-prone (type 1) diabetics. Furthermore, these agents should not be used as the initial form of treatment for ketosis-resistant diabetics except

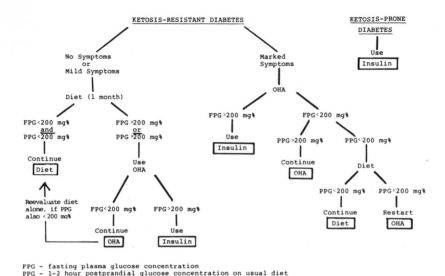

FPG – fasting plasma glucose concentration
PPG – 1-2 hour postprandial glucose concentration on usual diet
OHA – oral hypoglycemic agents

Figure 5-9. General guidelines for use of the sulfonylurea agents.

for those who are symptomatic, with polydipsia, polyuria, and weight loss. In the latter patients, oral hypoglycemic agents can be utilized without a previous trial of dietary therapy. However, if a sulfonylurea agent proves to be effective, the dose should then be gradually decreased in order to determine whether control can be maintained by means of diet alone. As discussed in chapter 4, once control improves, patients may become more sensitive to insulin (endogenous in this instance) and therefore may be able to maintain control without the aid of a drug. This is often the case in obese symptomatic patients who lose weight while following an appropriate diet and taking an oral hypoglycemic agent. However, as the dose of drug is decreased, a level is often reached at which the 1- to 2-hour PPG concentration cannot be kept below 200 mg/100 ml. At this point, the dose should be increased again until this degree of control can be consistently maintained. Thus, patients will not be exposed unnecessarily to the risk of adverse effects of these drugs.

Most newly diagnosed, type 2 diabetics are relatively asymptomatic and should be treated by means of diet alone for at least a month. A follow-up visit 2 weeks after institution of the diet is useful in monitoring patients' understanding of the diet, their compliance with it, and their metabolic response to it. The diet should be continued for another 2 weeks after the follow-up visit. If at this time the fasting plasma glucose (FPG) concentration remains above 200 mg/100 ml, an oral hypoglycemic agent should be considered. Since lean ketosis-resistant patients (those within 10% of their ideal body weight) are less likely than obese patients to respond to dietary therapy alone, I routinely add a sulfonylurea agent to their regimen at this point. If the FPG concentration exceeds 300 mg/100 ml in obese patients, we also initiate drug therapy. However, since dietary therapy is most effective in the latter group, I often continue to use it exclusively for another month if the FPG concentration has shown a definite response and is between 200 and 300 mg/100 ml. I may also extend dietary therapy for another month in a noncompliant obese diabetic, regardless of the FPG level. However, after an 8-week trial of dietary therapy, treatment with sulfonylurea agents is started in most patients if the FPG level remains above 200 mg/100 ml. A few individuals who are initially noncompliant but begin to respond to dietary therapy during the second month are allowed to continue without drugs for a third month in order to determine whether their FPG levels will fall below 200 mg/100 ml. However, this situation is somewhat unusual since, with most obese patients, dietary compliance is maximal at first and tapers off subsequently.

Eventually, all ketosis-resistant patients whose FPG concentrations remain above 200 mg/100 ml with dietary therapy alone should be given sulfonylurea agents. The dose of the drug should be increased until either the FPG level drops below 200 mg/100 ml or the maximal dose is being given. If the FPG level remains above 200 mg/100 ml despite administration of the maximal dose of the two more potent sulfonylurea agents (tolazamide or chlorpropamide), the patient should be switched to insulin (see chapter 4).

If, on the other hand, the FPG decreases to less than 200 mg/100 ml, the 1- to 2-hour PPG concentration is then monitored. If that value remains above 200 mg/100 ml, the dose of the drug is increased until either the PPG level falls below 200 mg/100 ml or the maximal dose is being given. If the PPG value remains above 200 mg/100 ml despite administration of the maximal dose of the most potent sulfonylurea agent, I continue to encourage the patient concerning dietary therapy but do not prescribe insulin. As long as the FPG value remains at less than 200 mg/100 ml, the patient continues to take the maximal dose of the most potent sulfonylurea agent. Although I do believe in tight diabetic control (see chapter 2), insulin therapy is no panacea and in many cases does not lead to better control than that already attained (especially in obese patients).

Let us now return to the newly diagnosed, ketosis-resistant, relatively asymptomatic diabetic in whom the FPG concentration either falls below 200 mg/100 ml in response to dietary therapy or was never elevated to that level. The 1- to 2-hour PPG concentration determines the next step in therapy for such a patient. Most patients whose PPG level exceeds 200 mg/100 ml will be given a sulfonylurea agent. Certainly lean individuals and obese patients who have stopped losing weight will be treated in this manner. Obese patients who are continuing to lose weight and whose PPG values are falling but remain above 200 mg/100 ml can be monitored without drugs. However, if PPG concentrations stabilize above 200 mg/100 ml, treatment with a sulfonylurea agent should be started. The dose is increased until either the PPG concentration is maintained consistently below 200 mg/100 ml or the maximal dose of the most potent agent is being given, at which point no further therapeutic adjustments are made.

If the 1- to 2-hour PPG concentration can be consistently kept below 200 mg/100 ml by oral hypoglycemic agents, the physician should determine at least once during a patient's course whether these drugs are really necessary. Although this question is especially pertinent in the case of obese patients who have managed to lose weight gradually over an extended period, it should be answered for all patients with this degree of diabetic control. The dose of the sulfonylurea agent is decreased slowly until the PPG concentration exceeds 200 mg/100 ml, at which point a return to higher doses is indicated. Some patients, however, may be able to maintain their level of control without oral hypoglycemic agents. Discontinuation of drug therapy is preferred, of course, since unnecessary exposure to the risk of adverse effects of these drugs is thereby avoided. If continued testing reveals an increase of in 1- to 2-hour PPG levels to values that once again exceed 200 mg/100 ml, treatment with a sulfonylurea agent should be recommenced. It is not uncommon for the severity of the metabolic abnormality in diabetics to fluctuate over time (20).

Selecting a Regimen

The preparations of sulfonylurea agents currently available in the United States are listed in Table 5-8. Their pharmacology was discussed previously. The choice of agent is based on differences in cost, efficacy, and adverse effects. Obviously, the potency per milligram is clinically irrevelant. At present, the differences in the cost of these agents is generally not a determining factor. The relative effectiveness of the preparations can be determined in two ways. First, the proportion of newly diagnosed, ketosis-resistant diabetics who are controlled by each drug can be compared. (Theoretically, these patients should have failed to respond satisfactorily to dietary therapy alone.) The second and more rigorous method is to evaluate how many patients who fail to respond appropriately to maximal doses of one drug will respond to another one. Only tolbutamide and chlorpropamide, the first two sulfonylurea agents released, have been compared in this manner. By both criteria, chlorpropamide is clearly more effective than tolbutamide (21).

The later two oral hypoglycemic agents, acetohexamide and tolazamide, have not been evaluated by these criteria. Reports of their relative effectiveness are difficult to interpret because, in most cases, patients were not given maximal doses of one sulfonylurea agent before a second one was substituted. Furthermore, direct comparisons of the proportion of newly diagnosed, ketosis-resistant diabetics controlled by one of the two newer sulfonylurea agents with the proportion controlled by one of the two older agents have been limited to only a handful of patients. Finally, I could find no studies that assessed whether acetohexamide or tolazamide can be used successfully in patients who fail to respond to maximal doses of another sulfonylurea agent. My impression is that chlorpropamide, tolazamide, and acetohexamide are all more effective clinically than tolbutamide and that patients who have failed to respond to acetohexamide

Table 5-8. Selected Properties of Sulfonylurea Agents

Generic Name	Trade Name	Tablet Size(s) (mg)	Usual Daily Dose Range (mg)	Maximal Dose (mg)	Duration of Action (hrs)
Tolbutamide	Orinase	250, 500	500–2,000 (divided)	3,000	6–12
Chlorpropamide	Diabinese	100, 250	100–500 (single)	750	36+
Acetohexamide	Dymelor	250, 500	250–1,500 (single or divided)	1,500	12–24
Tolazamide	Tolinase	100, 250, 500	100–750 (single or divided)	1,000	12–24

181

often do respond to chlorpropamide. Although tolazamide is reported to be as potent as chlorpropamide, data from appropriate studies (as just defined) to substantiate that assertion are not available.

The recommended initial doses of the sulfonylurea agents are listed in Table 5-9. A symptomatic patient is given maximal doses of tolazamide or chlorpropamide. Symptoms should improve discernibly within a week. If they do not, the drug should be discontinued and insulin started. If the symptoms have improved, the patient should be monitored for another 1 or 2 weeks. If symptoms of uncontrolled diabetes are still noted after this interval, the sulfonylurea agent should be abandoned and the patient switched to insulin. If the patient has been obese but loses a significant amount of weight in the future with a demonstrable increase in insulin sensitivity as evidenced by diminishing insulin requirements, therapy with an oral hypoglycemic agent should be reconsidered.

On the other hand, if the symptoms disappear entirely, maximal doses of the sulfonylurea agent are continued for another month even if the FPG remains above 200 mg/100 ml. If the FPG concentration is still above 200 mg/100 ml, at that time, insulin therapy should be instituted. A possible exception would be the obese patient who is losing weight but whose FPG level, although decreasing, still exceeds 200 mg/100 ml. As described earlier, one might delay the initiation of insulin therapy in this situation in anticipation of continued weight loss and increasing insulin sensitivity. However, if FPG concentrations stabilize above 200 mg/100 ml, insulin treatment should be begun. At the other end of the spectrum, if both the FPG and 1- to 2-hour PPG levels drop below 200 mg/100 ml, the dose of the oral hypoglycemic agent should gradually be reduced as discussed previously.

Table 5-9. Recommended Initial Doses of Sulfonylurea Agents for Ketosis-Resistant Patients with Diabetes Mellitus

| | Initial Dose (mg) for Indicated Group | | |
| | Asymptomatic Diet Failures[a] with Indicated FPG | | |
Agent	<200 mg/100 ml	>200 mg/100 ml	Symptomatic Patients
Acetohexamide	250	500	
Tolazamide	100	250	1,000
Chlorpropamide	100	250	750

Abbreviation: FPG, fasting plasma glucose concentrations.

[a]Relatively asymptomatic patients who should be treated with diet alone initially. See text for full discussion.

The initial dose of an oral hypoglycemic agent in the asymptomatic ketosis-resistant diabetic for whom dietary therapy has failed depends on the prevailing FPG concentration. If this value is below 200 mg/100 ml, the lowest-strength tablet of any of the three sulfonylurea agents listed in Table 5-9 is used. If the value exceeds 200 mg/100 ml, the next highest tablet strength is chosen. The patient should be monitored every 2 to 4 weeks while the initial dosage adjustments are being made.

The therapeutic goals are depicted in Figure 5-9 and have already been discussed. The dose of the sulfonylurea agent is gradually increased until either the goals are achieved or the maximal allowable dose is being given. Chlorpropamide is always given once a day because of its long half-life. Up to 1 g of acetohexamide is taken in the morning, with the final 500 mg taken in the evening. For tolazamide, doses of up to 500 mg are taken in the morning and any additional amounts necessary are given in the evening. If therapy with acetohexamide fails, a switch to maximal doses of chlorpropamide or tolazamide will improve diabetic control in a significant number of patients although this control may not be maintained. If the patient is more than 60 years of age, the drug substituted should be tolazamide, not chlorpropamide, for reasons that will be discussed shortly. As already mentioned, there are not reliable data on how many patients in whom chlorpropamide or tolazamide therapy has failed are helped by switching to whichever drug has not been used. I have had little relevant personal experience. However, substitution of maximal doses of one drug for maximal doses of the other seems to be a reasonable step to take before abandoning sulfonylurea agent therapy in patients whose FPG concentration remains above 200 mg/100 ml. Additionally, those whose 1- to 2-hour PPG level stabilizes above 200 mg/100 ml when the FPG levels are below this value should be given a trial of the other drug.

Tolbutamide is not shown in Table 5-9 and acetohexamide is not included for the treatment of symptomatic ketosis-resistant diabetics for the following reasons. I use tolbutamide primarily in the unusual situation in which a ketosis-resistant patient with renal insufficiency is a candidate for therapy with a sulfonylurea agent. The decision not to use tolbutamide more routinely is based on the following points: (a) The necessity for more tablets increases the cost to the patient. (b) The drug is routinely given in divided doses, a regimen that reduces compliance by the patient. (c) Tolbutamide is the least effective of the sulfonylurea agents. Acetohexamide is not recommended for symptomatic ketosis-resistant diabetics since the chance of successful treatment seems less than with tolazamide or chlorpropamide.

Chlorpropamide should not be the first drug given to patients over the age of 60 years. Although hypoglycemia may occur with any sulfonylurea agent, the problem may be more severe with chlorpropamide therapy in the elderly. Since the half-life of this drug is about 36 hours and its biologic effectiveness may last for up to 60 hours, patients who become hypoglycemic while taking it have to be admitted to the hospital and monitored carefully for at least several days. In addition, the symptoms of hypoglycemia in elderly patients may be difficult to reverse, and inordinate amounts of glucose are often necessary. Since elderly patients, who frequently have irregular eating habits, are more likely to experience sulfonylurea-induced hypoglycemia than their younger counterparts (22), control with a relatively short-acting sulfonylurea agent seems preferable if possible. Second, as discussed previously, chlorpropamide occasionally causes inappropriate antidiuretic hormone secretion. This syndrome is much more likely to occur in older patients and especially in those taking diuretics. Therefore, chlorpropamide is used in this age group only if satisfactory control (i.e., 1- to 2-hour PPG levels of less than 200 mg/100 ml) is not attained with maximal doses of tolazamide.

Ketosis-resistant diabetics with renal insufficiency present a special problem. Although none of the sulfonylurea agents is recommended for these patients, insulin therapy occasionally is not feasible. There are no comparative studies of sulfonylurea agents in these patients. However, on the basis of the metabolic characteristics of these drugs, the following approach seems reasonable. Tolbutamide is preferred since it is metabolized in the liver and its degradation products are not hypoglycemic. If tolbutamide proves ineffective, tolazamide should be tried next since its degradation products (which are excreted by the kidney) are only 40% as hypoglycemic as the parent compound. Acetohexamide would be my third choice; its breakdown product is 2.4 times as hypoglycemic as the drug itself. Chlorpropamide should be tried last because of its very long biologically effective half-life and its renal excretion. The lowest doses of the selected agent should be used initially and increased cautiously. I usually attempt to control glucose levels in these patients with oral hypoglycemic agents before using insulin therapy. Patients experiencing renal failure are often unusually sensitive to insulin, presumably because the degradation of insulin by the kidney is impaired and its half-life is prolonged. Therefore, hypoglycemia is always a potential problem for these patients, regardless of the therapeutic approach. In addition, chronic renal failure itself is sometimes associated with fasting hypoglycemia (see chapter 10).

Discussions of the sulfonylurea agents usually include comments on the percentage of patients who experience primary and secondary failure with this form of therapy and refer (somewhat snidely) to the number of patients who did just as well when drug treatment was discontinued. The percentage of primary failure (i.e., patients who never respond satisfactorily to the drug) ranges from 5% to 40%, and secondary failure (i.e., patients who initially respond but later become refractory) ranges from 3% to 30%. Many of these data were generated before the proper criteria for selection of appropriate patients to receive sulfonylurea agents were established. Therefore, they have little bearing on the decision about whether to use these drugs in an individual patient. If the criteria outlined in Figure 5-9 for selection candidates for treatment with oral hypoglycemic agents are utilized, patients who will certainly be unresponsive (i.e., ketosis-prone patients) and those whose diabetes can be controlled by dietary therapy alone will be eliminated from consideration. Thus, the risk of primary failure will be minimized, and unnecessary exposure to the sulfonylurea agents will be avoided. Even though there seems to be a persistent incidence of secondary failure, it does not, in my view, invalidate the use of the sulfonylurea agents. For whatever period type 2 diabetics can be controlled satisfactorily with sulfonylurea agents, they will be able to avoid the inconvenience, pain, and relative inflexibility of meal and activity patterns required by insulin therapy. If the guidelines in Figure 5-9 are followed, patients in whom these drugs fail will have glucose levels that are out of control for only a short period before insulin is started.

One final comment can be made about Figure 5-9. The cutoff value of 200 mg/100 ml, both in the fasting state and 1 to 2 hours after eating, is only a guide to aid the clinician in deciding among the various therapies available for patients with diabetes mellitus. If the renal threshold is relatively normal (which, of course, is not always the case), and if chemical measurements of blood sugar are not available, persistent glucosuria can be substituted for the plasma glucose value of 200 mg/100 ml. I use the value of 200 mg/100 ml only in deciding to change therapy. I attempt to obtain plasma glucose concentrations as near normal as possible without subjecting the individual to the risk of frequent or profound hypoglycemia. For instance, if a diabetic who takes insulin maintains an FPG concentration between 175 and 200 mg/100 ml, I will increase the dose in order to lower this value to less than 150 mg/100 ml. Similarly, if a patient taking 500 mg of tolazamide consistently has FPG and PPG levels between 150 and 200 mg/100 ml, I will increase the dose to 750 mg in an attempt to decrease both values to less than 150 mg/100 ml. If this patient has been taking maximal doses of acetohexamide, I will switch her or him to full doses of tolazamide or chlorpropamide.

Practical Summary

The four sulfonylurea agents currently available in the United States are listed in Table 5-8. After rapid absorption from the gastrointestinal tract, all four are bound to serum proteins. Tolbutamide (Orinase) is catabolized by the liver to inactive products and has a short half-life. Therefore, it is usually given 2 or 3 times a day. Chlorpropamide (Diabinese) was originally thought to be excreted by the kidneys in an unchanged form, although more recent evidence points to some hepatic metabolism. On a clinical basis, the drug has a half-life of approximately 36 hours, and its pharmacologic effect may last for up to 60 hours. Therefore, it is taken only once a day. Because of its long half-life, however, steady-state levels are not attained until 7 to 10 days after initiation of therapy. Acetohexamide (Dymelor) is metabolized in the liver, but its metabolites, which are excreted in the urine, are more potent hypoglycemic agents than the parent compound. The combined pharmacologic effect of acetohexamide and its metabolites lasts from 12 to 24 hours. Up to 1,000 mg of the drug is given in the morning and the remainder (if any) is taken in the evening. Tolazamide (Tolinase) is also catabolized by the liver, and its breakdown products exert less potent hypoglycemic effects than the parent compound. The combined duration of action of tolazamide and its breakdown products is also 12 to 24 hours. The first 500 mg is given in the morning and any additional amounts (if necessary) in the evening.

Sulfonylurea agents lower glucose concentrations only in the presence of endogenous insulin. During the first several weeks of drug administration, increased insulin concentrations are noted. Therefore, the mechanism of action of these oral hypoglycemic agents has been widely held to be the stimulation of insulin secretion. However, after this initial period, diabetic control is still improved while insulin concentrations return to basal (predrug) levels or even lower. One explanation is that the sulfonylurea agents sensitize the pancreatic β-cell to respond to lower glucose concentrations than before. On the other hand, recent evidence strongly suggests that these drugs lower glucose levels by potentiating the effect of insulin. The mechanism of potentiation may be the enhancement of the binding of insulin to its tissue receptor—the critical first step in insulin action.

The incidence of adverse effects with the sulfonylurea agents is approximately 5%, and the drugs must be discontinued in only 2% of patients. (Hypoglycemia, although considered to be an adverse effect, is actually an extension of the pharmacologic effect of the sulfonylurea agents.) The most common adverse effects are gastrointestinal and cutaneous. The gastrointestinal effects are dose-related and may disappear when the dose is reduced. In fact, these problems often abate within several weeks even if the dose is not reduced. The gastrointestinal symptoms include anorexia, heartburn, nausea with occasional vomiting, feelings of abdominal fullness, and flatulence. The common adverse cutaneous effects are morbilliform, maculopapular, or urticarial rashes, which are often characterized by erythema and pruritus. There may be some cross-reactivity among the sulfonylurea agents. A disulfiram-like reaction (flushing, headache, and possibly nausea) after the ingestion of alcohol is sometimes noted by patients taking these drugs.

Other adverse effects are uncommon (<1%) or rare (occasional case reports). Other skin reactions include photosensitivity, erythema multiforme, and exfoliative dermatitis. Adverse hematologic effects may include leukopenia, agranulocytosis, thrombocytopenia, hemolytic or aplastic anemia, and pancytopenia. Reversible cholestatic jaundice may also occur. The risk of this uncommon adverse effect seems lowest with tolbutamide and highest with chlorpropamide. Chlorpropamide and tolbutamide, but not the other two sulfonylurea agents, occasionally cause inappropriate antidiuretic hormone secretion, a problem that has been reported most commonly with chlorpropamide therapy. This syndrome is characterized by hyponatremia, headache, and lethargy and may progress to stupor, coma, and seizures. Elderly patients and those taking diuretics are much more susceptible to this condition than are other patients. Finally, there are isolated case reports of fever, eosinophilia, nonspecific proctocolitis, hepatic porphyria, and porphyria cutanea tarda associated with sulfonylurea agent therapy. These drugs may also decrease slightly the thyroidal uptake of radio-active iodine, but they do not cause goiters or hypothyroidism.

Sulfonylurea agents interact with certain other drugs. These interactions can be classified as indirect or direct. An indirect interaction occurs with drugs that either decrease glucose tolerance (chapter 1) or cause hypoglycemia (chapter 10); they would be expected to impair or enhance the effect of the sulfonylurea agents. Common examples of drugs that can impair the action of these agents are potassium-losing diuretics, glucocorticoids, estrogen compounds, and diphen-ylhydantoin (Dilantin). Conversely, salicylates, propranolol, monoamine oxidase inhibitors, oxytetracycline, and ethanol can potentiate the hypoglycemic effect of the sulfonylurea agents. A direct interaction is an interference with the absorp-tion, distribution, metabolism, or excretion of a sulfonylurea compound by another drug. Only potentiation (not impairment) of the effects of the oral hypoglycemic agents has been reported to occur as a result of direct interactions. The drugs involved are listed in Table 5-2.

In the early 1960s, a study was initiated by the UGDP in order to ascertain whether tolbutamide therapy (and presumably better diabetic control) would be associated with fewer and less marked chronic complications of diabetes. More than 800 ketosis-resistant (type 2) diabetic patients were randomized into four treatment groups that received tolbutamide (1.5 g per day in divided doses), placebo tablets, insulin variable (a dose varied to control glucose concentrations), and insulin standard (a small fixed dose as a control for possible effects of insulin not mediated through its hypoglycemic action), respectively.

Eight years after the study was begun, the use of tolbutamide was discon-tinued because of an apparently higher mortality from cardiovascular causes among patients treated with this drug than among patients given the placebo. A spirited controversy concerning the validity of this conclusion has raged ever since. After a careful review of the UGDP publications, the articles defending and attacking the UGDP study, and the results of four other (similar but not identical) prospective studies of tolbutamide, I have concluded that oral sulfo-nylurea agents are not associated with an increase in mortality from cardiovascular causes. The reasons for my conclusion are as follows.

In the UGDP study, the prevalence of baseline cardiovascular risk factors was higher in the tolbutamide group than in the placebo group. In addition, mortality from cardiovascular causes in the placebo group was spuriously low during the early part of the study, the period in which tolbutamide was compared with placebo. (Cardiovascular mortality did return to expected levels during the latter part of the study, when tolbutamide had already been discontinued.) Subsequent events involving subjects who had dropped out of the study or whose medication had been changed were ascribed to the original treatment. Thus, deaths were sometimes attributed to tolbutamide in instances where a patient had not been exposed to the drug for a number of years before her or his death.

The increase in cardiovascular mortality was restricted to those patients who were taking tolbutamide but whose diabetes remained uncontrolled (fasting blood sugar level, >200 mg/100 ml). Since sound medical practice would dictate a change of therapy for such patients, generalization from this subset to all patients taking sulfonylurea agents seems unwarranted.

Finally, three other prospective studies evaluated nearly 400 subjects taking tolbutamide (some of whom had had documented myocardial infarctions) for periods ranging from 5 to 8 years. No increase in cardiovascular mortality was noted. Furthermore, cardiovascular mortality in type 2 diabetics monitored for 16 years in the Framingham study was lower among patients receiving sulfonylurea agents than among those treated by means of diet alone. The American Diabetes Association seems to agree that the conclusion of the UGDP investigators regarding the cardiovascular toxicity of tolbutamide is not valid, since it recently withdrew its original endorsement of the study.

The general guidelines for the clinical use of the sulfonylurea agents are depicted in Figure 5-9. These drugs are ineffective in ketosis-prone (type 1) diabetics and should not be used in these patients. Most ketosis-resistant (type 2) diabetics should be treated initially with a dietary prescription alone. However, a minority of these patients present with symptoms of polyuria, polydipsia, and weight loss and should be treated initially with maximal doses of tolazamide or chlorpropamide (Table 5-9). An appropriate diet (chapter 3) should also be prescribed. If the symptoms do not begin to abate within 1 or 2 weeks, the patients should be switched to insulin. If the symptoms disappear, the fasting plasma glucose (FPG) concentration determines the choice of subsequent therapy. If this value remains above 200 mg/100 ml after approximately 1 month, the sulfonylurea agent should be discontinued and therapy with insulin started. One exception to this rule might be an obese patient who is losing weight and whose FPG value, although falling, still exceeds 200 mg/100 ml. In this situation, an additional month of oral hypoglycemic therapy might be indicated in anticipation of increasing insulin sensitivity secondary to weight loss and a satisfactory response to the sulfonylurea agent. However, if the FPG level stabilizes above 200 mg/100 ml, insulin therapy should be initiated.

If, on the other hand, the FPG falls below 200 mg/100 ml, treatment with the oral hypoglycemic agent should be continued. At this point, the 1- to 2-hour postprandial glucose (PPG) concentration determines the choice of subsequent therapy. If this value remains above 200 mg/100 ml, the maximal dose of the drug is continued. If the PPG level drops below 200 mg/100 ml, the dose of the drug is gradually decreased until that value rises above 200 mg/100 ml. At this point, the dose is increased again until 1- to 2-hour PPG concentrations can be consistently kept below 200 mg/100 ml. In some patients, the dose can continue to be decreased and the drug can finally be discontinued without an increase in the PPG level to greater than 200 mg/100 ml. These individuals are then treated by means of diet alone.

Most ketosis-resistant diabetics are relatively asymptomatic, and dietary therapy alone should be tried for at least 1 month. If the FPG level *or* the 1- to

2-hour PPG concentration exceeds 200 mg/100 ml at this point, treatment with a sulfonylurea agent is started. As described above, a further trial of dietary therapy alone may be indicated for obese patients who are losing weight and whose FPG values are decreasing (although still exceed 200 mg/100 ml). Should these levels stabilize above 200 mg/100 ml, however, drug therapy is begun.

The initial doses of the three sulfonylurea agents that I recommend are shown in Table 5-9. The goal of therapy is to reduce both the FPG and the PPG levels to below 200 mg/100 ml. The dose of the oral hypoglycemic agent selected should be gradually increased until this goal is achieved or maximal doses are reached. In the latter instance, if acetohexamide was used initially, the patient should be switched to maximal doses of tolazamide or chlorpropamide since these compounds are probably more potent. Tolazamide is preferred in individuals over 60 years of age because of the propensity of chlorpropamide to cause inappropriate antidiuretic hormone secretion and more serious hypoglycemia in elderly diabetics. If therapy with maximal doses of either tolazamide or chlorpropamide fails, the other agent may be tried, but a successful outcome is less likely.

If the FPG concentration exceeds 200 mg/100 ml despite the administration of maximal doses, the sulfonylurea agents are discontinued and insulin therapy is initiated. If the FPG level is below 200 mg/100 ml but the 1- to 2-hour PPG concentration remains above this value, the patient continues with oral drug therapy. If the 1- to 2-hour PPG value is kept consistently below 200 mg/100 ml by either maximal or submaximal amounts of an oral hypoglycemic agent, the physician should determine at least once in the patient's course whether drug therapy is really needed. The dose should be decreased gradually either until the drug can be discontinued or until the 1- to 2-hour PPG concentration rises above 200 mg/100 ml. At this point, the dose is increased again until the value again falls below 200 mg/100 ml. In this way, unnecessary exposure to the drug is avoided. This approach is especially pertinent in obese patients who have gradually lost weight over an extended period.

One final comment is offered about the goal of achieving FPG and PPG concentrations of less than 200 mg/100 ml. This value serves only as a guide for the physician in choosing among the various therapies available for type 2 diabetics, and highlights the point at which therapy should be changed. I like to have glucose levels as near normal as possible without subjecting the patient to profound or frequent hypoglycemia. To that end, if the FPG and/or PPG values are between 150 and 200 mg/100 ml, I will increase doses (up to the maximum) or switch to a more potent agent in order to lower these concentrations to less than 150 mg/100 ml.

References

1. Clarke BF, Campbell IW: Long-term comparative trial of glibenclamide and chlorpropamide in diet-failed, maturity-onset diabetes. Lancet 1:246–248, 1975

2. Chu PC, Conway MJ, Krouse HA, Goodner CJ: The pattern of response of plasma insulin and glucose to meals and fasting during chlorpropamide therapy. Ann Intern Med 68:757-769, 1968

3. Lebovitz HE, Feinglos MN: Sulfonylurea drugs: mechanism of antidiabetic action and therapeutic usefulness. Diabetes Care 1:189-198, 1978

4. Feldman JM, Lebovitz HE: Appraisal of the extrapancreatic actions of sulfonylureas. Arch Intern Med 123:314-321, 1969

5. Davidson MB: Insulin binding in diabetes mellitus and the effect of treatment with diet and sulfonylurea agents. In *The Role of Sulfonylureas in the Treatment of Insulin-Independent Diabetes, 1980.* Edited by Reaven GM. Science and Medicine, Inc, New York, 1980, pp 24-30

6. Scott J, Poffenbarger PL: Pharmacogenetics of tolbutamide metabolism in humans. Diabetes 28:41-51, 1979

7. Thomas RC, Judy RW: Metabolic fate of chlorpropamide in man and in the rat. J Med Chem 15:964-968, 1972

8. Yu TF, Berger L, Gutman AB: Hypoglycemic and uricosuric properties of acetohexamide and hydroxyhexamide. Metabolism 17:309-316, 1968

9. Garcia M, Miller M, Moses AM: Chlorpropamide-induced water retention in patients with diabetes mellitus. Ann Intern Med 75:549-554, 1971

10. Hansen JM, Christensen LK: Drug interactions with oral sulphonylurea hypoglycaemic drugs. Drugs 13:24-34, 1977

11. University Group Diabetes Program: A study of the effects of hypoglycemic agents on vascular complications in patients with adult-onset diabetes. I. Design, methods and baseline results. Diabetes 19(Suppl 2):747-783, 1970

12. University Group Diabetes Program: A study of the effects of hypoglycemic agents on vascular complications in patients with adult-onset diabetes. II. Mortality results. Diabetes 19(Suppl 2):789-830, 1970

13. Feinstein AR: Clinical biostatistics. XXXV. The persistent clinical failures and fallacies of the UGDP study. Clin Pharmacol Ther 19:78-93, 1976

14. Kilo C, Miller JP, Williamson JR: The Achilles heel of the University Group Diabetes Program. JAMA 243:450-457, 1980

15. Garcia MJ, McNamara PM, Gordon T, Kannell WB: Morbidity and mortality in diabetics in the Framingham population. Sixteen year follow-up study. Diabetes 23:105-111, 1974

16. Whitehouse FW, Arky RA, Bell DI, et al: The UGDP controversy (policy statement). Diabetes 28:168-170, 1979

17. Keen H, Jarrett RJ, Fuller JH: Tolbutamide and arterial disease in borderline diabetics. In *Proceedings of the Ninth Congress of the International Diabetes Federation.* Edited by Malaisse WJ, Pirart J. Excerpta Medica, Amsterdam, 1974, pp 588-602

18. Paasikivi J, Wahlberg F: Preventive tolbutamide treatment and arterial disease in mild hyperglycaemia. Diabetologia 7:323-327, 1971

19. Feldman R, Crawford D, Elashoff R, Glass A: Oral hypoglycemia during prophylaxis in asymptomatic diabetes. In *Proceedings of the Ninth Congress of the International Diabetes Federation*. Edited by Malaisse WJ, Pirart J. Excerpta Medica, Amsterdam, 1974, pp 574-587

20. Pirart J: Diabetes mellitus and its degenerative complication: a prospective study of 4,400 patients observed between 1947 and 1973. Diabetes Care 1:168-188, 1978

21. Katz HM, Bissel G: Blood sugar lowering effects of chlorpropamide and tolbutamide. A double blind cooperative study. Diabetes 14:650-657, 1965

22. Frey HMM, Rosenlund B: Studies in patients with chlorpropamide-induced hypoglycemia. Diabetes 19:930-937, 1970

Chapter 6
Diabetic Ketoacidosis and Hyperosmolar Nonketotic Coma

Diabetic Ketoacidosis

Pathophysiology

Diabetic ketoacidosis (DKA) is caused by a profound lack of effective insulin. Published studies routinely report some measurable insulin concentrations, but these low levels (usually <10 μU/ml) are clearly inadequate in the metabolic milieu of marked hyperglycemia, ketosis, and acidosis. Although levels of the contrainsulin hormones (catecholamines, glucagon, growth hormone, and cortisol) are elevated as the result of stress, such elevations do not *cause* the metabolic derangements that lead to DKA. Elevated levels of these hormones may potentiate the effect of a lack of insulin but patients can become ketoacidotic in the absence of high levels of these hormones.

The clinical hallmarks of DKA are acidosis, dehydration, and electrolyte depletion. The mechanisms behind these conditions are outlined in Figure 6-1. The effect of a lack of insulin on all three general areas of metabolism—carbohydrate, protein, and fat—figures prominently in the pathophysiology of DKA. In the absence of effective insulin, ingested carbohydrate is not utilized by the three insulin-sensitive tissues (liver, muscle, and adipose tissues). This impairment of glucose uptake causes hyperglycemia. Not shown in Figure 6-1 is the effect of a lack of insulin on glucose production by the liver. In the late postprandial state, after the carbohydrate content of the diet has been stored, insulin is critically important in the modulation of glucose production by the liver. In the absence of insulin, unchecked hepatic glucose production further increases the already-elevated glucose concentrations. Hyperglycemia, in turn, causes an osmotic diuresis that results in water and electrolyte depletion. The water and electrolyte losses cause dehydration, which is clinically manifest as intravascular

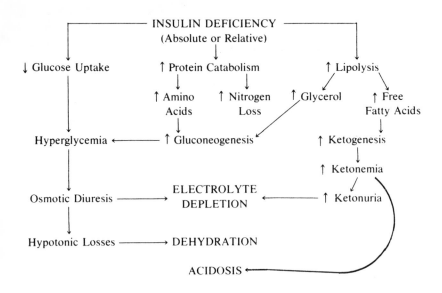

Figure 6-1. Pathophysiology of DKA.

volume depletion. The fluid losses are hypotonic to plasma, and a hyperosmolar state therefore develops.

In protein metabolism, a lack of insulin reinforces fluid and electrolyte depletion. In the absence of effective insulin, the transport of amino acids into cells and the incorporation of these intracellular amino acids into protein are decreased. In addition, the inhibition of protein degradation by insulin is reversed. Therefore, the effects of a lack of insulin on amino acid transport, protein synthesis, and protein degradation all cause protein catabolism, which results in increased release of amino acids from muscle tissue. Some of these amino acids are gluconeogenic precursors and are converted to glucose by the liver. The rate of gluconeogenesis is controlled by the amount of appropriate substrates delivered to the liver. Therefore, the increased flux of amino acids from muscle contributes significantly to hyperglycemia, with its attendant fluid and electrolyte losses. The amino acids not utilized for gluconeogenesis are metabolized by the liver in order to fulfill energy demands. This increased nitrogen loss leads to a depletion of lean body mass, which is an important component of the weight loss suffered by the affected patients.

In the case of fat metabolism, the lack of effective insulin also contributes to fluid and electrolyte depletion. However, ketosis and eventual acidosis are solely attributable to the lack of an insulin effect on adipose tissue. A critical aspect of insulin action on this tissue is an inhibition of the breakdown of triglycerides, a pathway termed *lipolysis* (see chapter 2). Increased lipolysis results in elevated concentrations of glycerol and free fatty acids (FFA) in plasma. Because glycerol is a gluconeogenic precursor, its increased flux from adipose tissue enhances gluconeogenesis even further. This enhancement, of course, leads to more pronounced hyperglycemia and greater fluid and electrolyte losses. Some of the FFA can be utilized by tissues for energy purposes or reconstituted as hepatic triglycerides. However, as discussed in chapter 2, the most important determinant of ketone body formation (ketogenesis) is the amount of FFA delivered to the liver. The ketogenic pathway is further activated by the presence of the low insulin and high glucagon concentrations that characterize DKA. The ketone bodies (acetoacetate and β-hydroxybutyrate) are weak acids that must be buffered upon release by the liver into the circulation (ketonemia). As more and more ketone bodies are produced, the body bases become depleted and acidosis ensues. In addition to causing acidosis, the ketone bodies also contribute to the loss of electrolytes. Although they can be utilized to some extent by various body tissues, the capacity to metabolize ketone bodies is soon exceeded, and they are excreted into the urine (ketonuria). This event exacerbates electrolyte depletion as cations must be excreted with the ketone bodies. These are the mechanisms, then, by which a lack of insulin affects carbohydrate, protein, and fat metabolism and leads to the dehydration, electrolyte depletion, and acidosis that characterize DKA.

Losses

The usual fluid and electrolyte losses sustained by patients experiencing DKA are marked, as shown in Figure 6-2. The values in this figure are derived from two kinds of studies. In one type of study, the use of insulin was discontinued in ketosis-prone diabetics, and the amounts of fluid and electrolytes lost over a 24-hour period were measured. In the other type, the amounts of fluid and electrolytes needed to treat patients experiencing DKA in the first 24-hour period were carefully tabulated. In a "typical" 70-kg individual, the fluid, sodium, potassium, and chloride losses depicted in Figure 6-2 are indeed impressive. Extracellular water represents 17% of body weight, or ~12 L in our reference subject. Therefore, over one half of the extracellular fluid compartment was lost. The amount of exchangeable sodium in a normal individual is 41 mEq/kg. The sodium loss in these diabetic subjects represented >15% of this total exchangeable pool. Similarly, the chloride loss was between 15% and 20% of the normal chloride pool (33 mEq/kg). Approximately 10% of total body potassium (50 to 54 mEq/kg) was excreted by these subjects. Of the total exchangeable magnesium pool (10 mEq/kg), 7% was lost under these circumstances.

The situation with regard to phosphorus is more complicated. The body of a 70-kg man, for example, contains ~712 g, or 23,000 mmol, of phosphorus. Of this amount, 80% is in bone and 9% in muscle. However, the bulk of the intracellular phosphorus is in organic form, and only a small fraction is inorganic. Thus, although the amount of phosphorus lost in the urine of these diabetic subjects over a 24-hour period is a minuscule percentage of total body phosphorus, it represents a relatively substantial part of the available inorganic phosphorus pool. Balance studies done during several weeks after recovery from DKA have demonstrated substantial retention of phosphorus (up to 400 mmol).

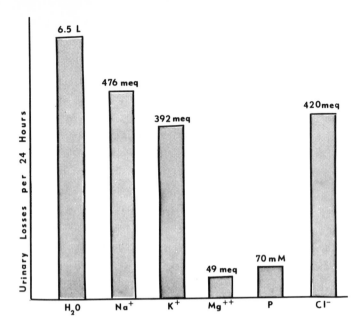

Figure 6-2. Urinary losses of water and electrolytes in patients with DKA.

These studies probably underestimate net phosphorus losses since they were completed before the pre-DKA weight had been regained. The problems of phosphorus homeostasis in the treatment of DKA have recently emerged again and will be discussed in greater detail later.

Causes

The precipitating causes of 100 consecutive admissions for DKA in an English population (1) are listed in Table 6-1. Approximately 25% of these admissions resulted from an omission or reduction of insulin doses, in many cases by health professionals caring for these patients! Diabetic ketoacidosis was the initial manifestation of diabetes in roughly another 25%. In still another 25%, DKA was precipitated by an infection. In the remaining 25%, no easily identifiable precipitating cause could be found. Thus, in this series, one half of the episodes of DKA were potentially preventable (those associated with decreased insulin doses and those related to infection), while the other half were not.

Symptoms

The symptoms of DKA are listed in Table 6-2. Polyuria and polydipsia are simply manifestations of osmotic diuresis secondary to hyperglycemia. Weakness,

Table 6-1. Causes of DKA in 100 Consecutive Cases[a]

Cause		No. of Cases
Omission or reduction of insulin		27
By patient	20	
By clinic	4	
By doctor	3	
Initial manifestation of diabetes		22
Infection		22
Respiratory	9	
Urinary tract	5	
Gastroenteritis	6	
Other	2	
Acute pancreatitis		5
Uremia		2
Insulin resistance		2
Digitalis intoxication		1
Unknown		19

[a]Adapted with permission from Sheldon J, Pyke DA: Severe diabetic ketosis: precoma and coma. In *Clinical Diabetes and Its Biochemical Basis*. Edited by Oakly WG, Pyke DA, Taylor KW. Blackwell Scientific Publications, Oxford, 1968, p 423.

Table 6-2. Symptoms of DKA

Polyuria	Anorexia
Polydipsia	Nausea
Weakness	Vomiting
Lethargy	Abdominal pain
Myalgia	"Dyspnea"
Headache	

lethargy, headache, and myalgia are relatively nonspecific symptoms. The gastrointestinal and respiratory symptoms, however, are specifically related to DKA.

Although documentation is difficult, ketosis is probably responsible for many of the gastrointestinal symptoms. (Ketosis secondary to a low carbohydrate intake—i.e., starvation ketosis—is associated with anorexia, nausea, and occasionally vomiting.) In any event, nausea, vomiting, and abdominal pain are often noted in patients with DKA. The abdominal pain can be quite severe and may even suggest an intraabdominal process requiring surgery.

When questioned more closely, patients who complain of "dyspnea" (shortness of breath on exertion) are found actually to be having difficulty in catching their breath even while sitting or lying quietly. This symptom, of course, represents hyperventilation, which is the ventilatory response to metabolic acidosis originally described by Kussmaul.

Signs

The signs of DKA are listed in Table 6-3. It is not generally recognized that low body temperatures are characteristic of patients experiencing DKA. Hyperpnea (Kussmaul respirations) is usually seen when the pH of the blood is <7.2 and the bicarbonate concentration ($[HCO_3]$) is <12 mEq/L. The depth of respiration, not the rate, characterizes Kussmaul respirations. Often patients have a normal respiratory rate but on closer inspection are noted to be breathing very deeply. The signal for this hyperventilation is acidosis, which stimulates the respiratory center in the brain. The resulting respiratory alkalosis offsets metabolic acidosis to some extent but cannot compensate for it entirely in the absence of treatment.

The structure of and relation among the ketone bodies are depicted in Figure 6-3. Acetoacetate is irreversibly converted to acetone, which is excreted by the lungs. Acetone has a fruity odor that is often apparent on the patient's breath, although not all observers can distinguish this odor.

Although the term *dehydration* is often used to describe patients experiencing DKA, the symptoms really result from intravascular volume depletion. In adults, the most sensitive sign of intravascular volume depletion is a change in the way in which the neck veins fill. When normally hydrated subjects lie entirely horizontally (i.e., without a pillow), the neck veins fill from below up to a point near the angle of the mandible. This sign is essentially a clinical measurement of venous pressure, which is normally ~7 cm of H_2O. In order to ascertain whether

Table 6-3. Signs of DKA

Hypothermia
Hyperpnea (Kussmaul respirations)
Acetone breath
"Dehydration" (intravascular volume depletion)
Hyporeflexia
"Acute abdomen"
Stupor (→ coma)
Hypotonia
Uncoordinated ocular movements
Fixed, dilated pupils

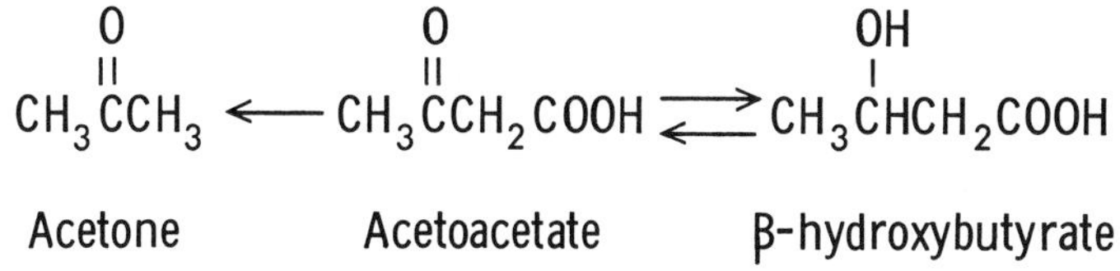

$$\underset{\text{Acetone}}{CH_3\overset{\displaystyle O}{\overset{\|}{C}}CH_3} \longleftarrow \underset{\text{Acetoacetate}}{CH_3\overset{\displaystyle O}{\overset{\|}{C}}CH_2COOH} \rightleftarrows \underset{\beta\text{-hydroxybutyrate}}{CH_3\overset{\displaystyle OH}{\overset{|}{C}H}CH_2COOH}$$

Figure 6-3. Structure of and relation among the ketone bodies.

the jugular veins are filling from above, the vein near the clavicle should first be occluded so that its course can be delineated as it fills from above. Next, the vein near the angle of the jaw should be occluded in order to determine how far over the clavicle it fills from below. It is helpful to empty the vein by "milking" it while it is occluded from above so that the column of blood can actually be seen as the vein is subsequently filled from beneath the clavicle. If the vein is not filled from below or is filled to less than one half of the distance to the angle of the mandible, the intravascular volume is significantly reduced.

The only other reliable sign of intravascular depletion is a fall of systolic blood pressure by 20 mm Hg or greater when the patient moves from a lying to a sitting or standing position. So that equilibrium is ensured, at least 1 minute should elapse before the semivertical or vertical blood pressure is recorded. This orthostatic change in systolic blood pressure is a less sensitive measurement than decreased filling of the neck veins and thus represents a more marked deficit in intravascular volume. (It must be kept in mind, however, that diabetics with dysfunction of the autonomic nervous system may manifest orthostatic changes in blood pressure in the absence of any fluid loss.)

The other signs often considered in the determination of dehydration are really not very helpful. Dry mucous membranes are noted in patients who breathe with their mouth open. Soft eyeballs and poor skin turgor are seen, at least in adults, only with profound dehydration.

Hyporeflexia may be noted in patients experiencing DKA. If not present initially, it often develops during treatment as the potassium concentration ([K]) falls. (The response of potassium to therapy will be discussed later.)

An abdominal examination of patients experiencing DKA can yield striking results. Abdominal tenderness to palpation and muscle guarding are usual. Bowel sounds may be diminished or even absent. Rebound tenderness is often noted. In an occasional patient, a boardlike abdomen with no bowel sounds and rebound tenderness may suggest a catastrophic intraabdominal process requiring immediate surgery. However, this whole syndrome is caused by DKA, although the mechanism behind it is unknown. Except for the very rare patient in whom DKA may be precipitated by such an event, these signs will clear as the patient's biochemical status improves. In any event, since surgery is contraindicated in patients with DKA because of the extremely high related mortality, treatment of DKA must precede surgical intervention, and signs suggesting the need for surgery almost invariably disappear with treatment.

The mental status of patients experiencing DKA ranges from completely alert to comatose and is not related to the degree of ketosis or acidosis. In fact, the patient's mental status seems best correlated with plasma osmolality (Fig. 6-4). Various degrees of lethargy, stupor, and coma are seen in most patients, and altered mental status is an important sign of DKA.

Hypotonia, uncoordinated ocular movements, and fixed, dilated pupils are (fortunately) unusual symptoms that are associated with a poor prognosis (as is very deep coma).

Differential Diagnosis

The diagnosis of DKA is simple if it is considered in the differential. A urine sample showing marked glucosuria and ketonuria or an undiluted plasma sample giving a strongly positive result in the nitroprusside test for acetoacetate is sufficient for the diagnosis. However, too often, these tests are not performed and the diagnosis is regrettably delayed.

Other conditions that may mimic DKA to various degrees and the clinical similarities between these conditions and DKA are listed in Table 6-4. Although coma is certainly seen in DKA, most diabetics who present in coma will be found to have suffered cerebral vascular accidents, simply because many more diabetics have strokes than have episodes of DKA.

A brainstem hemorrhage may be confused with DKA because both conditions may be associated with glucosuria and hyperventilation. The hyperventilation in brainstem hemorrhage is explained by the fact that the respiratory center is located in the brainstem. In the nineteenth century, Claude Bernard showed that stimulation of an area in the brainstem resulted in glucosuria, or "piqûre" diabetes.

The many features that distinguish DKA from hypoglycemia are listed in Table 6-5. In hypoglycemia, the onset is rapid (within minutes), gastrointestinal symptoms are lacking, signs of intravascular volume depletion are absent, and respiration is normal. In DKA, in contrast, the onset is slow (over a period of hours), gastrointestinal symptoms and signs of intravascular volume depletion are prominent, and Kussmaul respirations are noted. In DKA, tachycardia is present secondary to intravascular volume depletion. In hypoglycemia, the sympathetic nervous system is fully activated, and, in addition to tachycardia, the patient may exhibit tremors, anxiety, hunger, tingling of the fingers and around the mouth, palpitations, and sweating. Sweating leads to cool, wet skin that contrasts with the dry, flushed skin of DKA. Although glucosuria is usually minimal or absent in hypoglycemia, the test can be positive if the bladder contains urine formed during a hyperglycemic period preceding the onset of hypoglycemia. The presence of ketonuria establishes the diagnosis of DKA, while its absence indicates a diagnosis of hypoglycemia. The diagnosis of DKA is clearly untenable in the absence of ketonuria.

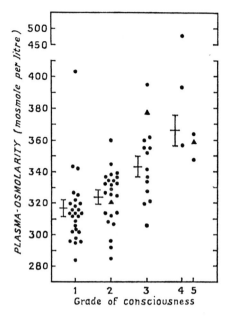

Figure 6-4. Relation between state of consciousness and calculated plasma osmolarity in 70 episodes of DKA. The means (horizontal line) are shown, and ± 1 SEM is enclosed by brackets. The three triangles refer to three values reported as exceeding those shown. States of consciousness were defined as follows: (1) awake or mildly drowsy (26 episodes); (2) moderately drowsy but easily arousable and fully oriented (24 episodes); (3) very drowsy but arousable by loud questioning and then partially oriented (14 episodes); (4) stuporous, barely responsive, and then not oriented (3 episodes); and (5) comatose (4 episodes). (Reprinted with permission from Fulop M, Tannenbaum H, and Dreyer N: Hyperosmolar coma. Lancet 2:635–639, 1973.)

The other conditions listed—metabolic acidosis, gastroenteritis, and pneumonia—can all be ruled out by the absence of significant ketosis. Although ketonuria may be present if carbohydrate intake has been poor, a less than strongly positive result in the nitroprusside test for ketone bodies in undiluted plasma effectively rules out DKA.

Initial Laboratory Values

The results of pertinent laboratory tests in patients presenting with DKA are listed in Table 6-6. Glucose concentrations obviously can vary considerably, and a substantial number of patients experiencing DKA have initial glucose values of <300 mg/100 ml (2). In a series of 211 episodes of DKA, 37 patients had severe acidosis—i.e., [HCO_3] <10 mEq/L—and "euglycemia." Glucose concentrations

Table 6-4. Differential Diagnosis of DKA

Cerebrovascular accident (altered mental status)[a]

Brainstem hemorrhage (hyperventilation, glucosuria)

Hypoglycemia

Metabolic acidosis (hyperventilation, anion gap, acidosis)
  Uremia
  Salicylates
  Methanol
  Ethylene glycol

Gastroenteritis (nausea, vomiting, abdominal pain)

Pneumonia (hyperventilation)

---

[a]Clinical similarities to DKA are listed in parentheses.

Table 6-5. Features Distinguishing DKA from Hypoglycemia

	Condition	
Feature	*DKA*	*Hypoglycemia*
Onset	Slow	Fast
Gastrointestinal symptoms	Yes	No
Intravascular volume depletion	Yes	No
Respiration	Deep	Normal
Sympathetic nervous system signs and symptoms	Tachycardia only	Yes
Glucosuria	$\geq 2\%$	$\pm$
Ketonuria	Strong	Negative

were between 200 and 300 mg/100 ml in 21 patients, between 100 and 200 mg/100 ml in 9, and <100 mg/100 ml in 7! Thus, 17.5% of patients in this report presented with glucose levels of <300 mg/100 ml although they were experiencing severe DKA (2). Obviously, glucose concentrations are not a good index of the severity of metabolic derangement.

The nitroprusside test for ketone bodies yields strongly positive results in undiluted plasma, and these results most often remain strongly positive through several dilutions. The result of this test does not represent the full extent of the ketosis, however, since the nitroprusside reagent measures only acetoacetate and not β-hydroxybutyrate. (Actually, acetone is also measured, but it is only 0.05%

Table 6-6. Initial Laboratory Values for Patients Experiencing DKA

Test	Result	Remarks
Glucose	300–800 mg/100 ml	Concentration not related to severity of DKA
Ketone bodies	Strong at least in undiluted plasma	Measures only acetoacetate, not β-hydroxybutyrate
[HCO_3]	0–15 mEq/L	
pH	6.8–7.3	
[Na]	Low, normal, or high	Total body depletion; concentration dependent on relative H_2O loss
[K]	Low, normal, or high	Total body depletion; heart responsive to extra-cellular concentrations
Phosphate	Usually normal or slightly elevated; occasionally slightly low	Associated with phosphaturia; marked decrease with treatment in levels of both serum and urine phosphates
Creatinine, BUN	Usually mildly increased	May be prerenal
WBC count	Usually increased	Possibility of leukemoid reaction (even in absence of infection)
Amylase	Often increased	Predominant form of salivary gland origin
Hemoglobin, hematocrit, total protein	Often increased	Secondary to contracted plasma volume
SGOT, SGPT, LDH	Can be elevated	Spurious increases due to acetoacetate interference in older colorimetric methods

Abbreviations: [HCO_3], concentration of bicarbonate; [Na], concentration of sodium; [K], concentration of potassium; BUN, blood urea nitrogen; WBC, white blood cell; SGOT, serum glutamic oxaloacetic transaminase; SGPT, serum glutamic pyruvic transaminase; LDH, lactic dehydrogenase.

as active as acetoacetate on a molar basis and occurs in patients with DKA at levels that are only 2 to 4 times higher than those of acetoacetate.) The ratio of β-hydroxybutyrate to acetoacetate varies greatly in DKA but may be as high as 3:1 to 5:1 (3).

The decreases in [HCO_3] and pH need no further explanation and obviously do reflect the severity of metabolic derangement.

Although there is total body depletion of sodium stores in DKA, the serum concentration of sodium ([Na]) may be low, normal, or high and depends on water balance. If hyperlipemia is present, the serum [Na] measured is falsely low. If hyperlipemia is absent, the serum [Na] is simply a measure of the relative amounts of the cation and body water. Since urinary fluid losses are hypotonic, plasma osmolality becomes elevated, and a high serum [Na] would be expected. However, polyuria leads to polydipsia and the amount of water ingested affects the [Na]. If an appropriate amount of water is consumed, the [Na] may be normal. If an excess amount is ingested, the [Na] decreases. Vomiting further complicates the relation between sodium and water. Finally, if intravascular volume depletion is profound, antidiuretic hormone is secreted in an attempt to restore the vascular volume, even at the expense of decreasing serum osmolality. This event lowers the [Na] even if it was decreased before the antidiuretic hormone response. The clinical lesson here is that affected patients need saline repletion to restore their vascular volume, regardless of the [Na]. (The rate and osmolality of the replacement solutions will be discussed under *Treatment*.)

Similar considerations pertain to the initial [K], which may be low, normal, or high. There is a profound total body depletion of potassium regardless of the serum concentration, and affected patients must have their stores replenished with potassium salts. The clinical situation with regard to potassium homeostasis in DKA is somewhat complicated and will be discussed in greater detail under *Treatment*.

Serum phosphorus concentrations are usually normal or even slightly elevated in untreated DKA. This finding is associated with marked phosphaturia (which accompanies all forms of metabolic acidosis). The explanation given is that acidosis leads to the breakdown of intracellular organic compounds and that inorganic phosphate is thus liberated, transferred into the plasma, and subsequently excreted in the urine. Treatment of DKA results in a gradual reduction of phosphaturia (over 8 to 10 hours) and a marked decrement of serum phosphorus concentrations, which may not reach their nadir for several days. The hypophosphatemia is presumably the result of the uptake of inorganic phosphorus by cells that had been phosphorus-deficient.

Creatinine and blood urea nitrogen (BUN) levels are usually increased in DKA. This increase often represents prerenal azotemia caused by diminished perfusion of the kidneys secondary to intravascular volume depletion. Therefore, a valid assessment of renal function must await resolution of DKA. In many cases, however, BUN and creatinine values do not return to normal, a result reflecting underlying diabetic nephropathy.

Not only is leukocytosis common in DKA, but leukemoid reactions with white blood cell (WBC) counts of 20,000 to 40,000/mm^3 are occasionally seen. The high WBC counts are associated with lymphopenia and eosinopenia. This leukocyte response to DKA is thought to reflect increased adrenal cortical activity and dehydration. Therefore, leukocytosis is not a reliable sign of infection in this setting, and independent evidence must be sought.

Amylase values are frequently elevated in patients with DKA. However, the increase in the majority of instances is in amylase of salivary origin rather than in that of pancreatic origin (4, 5). Furthermore, the levels and origin of amylase do not correlate with signs and symptoms suggestive of pancreatitis (4, 5). Thus, hyperamylasemia probably represents transient nonspecific leakage of this enzyme from its two tissues of origin and does not support a diagnosis of pancreatitis in DKA.

The frequent increases in hemoglobin, hematocrit, and total proteins in DKA simply reflect the decreased volume of plasma. Therefore, a low but normal or slightly decreased hematocrit or hemoglobin value on admission indicates a probable anemia that will require further evaluation after DKA is treated.

In the recent past, tests for the enzymes serum glutamic oxaloacetic transaminase (SGOT), serum glutamic pyruvic transaminase (SGPT), and lactic dehydrogenase (LDH) often gave falsely elevated results because of interference by acetoacetate in the colorimetric methods used. Many laboratories are now using kinetic procedures for the measurement of these enzymes; in these procedures, false-positive results are not a problem. If the level of any of these enzymes is found to be elevated in patients who are ketotic, the physician should ascertain that the methodology employed involves direct measurements of reduced nucleotides via changes in ultraviolet absorption rather than coupling with a diazonium salt (the colorimetric method). However, levels of serum enzymes such as SGOT, SGPT, creatine phosphokinase (CPK), and 5-nucleotidase are truly elevated in many patients with DKA. Severe abnormalities are usually explained by readily apparent clinical disease. Elevated levels are not related to the degree of abdominal symptoms, nor are they caused by acidosis per se. When no cause can be found, patients generally do well with treatment, and the enzyme levels return to normal.

Treatment

The treatment of DKA can be conveniently discussed under six separate categories: general therapeutic approaches, fluid replacement, insulin therapy, potassium replacement, phosphate replacement, and bicarbonate therapy. Obviously, all six areas must be considered in clinical decisions. Some of these areas of treatment are controversial, and valid arguments can be made on both sides of the issues. Indeed, in many cases, it is difficult to be certain that one course of action is distinctly better for a given patient.

General Considerations. The use of "all deliberate speed" is appropriate in the treatment of DKA. Obviously, therapy within minutes is not necessary, but a delay of treatment for several hours can be detrimental to the patient. Several general principles should be followed. First, only one physician should be in charge of the patient's care and assume full responsibility for therapeutic decisions. Second, a Diabetic Ketoacidosis Progress Record (Fig. 6-5) should be

(a) Enter as applicable: 1 = ALERT   2 = LETHARGIC (easily aroused)
3 = STUPOR (aroused with difficulty)   4 = COMA (unresponsive)

(b) Last strongly positive dilution

DATE	SIGNS				PLASMA									URINE		TREATMENT							
														GLUCOSE		INSULIN		FLUIDS					
TIME	BP (↑or↓)	RESP	(a) CNS	GLUCOSE	(b) KETONES	CO_2 pH	K	Na Cl	Hct BUN					KETONES		TIME START	AMT (U/hr)	TIME START	TYPE	AMT (L)	K (mEq)	HCO_3 (mEq)	

Figure 6–5. Sample Diabetic Ketoacidosis Progress Record. Bp, blood pressure; RESP, respiratory; CNS, central nervous system; Hct, hematocrit; BUN, blood urea nitrogen; Amt, amount.

started *as soon as therapy is initiated.* Too often, this record is constructed from memory many hours after treatment has begun. An accurate and updated progress record will enable any health professional involved in the care of the patient to quickly become familiar with the treatment given and the response to therapy. This progress record is extremely important in situations where responsibility for the patient's care is transferred—e.g., when house staff coverage in teaching hospitals or evening and weekend coverage in the private sector causes a transfer of responsibility to personnel not familiar with the case. At that juncture, it is wise for the two physicians involved to discuss the patient's progress record, what has transpired, and what is planned. Unfortunately, the physician taking over the patient's care is often unaware of important information because it is not on the progress record and has not been communicated by the doctor going off duty.

Third, and most obvious, an appropriate site for intravenous fluid administration is necessary. Some patients require "cut-downs" because of their contracted plasma volumes. Since many hours of fluid administration will be necessary, a needle tenuously placed in a peripheral vein should not be relied upon, and a catheter should be inserted via a cut-down.

Fourth, urine samples are necessary not only in making the diagnosis of DKA but in following the patient's response to therapy. In addition, it must be ascertained that the patient is not experiencing renal shutdown before potassium replacement is started. Therefore, if the patient does not urinate spontaneously, bladder catheterization, which is rarely done in diabetics, is indicated. In this instance, the initial bladder specimen should be cultured in order to ascertain whether the DKA is associated with (precipitated by "?") a urinary tract infection. Once the catheter is placed, the resulting pyuria will make such an assessment difficult.

Fifth, since the possibilities of pulmonary aspiration are enhanced considerably in the comatose patient, a nasogastric tube should be put in place and continuous suction applied until the patient becomes more responsive. In more alert patients, this maneuver is restricted to those with signs of gastric dilatation.

The sixth general principle concerns the ordering of laboratory tests and the timing of samples. This discussion will be limited to those tests that are concerned specifically with the diagnosis and treatment of DKA. I routinely order measurements of glucose, electrolytes, phosphate, and creatinine or BUN. Although the following tests are not absolutely necessary for either diagnosis or monitoring of the response to therapy, the initial arterial pH and the degree of ketosis may sometimes be used as a baseline measurement against which to judge the patient's status as treatment proceeds. If an arterial puncture cannot be done, a determination of venous pH is still useful as long as it is recognized that this value will be somewhat higher than that obtained with a concomitant arterial sample. The degree of ketosis should be recorded as the last dilution in which the nitroprusside test for acetoacetate yields a *strongly* positive result. Determination of the last dilution in which any reaction is noted is not particularly helpful. The advantage of measuring plasma ketone bodies by this semiquantitative technique is that the results are available immediately; with the other tests, which must be evaluated in the laboratory, a 1- to 2-hour wait is required. Of course, the nitroprusside test should be done near the patient's bedside by the physician or an appropriately trained person. Indeed, it makes little sense to send this test to the laboratory since, by the time the results are returned, they are of little value. Although the rapidity with which the results of the nitroprusside test are known would seem to make them very useful in therapeutic decisions, monitoring of the patient's response by this test is generally not helpful during the first 4 to 6 hours for reasons discussed later.

After treatment is started, glucose, electrolyte, and phosphate concentrations should be measured every 2 hours until the [HCO_3] reaches ~15 mEq/L; at this time, sampling every 4 hours becomes appropriate. If phosphate levels are elevated, calcium and magnesium concentrations in serum should also be measured. The BUN or creatinine test is repeated after the patient is adequately rehydrated.

Fluid Administration. Solutions containing dextrose should not be used initially because the additional glucose could not be utilized and would simply increase the degree of hyperglycemia. Since an occasional patient with DKA also has lactic acidosis (as described later), most diabetologists also avoid the use of solutions containing lactate. The controversy surrounding fluid administration involves the osmolality of the saline solution that should be used.

The patient experiencing DKA has two separate problems that are specifically treated by fluid administration. One is the hyperosmolar state of the circulation (secondary to hypotonic fluid losses) and the other is intravascular volume depletion. The first problem should be treated with hypoosmolal solutions, and the second requires saline to replenish the plasma volume. The argument against using a hypoosmolal solution (usually one-half normal or 0.45% saline) as the initial fluid replacement in DKA is that it will not reverse intravascular volume depletion as rapidly as will normal saline, and vital organs may continue to be underperfused for a longer period. On the other hand, the argument against the use of normal or isotonic (0.9%) saline as the initial fluid is its hyperosmolality (308 mOsm/kg) compared with normal plasma osmolality (285 mOsm/kg). Proponents of the use of normal saline point out that plasma osmolality in DKA is most often >310 mOsm/kg, and, therefore, a hyperosmolal solution is not really being infused. However, potassium and its anion (20 to 40 mEq of each) are often added to the first bottle (as described later) so that the osmolality is increased to 348 or 388 mOsm/kg. The need to reduce the plasma osmolality in DKA (and the possible danger of increasing it) is represented by the inverse relation between the patient's level of consciousness and plasma osmolality, as depicted in Figure 6-4.

Given these considerations, I use normal saline when intravascular volume depletion is profound and 0.45% saline when plasma volume contraction is more moderate. The two clinical signs of intravascular volume depletion (an orthostatic fall in systolic pressure of 20 mm Hg or greater and decreased neck-vein filling from below) are very helpful in making this clinical distinction. As long as the patient shows orthostatic changes, normal saline is the preferred solution. When the blood pressure can be maintained while the patient is sitting or standing but neck-vein filling is still low, the administration of 0.45% saline can be begun. An exception is a case in which the serum [Na] is <130 mEq/L; in this instance, the use of 0.9% saline is continued. When the neck veins fill appropriately, the patient is rehydrated, and further administration of iv fluid is unnecessary (unless, for some reason, oral intake is not feasible, in which case maintenance fluids are required). Patients with orthostatic changes in blood pressure secondary to dysfunction of the autonomic nervous system present a problem. For these patients, I first use 1 L of 0.9% saline and then switch to 0.45% saline.

The rate of fluid administration is important. A common cause of an apparent lack of response to insulin treatment is too slow a rate of fluid replacement. (A typical situation might involve an infusion rate of 200 to 300 ml per hour and glucose concentrations that remain within 50 mg/100 ml of their initial level for several hours.) It has even been suggested that insulin has little, if any, effect on hyperglycemia and that the reduced glucose concentrations are second-ary to rehydration, which results in urinary disposal of the excess glucose (6). One liter of fluid per hour should be given for at least the first 2 hours and even longer if orthostatic changes are noted. (The amount of fluid deficit shown in Figure 6-2 should be kept in mind. As the signs of intravascular volume depletion abate, the rate of fluid administration can be decreased appropriately, usually to 500 or 600 ml per hour. Intravenous administration of saline is usually continued until the intravascular volume has been fully restored, an event that is signified by normal filling of the neck veins.

Because it takes longer to correct acidosis than to correct hyperglycemia, it is almost always necessary to add dextrose to the fluids being administered at some point during treatment. When glucose concentrations have fallen to $\sim$250 mg/100 ml, 5% dextrose should be added to the infusion. The average decrement in glucose concentrations is $\sim$100 mg/100 ml per hour. Therefore, the time at which dextrose is needed can often be estimated if this rate of fall in glucose level can be documented during the early phase of treatment. Since the osmolality of 5% dextrose in water is 277 mOsm/kg, the appropriate fluid for infusion is 5% dextrose-0.45% saline. By the time dextrose is needed, most patients have been rehydrated to the point at which 0.45% saline is appropriate. However, if intravascular volume depletion is still severe, a 5% dextrose-0.9% saline solution should be used. The hyperosmolality of the infusate decreases appreciably as glucose is metabolized or excreted and leaves the vascular space.

Insulin Treatment. Although the efficacy of low doses of insulin in the treatment of DKA has been reported sporadically over the past 50 years, until recently, most authorities have recommended administration of high doses at frequent intervals. In 1974, three papers (7-9) stressed again the ease and effectiveness of using small amounts of insulin to reverse DKA. Soon thereafter, a direct comparison of high- and low-dose insulin was made (10). In the study depicted in Figure 6-6, the rate of fall of glucose concentrations was not significantly different in any period during the first 7 hours of therapy. Although the initial decrement in ketone bodies was delayed in patients receiving low-dose insulin, there was no difference between the two groups of patients by 7 hours. In several other direct comparisons of low- and high-dose insulin, no difference in the response of ketone bodies was detected (11, 12). Furthermore, patients treated with low doses of insulin had less hypoglycemia and hypokalemia than those given the higher "conventional" amounts (10-13).

These reports, however, were not universally accepted, and doubts were raised concerning the effectiveness of low-dose insulin treatment in patients with severe DKA—i.e., those presenting in coma (14). A recent report, however,

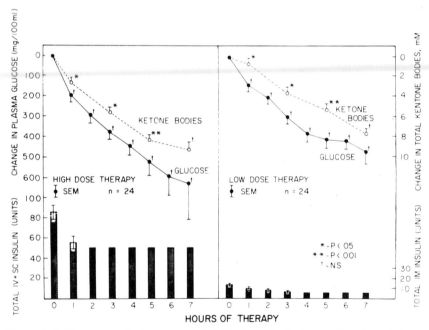

Figure 6-6. Response of glucose and total ketone body (sum of acetoacetate and β-hydroxybutyrate) concentrations to high- and low-dose insulin in patients with DKA. The amounts of insulin given are depicted at the bottom of the figure. Low-dose insulin was injected im, whereas the administration of high-dose insulin was split between the iv and sc routes. NS, not significant. (Reprinted with permission from Kitabchi AE, Ayyagari V, Guerra SMO, and Medical House Staff: The efficacy of low-dose versus conventional therapy of insulin for treatment of diabetic ketoacidosis. Ann Intern Med 84:633-638, 1976.)

compared the response to low-dose insulin therapy and that to high-dose therapy in comatose or stuporous patients (15). No differences were found in the rate of decrement of glucose concentrations, the control of acidosis, or the time elapsed before the patient became mentally alert.

Additional comparisons have demonstrated that the route of administration of low doses of insulin has little influence on the patient's response (16). In the study depicted in Figure 6-7, the group receiving iv insulin had a more rapid fall in concentrations of glucose and ketone bodies for the first 2 hours only. In other studies, a loading dose of insulin was used in some patients (7, 9-11) but not in others (8, 11-13). This loading dose seemed to have little effect, perhaps because the initial glucose response may be largely dependent on rehydration, as was discussed earlier.

Based on these data, I treat all patients who are experiencing DKA with a low-dose iv infusion of regular insulin. In order to simplify the protocol, I do not use a loading dose since there is no clinical evidence that it is necessary. I use the iv route of administration in order to minimize the trauma of repeated injections for the patient. The initial dose is 5 U per hour. A solution of 0.2 U/ml is prepared by addition of 100 U (1.0 ml of U-100 regular insulin) to 500 ml of 0.9% saline. Although insulin is adsorbed to the glass bottle and plastic

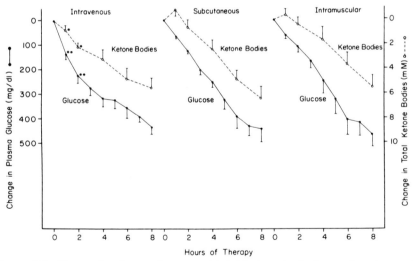

Figure 6-7. Change in plasma glucose and total ketone body (sum of acetoacetate and β-hydroxybutyrate) concentrations after iv, sc, or im administration of low-dose insulin. There were 15 patients in each group. *$P < .05$, iv versus sc and im; **$P < .01$, iv versus sc and im. Remaining periods are not significant in the three groups. (Reprinted with permission of the *New England Journal of Medicine* from Fisher JN, Shahshahani MN, Kitabchi AE: Diabetic Ketoacidosis: low-dose insulin therapy by various routes. N Engl J Med 297:238–241, 1977.)

tubing, it is not necessary to add albumin to this solution. Rather, to avoid the expense and time wasted in waiting for albumin to arrive from the pharmacy, 50 to 100 ml may simply be discarded into the sink (after the tubing is attached to the bottle). This procedure will saturate the adsorption sites, and the appropriate amount of insulin will be delivered to the patient (17). In our hospital, the insulin solution is administered via an infusion pump (IVAC 530/531) at a rate of 25 ml per hour (0.2 U/ml × 25 ml per hour = 5 U per hour). The insulin is either "piggybacked" onto the iv line delivering the rehydration fluid or administered via a separate vein. We avoid simply adding the insulin to the iv fluids because, as the rate of administration of these fluids changes, either the amount of insulin delivered will also change or new solutions with different insulin concentrations will have to be prepared. It is much simpler to control the rate of insulin delivery separately.

In most patients, this rate of insulin administration (5 U per hour) is effective. However, if the glucose concentration does not decrease by 10% from its initial level after 2 hours of administration at this rate (and if fluid replacement is adequate, as described earlier), the infusion rate of insulin should be doubled to 10 U per hour. This step is necessary in only a minority of cases and seems to be more commonly required (as expected) in obese and infected patients. When an occasional patient still does not respond and the glucose level fails to decrease by 10% from the initial level, the infusion rate should be doubled again (to 20 U per hour) at 4 hours. In fact, the infusion rate should be doubled every 2 hours until the patient starts to respond with a persistent lowering of the glucose concentration. Although infusion rates above 10 U per hour will be necessary in only an occasional patient, this approach will serve to identify early those few patients with DKA who are truly insulin-resistant; thus, they will be provided with increasing amounts of insulin. The highest infusion rate in my experience was 80 U per hour; this rate was used in an obese patient with severe DKA in whom immune-mediated insulin resistance (see chapter 4) was subsequently diagnosed.

An insulin concentration of 0.2 U/ml is particularly appropriate in this form of treatment of DKA. When 5 or 10 U of insulin per hour is required, the volume of fluid delivered in addition to the rehydration fluid is small enough (25 and 50 ml per hour, respectively) to be excluded from calculations of fluid balance. Only at an infusion rate of ⩾20 U of insulin per hour (which is rarely necessary) does the amount of additional fluid (100 ml per hour) become large enough to require consideration in the overall fluid balance. Conversely, after the metabolic derangements of DKA have mostly been reversed, patients often require infusion of insulin at a slower rate (1 to 3 U per hour) until the appropriate time for administration of intermediate-acting insulin (as described in the following paragraph). At a concentration of insulin of 0.2 U/ml, infusion rates of 5 to 15 ml per hour are required, and such infusions can be accurately delivered by an IVAC pump. (The possible need for these slow-rate infusions is why an infusion *pump*, rather than an infusion *controller* (IVAC 230/231), is recommended. The infusion controller has difficulty in accurately controlling infusion rates below 15 ml per hour.)

When the [HCO_3] is >18 to 20 mEq/L (however, see the following discussion of delayed return of [HCO_3] to normal) and the patient is able to drink and eat light foods, insulin infusion can be discontinued and administration of inter- mediate-acting (NPH or Lente) insulin started. It is helpful to give the first dose of intermediate-acting insulin in the morning or in the evening—i.e., at a time when the patient normally receives it. In this way, adjustments can be made in the manner described in chapter 4. Since patients recovering from DKA will probably not be eating the usual number of calories initially, the first dose of NPH insulin should be approximately two thirds of the usual amount. Patients in whom this episode is the initial manifestation of DKA should be given the usual starting doses of NPH insulin discussed in chapter 4. Although these patients will not be eating normally, these initial doses are usually lower than those that the patients eventually require and thus will not be excessive.

A question often arises concerning the interval between the discontinuation of regular insulin infusions and the administration of NPH insulin. If the patient eats at the time when NPH insulin is first administered, insulin infusion is con- tinued for 1 or 2 hours (with the interval determined by the size of the meal). This regular insulin will help dispose of the ingested calories during the 2- to 4- hour lag period before intermediate-acting insulin starts to act. On the other hand, if NPH insulin is injected when the patient is not eating, insulin infusion is stopped at the time of injection. In many patients, the regular insulin seems to exert some tissue effects for 1 or 2 hours after infusion is discontinued and thereby helps to control the glucose concentration during the lag period before NPH insulin begins to act.

In many instances, a number of hours elapse between the time that acidosis clears and the time appropriate for administration of NPH insulin (morning or evening). In this situation, insulin infusion should be continued, but at a slower rate (1 to 3 U per hour). Glucose concentrations should be measured every 4 hours, and the infusion rate should be titrated according to the patient's response. Plasma glucose levels under these circumstances will obviously depend on the rate of glucose administration. Once the patient has recovered from DKA, 5% dextrose in water should be infused at the same rate as in any other patient who is not taking oral nourishment—i.e., ~50 g of glucose during every 8-hour period, or 125 ml per hour. As just discussed, infusion of regular insulin is either discontinued at the time of injection of NPH insulin (if the patient is not eating) or continued for 1 or 2 hours (if the patient is eating). With these guidelines, the switch from insulin infusion to injection of intermediate-acting insulin after recovery from DKA is a relatively simple process.

Potassium Replacement. In considering potassium therapy, one is faced with a certain dilemma. Although the total body depletion of potassium is profound (Fig. 6-2), the heart responds to extracellular concentrations, which, as shown in Table 6-6, can be high as well as normal or low. Therefore, potassium replacement may be contraindicated initially. However, because all modes of therapy reduce the serum [K], unless the patient is anuric, potassium replacement will be required at some time (usually soon) after treatment is started.

Rehydration lowers the serum [K] in two ways. First, as the plasma volume is expanded, the [K] will fall simply through dilution. Second, an expanding intravascular volume will improve renal perfusion. Improved perfusion will increase urinary glucose excretion, and the resulting osmotic diuresis will enhance urinary potassium losses.

Insulin treatment lowers the serum [K] by three separate mechanisms. First, insulin directly stimulates the uptake of potassium by adipose tissue, muscle, and liver. Second, the entry of glucose into these tissues enhances further potassium uptake. The third mechanism is more complicated and is related to the correction of acidosis by insulin. As DKA develops and the supply of extracellular buffers becomes depleted, hydrogen ions are taken up by tissue to be buffered intracellularly. To maintain electrical neutrality, an equimolar amount of potassium leaves the cell and enters the extracellular space. This exchange helps to explain the hyperkalemia that is sometimes seen initially in DKA. Insulin corrects the acidosis by limiting the production of ketone bodies; its antilipolytic effect in adipose tissue restricts FFA generation (see chapter 2), and its hepatic effect reduces the activity of the ketogenic enzymes. With the production of fewer ketone bodies, the extracellular buffering capacity is not exceeded and begins to buffer the hydrogen ions that had gone intracellularly. The reverse exchange—intracellular hydrogen and extracellular potassium—sends potassium back into the cells and lowers the serum [K].

Although the [K] measured in the laboratory is obviously the ultimate criterion on which clinical decisions must be based, the electrocardiogram (ECG) provides a reasonable alternative in the interval before laboratory results are available. The effect of potassium on the T wave of the ECG is depicted in Figure 6-8. Hyperkalemia causes a tall, symmetrically peaked T wave, while hypokalemia is associated with low or flat T waves and the development of U waves if the [K] is low enough. The relation between the shape of the T wave and the serum [K] may vary among patients. Therefore, the actual [K] cannot be predicted by the T-wave configuration on the ECG. However, in a given patient, the changes in the T waves will be consistent and will predict corresponding changes in [K]. That is, a serum [K] of 6.0 mEq/L may be associated with abnormally tall and peaked T waves in one patient but with normal-appearing T waves in another. In both patients, however, the T wave will decrease in amplitude during treatment. By the same token, a serum [K] of 2.6 mEq/L may be associated with low T waves in one patient and flat T waves in another. Treatment (without appropriate potassium replacement) will flatten out the T waves in the first patient and will cause the appearance of U waves in the second. Thus, no matter what the actual configuration of the T wave at the beginning of treatment, the change from the initial serum [K] can be predicted by a corresponding change in the T wave.

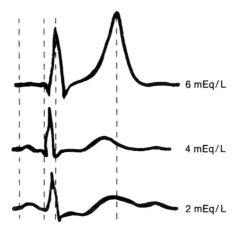

6 mEq/L

4 mEq/L

2 mEq/L

Figure 6-8. Relation between serum concentration of potassium [K] and T-wave configurations. (Reprinted with permission from *Current Concepts. Coma in the Diabetic*. The Upjohn Co., Kalamazoo, MI, 1974, p. 39.)

Since both hyperkalemia and hypokalemia have detrimental effects on the cardiovascular and respiratory systems, the goal of potassium replacement is to maintain the serum [K] within the normal range. If a patient presents with hyperkalemia, potassium replacement should be delayed until the serum [K] has fallen into the normal range. If the initial serum [K] is normal, the goal of potassium replacement should be to maintain this normal level. If hypokalemia is initially noted, potassium replacement should restore the serum [K] to normal relatively quickly; however, the patient's cardiovascular system must not be jeopardized by too-rapid administration of potassium.

For the accomplishment of these goals, the following approach is recommended. An ECG is done as soon as is feasible, and lead II, V_1 or V_2 is placed either in the patient's chart or posted at the bedside for further comparisons. Potassium replacement is not begun if the patient is anuric or if the T waves either are abnormally tall and peaked or have a high normal configuration. If the T waves are normal, 20 mEq of potassium (with an appropriate anion, which will be discussed later) is added to the first liter of replacement fluid. If the T waves are low or flat, 40 mEq of potassium is added. An ECG tracing of the same lead is taken every 1 or 2 hours, and appropriate changes in the potassium replacement regimen are made if necessary. For instance, when the abnormally tall or high normal T wave falls into a normal configuration, 20 mEq of potassium is added to the infused fluids. If the patient had a normal T wave on the previous EKG and was receiving 20 mEq of potassium/L and the current tracing shows a low or flat T wave, the potassium content of the replacement fluid should be increased to 40 mEq/L. Increases above this concentration should not be based on ECG changes alone. However, if the serum [K] is <2.5 mEq/L, the potassium content of the replacement fluid should be increased to 60 mEq/L. In the rare instance when the serum [K] is <2.0 mEq/L, 80 mEq of potassium/L can be given. These larger amounts, however, should be administered only with electrocardiographic monitoring. Furthermore, since administration of these high concentrations of potassium may be extremely irritating to the peripheral vein, use of more than one access route may be necessary or (if more than one route is impractical) a central line may need to be established.

As treatment continues, it may be possible to decrease the rate of potassium administration as the low T waves return to normal and the serum [K] rises. There is no need to replace the entire potassium deficit by the iv route. After the patient is able to eat, potassium should be supplied by the oral route. Although I do not routinely follow this recommendation, if the serum [K] remains normal, it has been suggested that patients recovering from DKA should be given several weeks of oral potassium supplementation (12 to 15 mEq three times a day with meals).

Phosphate Replacement. Although phosphorus depletion and hypophosphatemia in DKA (18) were investigated quite actively before the mid-1940s, the recognition at that time of the problems associated with potassium homeostasis in DKA lowered the level of interest in phosphorus metabolism. Ditzel and Standl (19) have recently reemphasized the profound hypophosphatemia that accompanies the treatment of DKA (Fig. 6-9) and have pointed out its possible consequences. A discussion of the clinical ramifications requires an understanding of red blood cell (RBC) metabolism and its relation to cell function—i.e., delivery of oxygen to the tissues.

The oxygen-hemoglobin dissociation curve is shown in Figure 6-10, which depicts the relation between the partial pressure of oxygen and the percentage saturation of hemoglobin. This sigmoidal curve reflects the affinity of hemoglobin for oxygen as the partial pressure of the gas changes. It is important to recognize the *inverse* relation between the delivery of oxygen to tissues and the affinity of oxygen for hemoglobin. That is, when the affinity of hemoglobin for oxygen is reduced, more oxygen is released to the tissues at a given oxygen tension, and vice versa. For instance, at a partial pressure or oxygen tension of 40 mm Hg, 25% of the oxygen is delivered to the tissues under normal conditions (Fig. 6-10). If the relation between oxygen tension and hemoglobin saturation is altered, changes also occur in oxygen delivery to tissues. The thin, dashed curve beneath the normal sigmoidal curve in Figure 6-10 represents the situation in which the affinity of oxygen for hemoglobin is reduced. Thus, oxygen delivery to the tissues should be increased, and, indeed, at an oxygen tension of 40 mm Hg, 40% of the oxygen is delivered to the tissues Conversely, the thin, dashed curve above the normal sigmoidal curve depicts the situation in which the affinity of oxygen for hemoglobin is increased. Under these circumstances, oxygen delivery to the tissues should decrease, and in fact, at 40 mm Hg, only 15% of the oxygen is extracted by the tissues.

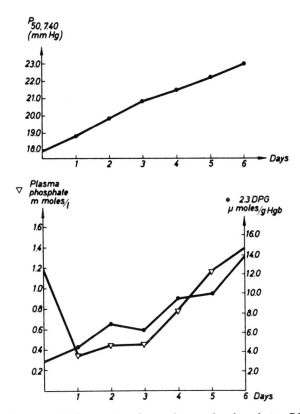

Figure 6-9. Pattern of changes in plasma inorganic phosphate, RBC 2, 3-DPG, and P_{50} (measured at a pH of 7.40) of the oxygen-hemoglobin dissociation curve in diabetic ketoacidosis. Hgb, hemoglobin. (Reprinted with permission from Ditzel J, Standl E: The problem of tissue oxygenation in diabetes mellitus. II. Evidence of disordered oxygen release from the erythrocytes of diabetics in various conditions of metabolic control. Acta Med Scand 578(Suppl):59-68, 1975.)

A convenient way to express the varying relations between oxygen tension and hemoglobin saturation is in terms of how much the curve is shifted and in which direction. When the affinity of oxygen for hemoglobin is decreased, the curve shifts to the right (and oxygen delivery to the tissues is increased). A leftward shift signifies an increased affinity of hemoglobin for oxygen (and less oxygen delivery). One can appreciate these shifts by focusing on a specific percentage saturation of oxygen and determining at which oxygen tension these shifts occur. For instance, under normal conditions, hemoglobin is 50% saturated with oxygen at a partial pressure of 26 mm Hg (Fig. 6-10). This is termed the P_{50} value or the whole-blood oxygen tension of 50% oxygen saturation. When hemoglobin has an increased affinity for oxygen, the P_{50} value is ~20mm Hg, as

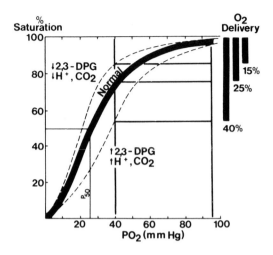

Figure 6-10. The normal oxygen-hemoglobin dissociation curve and the effects of changes of RBC 2,3-DPG, hydrogen ion, and carbon dioxide delivery of oxygen to the tissues. (Reprinted with permission from Ditzel J, Standl E: The problem of tissue oxygenation in diabetes mellitus. I. Its relation to the early functional changes in the microcirculation of diabetic subjects. Acta Med Scand 578(Suppl):49–58, 1975.)

in the example shown in Figure 6-10. Conversely, the P_{50} value is ~38 mm Hg in the circumstances of reduced affinity depicted in the figure. Thus, measurement of the P_{50} value will determine whether the curve has shifted and, if so, in which direction. This determination, in turn, furnishes direct data on the affinity of hemoglobin for oxygen and indirect information on oxygen delivery to the tissues.

Until fairly recently, it was assumed that only changes in temperature and pH can change the position of the oxygen-hemoglobin dissociation curve. For instance, acidosis shifts the curve to the right, while alkalosis shifts it to the left (Fig. 6-10). However, it was demonstrated in 1967 that the affinity of hemoglobin for oxygen could be decreased by its interaction with organic phosphates, the most important of which is 2,3-diphosphoglycerate (2,3-DPG). Approximately 60% of the organic phosphates in RBCs are in the form of 2,3-DPG; in other tissues, the concentration of this phosphate is <1% of that found in RBCs. The relation between 2,3-DPG and glycolysis in RBCs is depicted in Figure 6-11. The amount of 2,3-DPG is regulated by flow through the glycolytic pathway, which is impaired by two metabolic consequences of DKA and its treatment. Acidosis inhibits the enzyme phosphofructokinase (PFK), which slows the conversion of fructose-6-phosphate to fructose-1,6-diphosphate. This effect limits the production of the trioses, which eventually are converted into 2,3-DPG. In addition, inorganic phosphate is a cofactor for the enzyme glyceraldehyde-3-phosphate

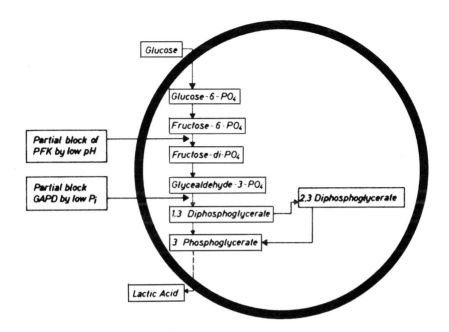

Figure 6-11. Effect of hypophosphatemia on RBC glycolysis and 2,3-DPG content. PFK, phosphofructokinase; GAPD, glyceraldehyde-3-phosphate dehydrogenase. (Reprinted with permission from Ditzel J, Standl E: The problem of tissue oxygenation in diabetes mellitus. I. Its relation to the early functional changes in the microcirculation of diabetic subjects. Acta Med Scand 578[Suppl]:49–58, 1975.)

dehydrogenase (GAPD), which is necessary for the production of the immediate precursor of 2,3-DPG. Therefore, the hypophosphatemia that usually occurs during the treatment of DKA (unless phosphate is replaced) will severely depress 2,3-DPG levels in RBCs, (Fig. 6-11).

What effect will these changes have on the oxygen-hemoglobin dissociation curve and oxygen delivery to tissues? Before treatment, the level of 2,3-DPG in RBCs is low; thus, the curve will shift to the left and oxygen delivery to the tissues will be impaired (Fig. 6-10). The acidosis, on the other hand, will cause the curve to shift to the right and oxygen delivery to the tissues will tend to increase. However, the acidosis is usually corrected within 6 to 12 hours, whereas reduced 2,3-DPG in RBCs persists for days, especially if phosphate is not replaced (Fig. 6-9). Thus, the impairment of oxygen delivery to the tissues (exemplified by a decreased P_{50} value) will be intensified shortly after institution of treatment and may persist for long periods. Such a course in one patient is depicted in Figure 6-9. Ditzel and Standl (19) have shown high correlation among serum phosphate concentration, levels of 2,3-DPG in RBCs, and P_{50} values in patients recovering from DKA.

This, then, is the argument for phosphate replacement. An increase in serum phosphate concentrations should cause an increase in 2,3-DPG levels in RBCs, and this change, in turn, will increase P_{50} values and enhance oxygen delivery to tissues. In addition, there are anecdotal reports that patients feel better more quickly if they receive phosphate. The issue is not clear-cut, however. Other workers (20, 21) have documented reduced levels of serum phosphate and RBC 2,3-DPG in patients undergoing treatment for DKA; although phosphate replacement increased RBC 2,3-DPG levels over those in controls not receiving phosphate, P_{50} values in the two groups did not differ (21). Furthermore, phosphate infusions are contraindicated for patients with renal insufficiency, and initially it is difficult to ascertain whether increased creatinine and BUN levels represent prerenal azotemia or true renal failure. Overly zealous administration of phosphate has been reported to cause symptomatic hypocalcemia (22, 23), although hypocalcemia does not routinely develop (21). Finally, since the prognosis in DKA is usually very good and the causes of death do not seem to be related to hypophosphatemia, it can be argued that the cost-benefit ratio does not favor phosphate replacement.

A comparison of regimens for potassium replacement—chloride alone, phosphate alone, or an equal mixture of the two as the anion—is shown in Figure 6-12. When KCl was given alone, the level of ionized calcium in plasma fell by only 7% but the level of plasma phosphate decreased by 26%. If phosphate was the anion used, the concentration of calcium dropped by 22% while that of phosphate increased slightly. Administration of an equal amount of phosphate and choloride yielded a 4% decrease in the plasma concentration of ionized calcium and a 39% increase in the plasma phosphate level. Although the numbers of patients studied in each group were small, the data seemed to indicate that the use of chloride and phosphate together avoided significant decreases in plasma calcium while correcting phosphate deficits.

On the basis of all of these considerations, I use the following approach. Potassium is replaced with the chloride anion unless the serum phosphate concentrations are initially in the low or the low normal range. In that case, half of the potassium is given as the chloride and half as the phosphate salt. In addition, I use phosphate for one half of the potassium replacement as soon as an initially high serum level drops into the normal range because of the likelihood of a continued fall unless phosphate is given. In any event, continued monitoring of serum phosphate levels is important in the prevention of unexpected hyperphosphatemia or very low values (<1.0 mg/100 ml), which can cause muscle weakness, respiratory failure, hemolytic anemia, hemorrhage, rhabdomyolysis, and neurologic dysfunction.

Inorganic phosphate exists in serum in two valence states, HPO_4^{2-} and $H_2PO_4^-$; the proportions vary with the pH. Therefore, the number of milliequivalents in 1 mmol of phosphate is not constant. In contrast, the amount of phosphate as expressed in millimoles does not vary, so phosphate replacement should be calculated in millimoles (24). Although potassium phosphate for injection is

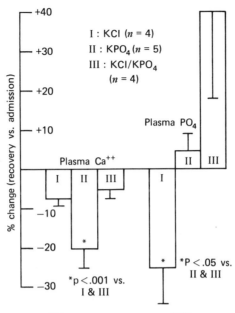

Values are means + or − SEM

Figure 6-12. Effect of replacement of potassium with chloride and/or phosphate as the anion on changes in plasma calcium (Ca^{++}) and phosphate (PO_4). (Reprinted with permission from Kappy MS, Plotnick LP, Aziz S: Effect of intravenous phosphate-containing fluids on plasma ionized calcium and phosphate in diabetic ketoacidosis. Clin Res 28:114, 1980.)

a mixture of two salts, KH_2PO_4 and K_2HPO_4, the important consideration is the total amount of phosphate being administered. Table 6-7 lists the concentrations of both phosphate (mmol/ml) and potassium (mEq/ml) in the three commercial preparations available. For a given amount of potassium replacement, the amount of phosphate administered will vary appreciably according to the preparation used. The physician needs to be aware of these differences.

Bicarbonate Therapy. The use of bicarbonate is another controversial area in the treatment of DKA. In my view, most patients experiencing DKA do not require and therefore should not receive bicarbonate therapy. Although many standard texts state that a pH of <7.0 is incompatible with life (or words to that effect), two important caveats must be issued. First, this assertion applies to a chronic situation, while DKA is an acute acidosis. Second, and probably more important, the acid-base status of the cerebrospinal fluid (CSF), not the pH of the systemic circulation, determines brain function (25). In contrast to respiratory acidosis, in which systemic pH and that of CSF fall in parallel (25), the pH of CSF is much higher than the systemic pH in DKA (26) for reasons that will be discussed later.

Table 6-7. Amounts of Potassium (K) and Phosphate (PO$_4$) in Commercial Preparations of Potassium Phosphates for Injection

Pharmaceutical Company	K (mEq/ml)	PO$_4$ (mmol/ml)	PO$_4$/K
Abbott	4.4	3.0	0.68
McGaw	2.0	1.1	0.55
Baxter	3.0	2.2	0.73

There are several cogent arguments against the administration of bicarbonate to patients with DKA. First, endogenous bicarbonate is generated during insulin treatment. Second, since bicarbonate administration usually reverses systemic acidosis relatively quickly, hypokalemia becomes much greater a problem. Indeed, before the relation between bicarbonate therapy and hypokalemia was recognized, a number of patients treated with alkali died from cardiac arrhythmias. Third, administration of bicarbonate enhances the paradoxical acidosis of the CSF that develops during the treatment of DKA. The mechanism of enhancement can be comprehended by means of the following arrangement of the Henderson-Hassalbach equation, which expresses the relation among pH, [HCO$_3$], and the partial pressure of carbon dioxide (pCO$_2$):

$$pH \, \alpha \, \frac{[HCO_3]}{pCO_2} \tag{1}$$

Because CO$_2$ crosses freely from blood to CSF and vice versa, it quickly equilibrates between the two. Bicarbonate, on the other hand, diffuses much more slowly across the blood-brain barrier; an active transport process has even been suggested (25). The difference between the rate of diffusion of CO$_2$ and that of bicarbonate explains both the higher pH of the CSF in DKA and the paradoxical fall of the pH of CSF during treatment. In the untreated state, as the [HCO$_3$] falls, it is lower in the systemic circulation than in the CSF because of the delayed attainment of equilibrium. Because CO$_2$, on the other hand, equilibrates rapidly between the blood and CSF, CO$_2$ tension is equal on both sides of the blood-brain barrier. As can be appreciated from the equation just cited, the pH will be higher in the CSF than in the plasma. As treatment progresses, both the pCO$_2$ and the [HCO$_3$] will increase in the plasma. In the CSF, the increase in the [HCO$_3$] will be delayed compared with that in the pCO$_2$, so that the pH actually falls. Bicarbonate therapy enhances this decrease in the pH of CSF (26, 27). Since mental status correlates with the pH of CSF rather than with systemic pH (25), bicarbonate therapy could be deleterious.

In several circumstances, however, I do add bicarbonate to the therapeutic regimen. Occasionally, lactic acidosis occurs in association with DKA. In such an instance, an anion gap acidosis persists after ketone bodies have almost disappeared from plasma. Under normal circumstances, the sum of the [Na] and the [K] is ~12 to 15 mEq/L greater than the sum of the [HCO_3] and the chloride concentration. This anion gap is a reflection of the unmeasured anions, such as phosphates, sulfates, proteins, and small amounts of lactate and ketone bodies. During DKA, the anion gap is much greater than 12 to 15 mEq/L and is caused by the accumulation of ketone bodies. As the ketone bodies are cleared and the acidosis is reversed, the anion gap returns to normal. If the ketone bodies disappear but acidosis persists, it is important to calculate the anion gap. If the anion gap remains increased, the unmeasured anions involved are probably lactate and the patient has lactic acidosis. This condition is potentially very serious and must be treated vigorously with bicarbonate therapy. However, since phenformin (DBI-TD) has been banned by the FDA, the incidence of lactic acidosis (with or without DKA) has decreased markedly.

Another circumstance in which bicarbonate therapy should be used is in severe acidosis (pH <7.2) and shock that is unresponsive to intravascular volume repletion. If rehydration with saline (which is distributed throughout the entire extracellular fluid compartment) is initially ineffective, the intravascular volume should be expanded with plasma, albumin, or even whole blood (all of which are contained within the vascular volume). If these measures do not restore the blood pressure, bicarbonate therapy is indicated. The rationale for the use of alkali under these circumstances is that severe, prolonged acidosis may impair left ventricular contractility, whereas a more rapid reversal of acidosis may improve cardiac output.

Bicarbonate therapy should also be considered in patients who are very tired from hyperventilating over a long period. More rapid reversal of acidosis will decrease their ventilatory effort and allow them to rest more comfortably. Finally, if the [HCO_3] remains below 10 mEq/L and the pH is <7.2 at 4 hours after the initiation of treatment, bicarbonate therapy may also be considered. However, if the patient is alert and not hypotensive, I usually do not use bicarbonate therapy at this time but rather reevaluate the situation at 6 hours.

If bicarbonate therapy is to be used to treat DKA, it should *never* be given in the form of an iv bolus. Death secondary to hypokalemia has occurred under these circumstances, even when the [K] was elevated at the time of administration. Bicarbonate should be added to 0.45% saline and infused into the patient over at least a 1-hour period. An ampule of $NaHCO_3$ contains 44 mEq of Na and HCO_3 each, or a total of 88 mEq. Therefore, the osmolality of a solution containing 1 ampule of $NaHCO_3$ in 1 L of 0.45% saline is 242 mOsm/kg. Addition of 20 mEq of potassium plus 20 mEq of an appropriate anion will yield a true isotonic solution (282 mOsm/kg). If more potassium replacement is indicated (and potassium administration should be generous when bicarbonate is infused), 40 mEq of potassium plus 40 mEq of appropriate anions should be added. The addition of these amounts of $NaHCO_3$ and potassium plus its anion to 0.45% saline gives a solution with an osmolality of 322 mOsm/kg (which is lower than that of isotonic saline plus potassium replacement). In the unusual situation where more alkali therapy is appropriate (for instance, if a patient is in shock with a profound acidosis), addition of 2 ampules of $NaHCO_3$ plus 40 mEq of potassium and 40 mEq of its anion to 1 L of *distilled water* gives a solution containing 256 mOsm/kg. Finally, in the rare instance in which potassium replacement is not indicated (because of hyperkalemia and/or anuria), addition of 2 ampules of $NaHCO_3$ to 1 L of 0.45% saline yields a solution containing 330 mOsm/kg.

Thus, various combinations of saline, bicarbonate, and potassium can be given, with the choice depending on the clinical situation. The following points should be emphasized: (*a*) Do not give boluses of bicarbonate. (*b*) Infuse $NaHCO_3$ over a period of hours. (*c*) Include generous amounts of potassium. (*d*) Use solutions with osmolalities of ~250 to 330 mOsm/kg. I do not attempt to calculate the amount of alkali that should be given in order to replenish the bicarbonate pool. Instead, I simply monitor the serum $[HCO_3]$ and usually discontinue bicarbonate therapy when the pH exceeds 7.30 or the $[HCO_3]$ reaches ~15 mEq/L.

Response to Therapy

Glucose concentrations fall at a rate of 75 to 100 mg/100 ml per hour in patients receiving low-dose insulin infusions for the treatment of DKA. In general, glucose levels reach 200 to 300 mg/100 ml within 4 to 5 hours. At this time, because of the continued need for insulin to treat the still-uncorrected ketosis and acidosis, dextrose must be added to the infusion in order to avoid hypoglycemia.

Ketosis is reversed in ~12 to 24 hours, although some patients may have detectable ketone bodies for several days. However, as shown in Figure 6-13, levels of β-hydroxybutyrate and acetoacetate do not change in a parallel fashion initially. As ketosis begins to be alleviated, the equilibrium between β-hydroxybutyrate and acetoacetate (which initially favors the former by a ratio of 3-1 to 5-1) shifts so that the concentration of the latter falls less rapidly (and may even increase early in treatment) than that of the former. This has important clinical ramifications if the patient's course is being monitored by the nitroprusside test for plasma ketone bodies. Since only acetoacetate is measured by this method, it may appear that the ketosis is not responding to treatment or even that it is worsening, although the total amount of ketone bodies is actually decreasing (hours 2 through 8 in Fig. 6-13).

Monitoring of the reversal of acidosis on the basis of changes in the $[HCO_3]$ may also be somewhat misleading. Frequently, the $[HCO_3]$ seems to remain low (between 12 and 18 mEq/L) after most other signs, symptoms, and biochemical abnormalities associated with DKA have markedly improved. If the pH is measured at this time, it is frequently >7.3, while both the $[HCO_3]$ and the pCO_2 are low (28). (The anion gap is usually normal, with chloride ion replacing the ketone bodies.) Thus, the metabolic acidosis has been fully compensated at this point by a respiratory alkalosis (see equation 1). Indeed, if patients are observed closely, deep respirations will be noted even though tachypnea is frequently

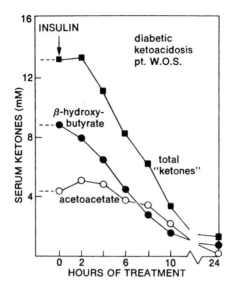

Figure 6-13. Response of serum ketone bodies to treatment in DKA. See text for discussion. (Reprinted with permission from *Current Concepts. Coma in the Diabetic.* The Upjohn Co., Kalamazoo, MI, 1974, p. 16.)

absent. This explains the discrepancy between the time when the pH returns to >7.3 (8 to 9 hours) and that when the [HCO_3] returns to normal (14 to 24 hours).

Full replacement of total body water may require 1 or 2 days and obviously can be completed by the oral route. Full repletion of intracellular electrolytes can take up to 10 days. Nitrogen balance may require several weeks to return to normal.

Mortality in DKA has been reported to be between 3% and 30%, although the more recent figures have been between 5% and 10%. No single factor seems to predict which patients will do poorly. The presence of a complicating condition is often associated with a poor outcome. Age and the duration and degree of unconsciousness have also been cited as relevant factors. The severity of hyperglycemia or acidosis does not seem to be of prognostic importance. Deaths are usually the results of infections, arterial thrombosis, or unrelenting shock (6). Since infection leads to death in only 2% of patients with DKA, routine antibiotic coverage is not indicated. On the other hand, a thorough evaluation for a source of infection is mandatory in every patient with DKA.

Death secondary to arterial thrombosis has been reported to be relatively common in all published studies of patients with DKA. The site may be ubiquitous and can involve any of the following arteries: coronary, carotid, mesenteric, iliac, renal, splenic, or pancreaticoduodenal. The clinical manifestations usually become apparent late in the course of treatment or even after recovery from DKA.

It has been suggested recently that the treatment itself may trigger a number of phenomena that increase the propensity of the patient with DKA to develop vascular thromboses.

Hypotension, azotemia, and oliguria leading to anuria as a result of severe intravascular volume depletion in combination with hyperosmolality are often associated with a poor prognosis (29). Like vascular thrombosis, irreversible shock frequently develops during the course of treatment. Thus, vigorous rehydration at the beginning of treatment may be helpful. Decreased cardiac output secondary to severe prolonged acidosis may also contribute to a poor outcome through impairment of left ventricular function. If acidosis does not improve in this situation, treatment with bicarbonate may be helpful. However, preexisting heart disease may also be a major and untreatable factor.

Although it is fortunately a rare cause of death, cerebral edema is particularly distressing. It most often occurs in patients less than 25 years of age, and, like vascular thromboses and shock, it occurs during the course of treatment. The usual setting is one in which the patient is showing marked clinical and biochemical improvement but then lapses back into a fatal coma while the metabolic abnormalities return completely to normal. At autopsy, cerebral edema is found. Some authorities (6) have recommended funduscopic examination every hour in patients under the age of 45 years. If the level of consciousness decreases during treatment or if edema or erythema of the optic disk develops, a lumbar puncture is performed. If the CSF pressure is increased in this situation, these authorities recommend treatment with glucocorticoids or mannitol and neurosurgical consultation. Although clinically evident cerebral edema is usually fatal, rapid recognition and treatment of this dreaded complication may save some patients.

Most patients undergoing treatment for DKA probably go through a stage of mild cerebral edema. In one study (30), CSF pressures were monitored continuously in 5 patients during the first 10 hours of therapy. In 4 of the 5 patients, the CSF pressure was normal before initiation of treatment but became elevated during the course of therapy. In the fifth patient, the CSF pressure was elevated initially and increased even further during treatment. The highest pressure recorded was 600 mm H_2O, and 4 of the 5 patients had sustained elevations in pressure for at least 2 hours. All of these patients were alert on admission but became drowsy during the interval when CSF pressure was above normal. One patient developed slurred speech and became semistuporous 3 hours after treatment was begun. Another patient became incoherent and agitated at 4 hours and semistuporous at 6 hours.

More recently, cerebral edema during the treatment of DKA with low-dose insulin infusions was evaluated by means of serial repeat echoencephalograms (31). A decrease in the width of the lateral ventricles was taken as an indication of cerebral edema. Nine of 11 patients showed significant decreases in lateral ventricle size at some time during the 15-hour period after treatment was started. By 20 hours, the size of the lateral ventricle had returned to normal in all patients. In this study, no patient exhibited clinical evidence of cerebral edema.

Why an occasional, relatively young patient develops fatal cerebral edema and how this unfortunate outcome can be prevented are unknown. The current explanation for the increased intracranial pressure during treatment of DKA involves the rate of fall of the plasma glucose concentration. Experiments in animals have demonstrated that a rapid drop of the plasma glucose concentration after a 4-hour period of marked hyperglycemia causes cerebral edema. The mechanism involved may be the delay in attainment of equilibrium between glucose levels in CSF and those in plasma. Glucose concentrations fall more rapidly in the blood than in the CSF during treatment. This discrepancy results in a less marked decrease in CSF osmolality than in plasma osmolality, so that fluid enters the CSF compartment. Since expansion of this compartment is limited by the cranium, increased pressure and cerebral edema develop. Greater decrements in glucose concentrations and osmolalities in plasma than in the CSF have been documented in patients undergoing treatment with standard high-dose insulin regimens (26, 27). These data from studies in animals and humans suggest that a more gradual lowering of plasma glucose levels may be helpful, and they support the use of low-dose insulin infusions with dextrose supplementation when plasma glucose concentrations reach ~250 mg/100 ml.

Hyposmolar Nonketotic Coma

Although hyperosmolar nonketotic coma (HNKC) was first described prior to 1900 and sporadic cases were reported in the first half of this century, this syndrome has received ever-increasing attention since 1957. The "pure" syndrome is characterized by severe hyperglycemia (glucose levels of >800 mg/100 ml) and hyperosmolality (>350 mOsm/kg) and by profound intravascular volume depletion in the absence of "significant" ketosis (usually defined as a nitroprusside reaction of ≥2+ in a 1:1 dilution of plasma). Often the plasma glucose values are even higher (ranging to >2,000 mg/100 ml), as is the hyperosmolality (sometimes >400 mOsm/kg). A depressed sensorium is frequently encountered, especially if the plasma osmolality is >350 mOsm/kg. The affected patients are usually older than those presenting with DKA. In practice, patients are often encountered who have these characteristics but who are also mildly ketotic and acidotic. Indeed, DKA and HNKC represent two ends of a continuous spectrum, and many patients have various aspects of each syndrome. As might be expected, the pathogenesis, clinical presentation, and treatment of HNKC are similar to those of DKA in most respects. There are, however, several important exceptions. The following discussion will briefly mention the similarities between the two conditions but will emphasize the differences.

Pathophysiology

As outlined in Figure 6-1, the lack of effective insulin in carbohydrate and protein metabolism leads to intravascular volume depletion ("dehydration") and electrolyte depletion. The unregulated lipolysis that results from a lack of effective insulin in fat metabolism causes ketosis and the resultant acidosis. If lipolysis were not increased, ketosis and acidosis would not ensue and the patient would manifest only depletion of intravascular volume and electrolytes. Since, in fact, only the latter two manifestations characterize patients in HNKC, the relatively normal lipolysis in this setting must be explained.

Two explanations have been offered. Since the regulation of lipolysis is so sensitive to insulin (see chapter 2), the levels of insulin in patients in HNKC may be sufficient to control this pathway but not to prevent catabolism in the carbohydrate and protein pathways. In general, however, plasma insulin concentrations have been similar in DKA and in HNKC when measured. On the other hand, FFA levels are generally lower in HNKC than in DKA, a finding that reinforces the view that lipolysis is better controlled in HNKC. Recent in vitro data suggest that hyperosmolality itself inhibits lipolysis. Thus, the combination of some effective insulin acting in an environment of greatly increased osmolality may account for the lack of ketosis and subsequent acidosis.

Losses

The losses sustained in DKA and depicted in Figure 6-2 are often exceeded in patients in HNKC. In the absence of ketosis and acidosis, which cause severe gastrointestinal symptoms in patients with DKA and force them to seek medical attention within 1 or 2 days, many patients tolerate polyuria and polydipsia for weeks, thus losing great quantities of fluid and electrolytes. In one series of 37 episodes of HNKC (32), the following were administered: 11.9 L of fluid, of which 9.1 L was retained; 512 mEq of sodium, of which 407 mEq was retained; and 215 mEq of potassium, of which 137 mEq was retained. Most of the patients in this series were found to have some degree of renal insufficiency after recovery, a factor that might explain why they required lower amounts of potassium than are needed in DKA.

Causes

Conditions associated with the onset of HNKC are listed in Table 6-8. The mechanism by which these conditions induce HNKC is evident in most, but not all, cases. Hyperosmolar nonketotic coma can be the initial manifestation of diabetes mellitus in older patients. Infection is well known to cause insulin antagonism. Inflammation or tumors of the pancreas probably reduce insulin secretion. The potent insulin antagonism of growth hormone and glucocorticoids explains the association of HNKC with acromegaly and Cushing's syndrome, respectively.

Table 6-8. Conditions Associated with the Onset of HNKC

Diseases	Drugs	Miscellaneous
Diabetes mellitus[a]	Diuretic (potassium-depleting)	Burns
Infections	Diazoxide	Hemodialysis
Acute pancreatitis	Dephenylhydantoin	Peritoneal dialysis
Pancreatic carcinoma	Propranolol	Hypothermia
Acromegaly	Glucocorticoids	Heat stroke
Cushing's syndrome	Hypertonic $NaHCO_3$	
Thyrotoxicosis		
Subdural hematoma		
Uremia (with vomiting)		

[a]Initial manifestation without known precipitating cause.

The relation between HNKC and thyrotoxicosis, subdural hematoma, and uremia associated with vomiting is not readily apparent.

The mechanism by which the drugs listed in Table 6-8 cause HNKC is clear. Diazoxide and diphenylhydantoin (Dilantin) directly inhibit insulin secretion, as does hypokalemia. Propranolol, a β-adrenergic blocker, inhibits lipolysis. As was just mentioned, glucocorticoids are potent insulin antagonists. Finally, HNKC has been found to occur in patients treated for cardiac arrest with 7.5% $NaHCO_3$. The injection of a hypertonic solution in a situation of overwhelming stress (in which levels of all of the contrainsulin hormones were no doubt extremely elevated) would explain this association.

Several of the miscellaneous conditions listed in Table 6-8 would be expected to cause stress-related secretion of growth hormone, catecholamines, cortisol, and glucagon. These conditions include extensive burns, hypothermia, and heat stroke. Hyperosmolar nonketotic coma in burned patients is often associated with high carbohydrate intake, either orally or iv. Dialysis patients have usually received hypertonic glucose or sorbitol in the dialysate.

Symptoms

Except for "dyspnea," all of the symptoms of DKA listed in Table 6-2 also apply to HNKC. Polyuria and polydipsia are very intense for 3 to 7 days before treatment and have often been present for several weeks. Although less prevalent than in DKA, abdominal pain, nausea, and vomiting do occur in HNKC. However, the usual reason for which patients in HNKC are brought to a medical facility is their lack of responsiveness. Many also present with focal neurologic symptoms, which will be discussed in more detail in the next section.

Signs

Many of the signs of DKA (Table 6-3) do not apply to HNKC. Patients in HNKC often have an elevated temperature. Since marked ketosis and acidosis are not present, hyperpnea, acetone breath, and signs of an "acute abdomen" are lacking. Intravascular volume depletion is usually profound, and the related signs are therefore uniformly present.

The neurologic picture in HNKC differs dramatically from that in DKA in many patients. Although a depressed sensorium is common to both syndromes, focal neurologic signs and symptoms are frequently noted in patients in HNKC (33, 34). Seizures, often resistant to anticonvulsant therapy, are frequent (occurring in 10% to 15% of patients), and hallucinations and psychic disturbances are not uncommon. Focal dysfunctions include aphasia, homonymous hemianopsia, hemiparesis, hemisensory defects, unilateral hyperreflexia, and unilateral Babinski signs; all of these focal dysfunctions may be postictal but may also occur independently of seizures. Abnormal muscle tone, tonic eye deviations, and nystagmus are less frequent. Hyperpnea (in the absence of acidosis) is common and probably reflects stimulation of the medullary centers by non-acid-base parameters. In contrast to the Kussmaul respirations of DKA, in which both inspiratory and expiratory phases are increased, the hyperpnea of HNKC is reported to affect the expiratory phase only. Hyperthermia is a terminal event. Signs of nuchal rigidity have been reported in patients in HNKC even though meningitis was found to be absent by means of appropriate tests. Abnormalities in electroencephalograms are seen and are unaffected by treatment with anticonvulsant agents. These abnormalities disappear completely when hypotonic fluids are given.

Differential Diagnosis

As with DKA, the diagnosis of HNKC is easily made once it is considered. The usual difficulty is that only various neurologic possibilities are considered initially. Patients in HNKC are commonly admitted to the neurology or neurosurgical service, and the diagnosis of HNKC is made only when the results of routine urine and blood tests are known. This delay in the institution of appropriate treatment is partially responsible for the much poorer prognosis in HNKC than in DKA.

Initial Laboratory Values

The similarities and differences between the initial laboratory values in DKA (listed in Table 6-6) and those in HNKC should be apparent from the foregoing discussion. Glucose concentrations are generally higher in HNKC. Although the [Na] and [K] can be low, normal, or high in both syndromes, the [Na] in HNKC is more likely to be high. Serum osmolality is also higher in HNKC than in DKA. The *total* serum osmolality can be calculated as follows:

$$\text{osmolality} = 2[\text{Na} + \text{K}] + \frac{[\text{glucose}]}{18} + \frac{[\text{BUN}]}{2.8} \qquad (2)$$

In order to determine the *effective* serum osmolality, the final term is dropped from equation 2 because urea is freely distributed between the extracellular and intracellular compartments. However, the calculated *total* osmolality will correspond better with the measured serum osmolality values. Both [HCO₃] and pH values are normal in the pure syndrome of HNKC. The biochemical indices of plasma volume concentration (BUN, creatinine, hematocrit, hemoglobin, and total protein) are generally higher in HNKC because intravascular volume depletion is usually greater. Phosphate concentration, amylase levels, WBC counts, and serum enzyme changes have not been systematically reported in HNKC. The latter two values, of course, would depend on the presence of associated conditions.

Treatment

The points discussed under *General Considerations* in the treatment of DKA apply for the most part of HNKC, with several modifications. With regard to laboratory tests, if significant ketosis is absent, an initial measurement of pH is unnecessary. In the unusual event that the [HCO₃] is low (<15 mEq/L), pH can be measured. Since most patients in HNKC are relatively old and many have preexisting heart disease, monitoring of their cardiovascular status during fluid replacement is critically important. For this reason, placement of a central venous pressure line or, if possible, a right heart catheter that will measure pulmonary capillary wedge pressure should be considered in patients with a history of congestive heart failure.

The same controversy surrounding fluid administration in DKA exists in relation to HNKC. Because the correlation between plasma osmolality and depression of sensorium is even higher in HNKC (Fig. 6-14) than in DKA (Fig. 6-4), some investigators argue that hypotonic solutions should be used and plasma osmolality reduced fairly rapidly. Others point out that patients in HNKC are even more vulnerable to the effects of intravascular volume depletion than are those with DKA and thus that rehydration with 0.9% saline should take precedence. Since there are few scientific data on which to base a choice between these two philosophies, I use the same approach in both HNKC and DKA with regard to fluid administration. If intravascular volume depletion is severe, as evidenced by orthostatic changes, 0.9% saline is the basic solution used. However, if the serum [Na] is >150 mEq/L, a hypotonic solution is given regardless of intravascular volume. Once orthostatic changes have been reversed,

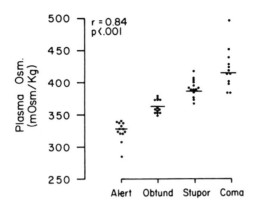

Figure 6-14. Relation between state of consciousness and measured plasma osmolality in 53 patients in HNKC. States of consciousness were defined as follows: (1) alert—the patient responds immediately and appropriately to normal stimuli; (2) obtundation—the patient is in a state of dull indifference in which increased stimulation is required to evoke a response; (3) stupor—the patient can be aroused only by vigorous and continuous stimulation; and (4) coma—the patient exhibits little or no response to stimulation. For calculation of the correlation coefficient (r), scores of 1 through 4 were given for each state of consciousness, respectively. For each group, Plasma osmolality was significantly different ($P < 0.01$) from that of the adjacent group(s). (Reprinted with permission from Arieff, AI, Caroll, H: Cerebral edema and depression of sensorium in nonketotic hyperosmolar coma. Diabetes 23:525–531, 1974.)

0.45% saline is substituted. As was just mentioned, precipitation of congestive heart failure during saline administration is all too common in patients in HNKC. Frequent monitoring of their cardiovascular status by physical examination and hemodynamic methods (if available) is extremely important to a successful outcome.

Insulin is given to patients in HNKC in the same manner as to those with DKA. When the glucose concentration falls to ~250 mg/100 ml, dextrose is added to the administered fluid. Cerebral edema is much less common in HNKC than in DKA. In the few reported cases, the symptoms began when the glucose concentration was well below 250 mg/100 ml (34).

Since patients in HNKC are not experiencing ketosis or acidosis, the glucose level is the sole biochemical endpoint. However, it will often be many hours or even a few days before these patients are able to tolerate oral intake because of their mental status and/or associated conditions. Under these circumstances, 50 g of dextrose should be administered every 8 hours, and the dose of insulin infused should be decreased appropriately (1 to 3 U per hour) on the basis of plasma glucose determinations every 4 to 6 hours. The transition from insulin infusion to sc administration of insulin is made as described for DKA.

The same considerations for potassium replacement that apply to patients with DKA are pertinent to those in HNKC, with three caveats. First, since no acidosis is involved, intracellular shifts of potassium in exchange for hydrogen ions will not occur. Secondly, because more patients in HNKC may have underlying renal disease, urinary potassium losses may be lower. Finally, bicarbonate therapy is inappropriate for patients in HNKC. All of these factors will lessen the possibility of hypokalemia. However, because patients with preexisting heart disease may be more susceptible to the effects of potassium, potassium replacement must still be monitored carefully.

Although phosphate homeostasis has not been evaluated in any detail in HNKC, it should follow a pattern similar to that seen in DKA. Since there is no acidosis to shift the oxygen-hemoglobin dissociation curve to the right initially (a change that increases oxygen delivery to the tissues), any tissue hypoxia caused by hypophosphatemia (via a decrease in levels of 2,3-DPG in RBCs, leading to a fall in the P_{50} value and a shifting of the curve to the left) will not be counterbalanced (Fig. 6-10). Tissue hypoxia leads to an increase in cardiac output that often cannot be sustained in these patients and therefore further compromises their cardiovascular status. In addition, tissue hypoxia may contribute to lactic acidosis, which has been reported in HNKC. Although these are theoretical considerations, the tenuous cardiovascular status of many patients in HNKC demands careful consideration of any factor (i.e., phosphate replacement) that may improve their prognosis. On the other hand, since many of these patients also have underlying renal disease, close monitoring of phosphate concentrations is required. The same approach for phosphate replacement in HNKC as in DKA should be used.

Prognosis

The prognosis for patients in HNKC is worse than that for those with DKA. Mortality ranging from 15% to 60% has been reported, with most values between 30% and 50%. Mortality is related largely to the age of the patients and the severity of complicating illnesses, which are either present initially or develop during treatment in the vast majority of patients. The causes of death are usually related to these associated conditions rather than to the metabolic derangements per se. Gram-negative sepsis is particularly lethal to patients in HNKC. In addition to infections, vascular events in which renal failure plays a prominent role are frequent causes of death. The neurologic symptoms may take 3 to 5 days to clear completely even though the metabolic parameters may long since have returned to normal.

Finally, in contrast to patients with DKA, who all eventually require insulin therapy after recovery, many patients who recover from HNKC can be treated with sulfonylurea agents and/or dietary therapy. These approaches are particularly effective in patients whose initial manifestation of diabetes was HNKC.

Diabetic Ketoacidosis versus Hyperosmolar Nonketotic Coma

Some of the salient features of DKA and "pure" HNKC are compared in Table 6-9. However, in clinical practice, a patient often presents with some features of each syndrome. In some patients (usually those who are relatively young), acidosis will be predominant, with a more moderate rise in serum osmolality. In others (usually older patients), serum osmolality will be markedly increased in combination with either fully compensated acidosis (i.e., a slight decrease in [HCO_3] and a normal pH) or mild acidosis (i.e., a slight decrease in pH with a moderate fall in [HCO_3]). Whatever the balance between acidosis and hyperosmolality, the approach to treatment is similar for DKA and HNKC.

Practical Summary

Diabetic Ketoacidosis

Diabetic ketoacidosis is caused by the lack of effective insulin in carbohydrate, protein, and fat metabolism. This deficiency leads (through mechanisms depicted in Fig. 6-1) to intravascular volume depletion (dehydration), electrolyte depletion, and acidosis. Losses of water and electrolytes are profound (Fig. 6-2). The symptoms and signs of DKA are listed in Tables 6-2 and 6-3, respectively. The symptom labeled "dyspnea" is actually hyperventilation (Kussmaul respirations). Although various conditions may be confused with DKA (Table 6-4), the diagnosis is simple if it is considered in the differential. Glucosuria and ketonuria are occasionally noted in patients whose clinical situation is not the result of DKA. However, if results of the nitroprusside test (Acetest) are strongly positive in a 1:1 dilution of plasma, the diagnosis of DKA is certain. The initial laboratory results in DKA are listed in Table 6-6.

In terms of the general approach to treatment of DKA, the obvious requirements are the management of the patient by only one physician, a reliable iv access for blood sampling and fluid administration, and the availability of urine samples. A situation in which a patient with DKA fails to urinate spontaneously is one of the few instances in which bladder catheterization in a diabetic is indicated. An initial urine culture should be done in order to ascertain whether the patient has a urinary tract infection since, if so, subsequent pyuria secondary to an indwelling catheter will occur. An accurately kept flow sheet (Fig. 6-4) is extremely helpful in the monitoring of patients with DKA. Placement of a nasogastric tube attached to a suction mechanism is advisable in patients in coma or with signs of gastric dilatation. Initial laboratory tests should include measurements of glucose, electrolytes, phosphate, and creatinine or BUN. A pH determination may be helpful but is not necessary. Glucose, electrolyte, and phosphate measurements should be repeated every 2 hours. Measurement of creatinine or BUN should be repeated after the patient is fully rehydrated.

Table 6-9. Comparison of Some Salient Features of DKA and HNKC

Feature	Condition	
	DKA	*HNKC*
Age of patient	Usually <40 years	Usually >40 years
Duration of symptoms	Usually <2 days	Usually >5 days
[Glucose]	Usually <800 mg/100 ml	Usually >800 mg/100 ml
[Na]	More likely to be normal or low	More likely to be normal or high
[K]	High, normal, or low	High, normal, or low
[HCO_3]	Low	Normal
Ketone bodies	At least 4+ in 1:1 dilution	<2+ in 1:1 dilution
pH	Low	Normal
Serum osmolality	Usually <350 mOsm/kg	Usually >350 mOsm/kg
Cerebral edema	Often subclinical; occasionally clinical	Not evaluated if subclinical; rarely clinical
Prognosis	5% to 10% mortality	30% to 50% mortality
Subsequent course	Insulin therapy required in virtually all cases	Insulin therapy not required in many cases

Abbreviations: [Glucose], serum concentration of glucose; [Na], serum concentration of sodium; [HCO_3], serum concentration of bicarbonate; [K], serum concentration of potassium.

The situation with regard to ketone bodies deserves special comment. The two ketone bodies circulating in the plasma, acetoacetate and β-hydroxybutyrate (Fig. 6-3), are in a state of equilibrium in which β-hydroxybutyrate predominates. Unfortunately, the semiquantitative nitroprusside test measures only acetoacetate. Although this test for plasma ketone bodies is helpful diagnostically, it should not be used to monitor the patient's response to therapy. As ketosis is alleviated, the equilibrium shifts back toward acetoacetate, and although the total amount of ketone bodies decreases, acetoacetate levels remain stable or even increase (Fig. 6-13). Thus, results in the nitroprusside test will not reflect the improving biochemical status of the patient.

The initial replacement fluid to be used depends on the degree of intravascular volume depletion. If depletion is severe, as evidenced by an orthostatic fall in systolic blood pressure of 20 mm Hg or greater, 0.9% saline should be given. When the orthostatic changes are reversed or if they are not present initially,

0.45% saline should be infused. However, regardless of intravascular volume, 0.9% saline should be used if the serum [Na] is <130 mEq/L, and 0.45% saline should be used if the serum [Na] is >150 mEq/L. The initial rate of fluid administration should be ~1 L per hour for several hours. Subsequent rates are adjusted downward on the basis of the patient's response. Saline administration should be continued until the intravascular volume returns to normal, as evidenced by filling of the neck veins *from below* to between one half and two thirds of the way to the angle of the jaw while the patient is lying in a fully horizontal position (i.e., without a pillow).

Insulin is given as a low-dose (5 U per hour) iv infusion, either "piggybacked" onto the fluid administration line or into a separate vein. A solution of 0.2 U/ml is prepared by the addition of 100 U (1.0 ml of U-100 regular insulin) to 500 ml of saline. After iv tubing has been attached to the bottle, 50 to 100 ml is discarded into a sink. This initial bolus will saturate the adsorption sites for insulin on the tubing and ensure that the proper amount is received by the patient. An infusion rate of 25 ml per hour (monitored by an appropriate pump) will deliver 5 U per hour (0.2 U/ml × 25 ml per hour).

If the patient's plasma glucose concentration does not decrease by at least 10% in 2 hours, the infusion rate should be doubled to 50 ml (10 U) per hour. In fact, the infusion rate should be repeatedly doubled every 2 hours if the glucose level fails to fall by 10% from the initial level. This approach will be necessary only occasionally and will serve to identify early the rare patients with DKA who are truly insulin-resistant; thus, they can be provided with increasing amounts of insulin.

Because glucose concentrations decrease by 75 to 100 mg/100 ml per hour, they will return to nearly normal levels before acidosis is fully reversed. Therefore, when glucose concentrations are ~250 mg/100 ml, dextrose solutions should be added and insulin administration continued at the usual rate. When acidosis clears and when the patient can tolerate oral fluids and light food, intermediate-acting insulin (NPH or Lente) should be introduced. Since it is advantageous to give NPH insulin in the morning or the evening, administration of a 5% dextrose solution at a rate of 125 ml per hour should be continued until one of those times. The rate of insulin infusion must often be decreased (to 1 to 3 U per hour); such a change depends on the glucose concentration, which should be measured every 4 hours. If the patient receives no food when NPH insulin is first given, insulin infusion is discontinued. If the patient does eat, the insulin infusion is continued for 1 or 2 hours (according to the size of the meal) to help the patient handle the meal calories during the lag period before intermediate-acting insulin takes effect. If the patient has previously taken insulin, one half to two thirds of the usual dose should be given initially, and the amount should be increased gradually as oral intake improves. If the patient has not taken insulin before, 15 U (to lean individuals) or 25 U (to infected patients or to those weighing >125% of their ideal body weight) should be given. Insulin doses are then adjusted as described in chapter 4.

The T waves of lead II, V_1, or V_2 of the ECG are helpful in monitoring the need for and the response to potassium replacement (Fig. 6-8). No potassium is added to the fluids initially administered if the patient is anuric or if the T waves are in the high-normal range or peaked. If the T waves are normal (and the patient is urinating), 20 mEq of potassium plus 20 mEq of appropriate anions are added to the fluids. If the T waves are abnormally low or if U waves are present, 40 mEq of potassium plus 40 mEq of appropriate anions are given. The criteria for potassium replacement per liter of fluid are as follows: elevated [K], no replacement; normal [K], 20 mEq of potassium; low [K], 40 mEq; [K] <2.5 mEq/L, 60 mEq. Since treatment invariably lowers the serum [K], monitoring of T-wave configuration every hour will detect the need for increased potassium replacement before laboratory results become available. For instance, a potassium replacement of 20 mEq/L of fluid, based on normal T waves, should be increased to 40 mEq if the T waves become flat during treatment.

Serum phosphate concentrations often fall to very low levels after treatment is started. Because hypophosphatemia may possibly impair the delivery of oxygen to the tissues, half of the potassium replacement should be given as the phosphate salt and the other half as the chloride salt if the serum phosphate concentration is normal or low. The entire amount of potassium is given as the chloride salt as long as the serum phosphate concentration remains elevated. The three commercial preparations of potassium phosphate for injection have different amounts of potassium and phosphate (Table 6-7).

Although bicarbonate therapy is usually not necessary in the treatment of DKA, it is required if lactic acidosis is also present. Patients experiencing severe DKA (pH <7.2) with shock unresponsive to plasma expansion should also receive bicarbonate infusions. Bicarbonate therapy may also be considered in two other circumstances: (a) if, after 4 hours of appropriate treatment, the [HCO$_3$] is <10 mEq/L or the pH is <7.2; and (b) if the patient is extremely tired from hyperventilating.

If bicarbonate is administered, it should *never* be given as an iv bolus. One ampule (44 mEq of NaHCO$_3$) added to 1 L of 0.45% saline yields a solution with an osmolality of 242 mOsm/kg. Since bicarbonate administration enhances the usual tendency for [K] to fall, 20 to 40 mEq of potassium plus a corresponding amount of anion should also be added. (The resulting osmolality will still be appropriate.) In the unusual event that more alkali therapy is necessary (for instance, if the patient has profound acidosis and is in shock), 2 ampules of NaHCO$_3$ plus 40 mEq of potassium plus appropriate anions added to 1 L of distilled water yields a solution containing 256 mOsm/kg. Bicarbonate therapy should be discontinued when the pH exceeds 7.30 or the [HCO$_3$] is ~15 mEq/L.

Mortality figures for patients with DKA have recently been reported to be 5% to 10%. Deaths have usually been from infections, arterial thrombosis, or irreversible shock. Poor prognostic signs include age and depth and duration of coma but not degree of hyperglycemia or acidosis. Cerebral edema is an uncommon cause of death that usually affects patients <25 years of age. It is heralded by deepening coma after initial neurologic improvement with a sustained return of biochemical parameters toward normal.

Hyperosmolar Nonketotic Coma

Hyperosmolar nonketotic coma is compared with DKA in Table 6-9. It usually occurs in older patients and is characterized by higher glucose concentrations and serum osmolalities than in DKA. In the "pure" syndrome of HNKC, significant ketosis (defined as a reaction of $\geqslant 2+$ in the nitroprusside test in a 1:1 dilution of plasma) is absent, and [HCO_3] and pH values are normal. In practice, however, many patients in HNKC have some ketosis and mild acidosis. In HNKC a lack of effective insulin in carbohydrate and protein metabolism leads to depletion of intravascular volume and electrolytes (Fig. 6-1), but lipolysis is not increased; therefore, ketosis and acidosis are prevented. The blunting of lipolysis in this situation may be due to the action of a small amount of insulin working in an environment of hyperosmolality. (Hyperosmolality itself will impair lipolysis in vitro.)

Conditions associated with HNKC are listed in Table 6-8. Just as DKA is often the initial manifestation of ketosis-prone diabetes (Table 6-1), ketosis-resistant diabetics can present in HNKC. The other conditions in Table 6-8 precipitate HNKC by one or more of the following mechanisms: (a) inhibition of insulin secretion; (b) enhancement of insulin antagonism either directly or by stimulation of the release of contrainsulin (stress) hormones; or (c) presentation of a hypertonic solution that the patient is unable to handle.

The symptoms of HNKC are similar to those of DKA (Table 6-2) except that "dyspnea," or hyperventilation secondary to acidosis, is not seen. In addition, nausea, vomiting, and abdominal pain, while noted in a number of patients, are often less severe than in DKA. For this reason, patients tolerate their symptoms for longer periods, and many patients are brought to medical attention only when they become unresponsive. This longer prodromal period often results in greater losses in HNKC than those sustained in DKA (Fig. 6-2).

The predominant signs in patients in HNKC are intravascular volume depletion (an orthostatic fall in systolic blood pressure and a failure of neck veins to fill from below while the patient is lying flat) and neurologic abnormalities. Although a depressed sensorium is noted in both DKA and HNKC, focal neurologic signs are also commonly seen in the latter. These signs include seizures (unresponsive to anticonvulsant therapy), hallucinations, psychic disturbances, asphasia, homonymous hemianopsia, hemiparesis, hemisensory defects, unilateral hyperreflexia, and Babinski signs. Electroencephalograms are often abnormal. Although all of these signs are reversed when the metabolic derangements are reversed, the initial (incorrect) diagnosis is often a primary cerebrovascular accident.

Treatment for HNKC is similar to that for DKA, with several modifications. Placement of a central venous line or a right heart catheter for monitoring of pulmonary capillary wedge pressure is often helpful in these older patients, many of whom have preexisting heart disease and are about to receive large quantities of saline. Since there is little or no acidosis to be treated, bicarbonate therapy is inappropriate. The biochemical endpoint for insulin treatment is the glucose concentration, which should be lowered to ~250 mg/100 ml with a low-dose insulin infusion; when this goal is reached, dextrose solutions are added, as in DKA. Techniques of fluid, potassium, and phosphate replacement in HNKC are similar to those applied in DKA; however, patients in HNKC are usually older and more susceptible to the adverse effects of such therapies.

The prognosis for patients in HNKC (30% to 50% mortality) is worse than for those with DKA (5% to 10%). The major causes of death are complicating illnesses, with infection (especially gram-negative sepsis) and cardiovascular events playing a prominent role. Unlike patients recovering from DKA, virtually all of whom require maintenance insulin therapy, many survivors of HNKC can be treated with dietary therapy either alone or in combination with sulfonylurea agents. This approach is especially effective in patients whose initial manifestation of ketosis-resistant diabetes is HNKC.

References

1. Sheldon J, Pyke DA: Severe diabetic ketosis: precoma and coma. In *Clinical Diabetes and Its Biochemical Basis*. Edited by Oakly WG, Pyke DA, Taylor KW. Blackwell Scientific Publications, Oxford, 1968, p 423

2. Munro JF, Campbell IW, McCuish AC, Duncan LJP: Euglycaemic diabetic ketoacidosis. Br Med J 2:578–580, 1973

3. Stephens JM, Sulway MJ, Watkins PJ: Relationship of blood acetoacetate and 3-hydroxybutyrate in diatetes. Diabetes 20:485–489, 1971

4. Warshaw A, Feller ER, Lee KH: On the cause of raised serum-amylase in diabetic ketoacidosis. Lancet 1:929–931, 1977

5. Vinicor F, Lehrner LM, Karn RC, Merritt AD: Hyperamylasemia in diabetic ketoacidosis: sources and significance. Ann Intern Med 91:200–204, 1979

6. Clements RS Jr, Vourganti B: Fatal diabetic ketoacidosis: major causes and approaches to their prevention. Diabetes Care 1:314–325, 1978

7. Kidson W, Casey J, Kraegen E, Lazarus L: Treatment of severe diabetes mellitus by insulin infusion. Br Med J 2:691–694, 1974

8. Page MM, Alberti KGMM, Greenwood R, et al: Treatment of diabetic coma with continuous low-dose infusion of insulin. Br Med J 2:687–690, 1974

9. Semple PF, White C, Manderson WG: Continuous intravenous infusion of small doses of insulin in treatment of diabetic ketoacidosis. Br Med J 2:694–698, 1974

10. Kitabchi AE, Ayyagari V, Guerra SMO, and Medical House Staff: The efficacy of low-dose versus conventional therapy of insulin for treatment of diabetic ketoacidosis. Ann Intern Med 84:633–638, 1976

11. Piters KM, Kumar D, Pei E, Bessman AN: Comparison of continuous and intermittent intravenous insulin therapies for diabetic ketoacidosis. Diabetologia 13:317–321, 1977

12. Pfeifer MA, Samols E, Wolter CF, Winkler CF: Low-dose versus high-dose insulin therapy for diabetic ketoacidosis. South Med J 72:149–154, 1979

13. Soler NG, Wright AD, FitzGerald MG, Malins JM: Comparative study of different insulin regimens in management of diabetic ketoacidosis. Lancet 2:1221–1224, 1975

14. Madison LL: Low-dose insulin: a plea for caution. N Engl J Med 294: 393–394, 1976

15. Morris LR, Kitabchi AE: Efficacy of low-dose insulin therapy for severely obtunded patients in diabetic ketoacidosis. Diabetes Care 3:53–56, 1980

16. Fisher JN, Shahshahani MN, Kitabchi AE: Diabetic ketoacidosis: low-dose insulin therapy by various routes. N Engl J Med 297:238–241, 1977

17. Peterson L, Caldwell J, Hoffman J: Insulin adsorbance to polyvinylchloride surfaces with implications for constant-infusion therapy. Diabetes 25: 72–74, 1976

18. Knochel JP: The pathophysiology and clinical characteristics of severe hypophosphatemia. Arch Intern Med 137:203–220, 1977

19. Ditzel J, Standl E: The problem of tissue oxygenation in diabetes mellitus. Acta Med Scand 578 [Suppl] :49–83, 1975

20. Kanter Y, Gerson JR, Bessman AN: 2,3-Diphosphoglycerate, nucleotide phosphate, and organic and inorganic phosphate levels during the early phases of diabetic ketoacidosis. Diabetes 26:429–433, 1977

21. Gibby OM, Veale KEA, Hayes TM, et al: Oxygen availability from the blood and the effect of phosphate replacement on erythrocyte 2,3-diphosphoglycerate and haemoglobin-oxygen affinity in diabetic ketoacidosis. Diabetologia 15:381–385, 1978

22. Zipf WB, Bacon GE, Spencer ML, et al: Hypocalcemia, hypomagnesemia, and transient hypoparathyroidism during therapy with potassium phosphate in diabetic ketoacidosis. Diabetes Care 2:265–268, 1979

23. Lavis VR: Treatment of diabetic ketoacidosis (letter). Diabetes Care 2:385–386, 1979

24. Lentz RD, Brown DM, Kjellstrand CM: Treatment of severe hypophosphatemia. Ann Intern Med 89:941–944, 1978

25. Posner JB, Plum F: Spinal-fluid pH and neurologic symptoms in systemic acidosis. N Engl J Med 297:605–613, 1967

26. Ohman JL Jr, Marliss EB, Aoki TT, et al: The cerebrospinal fluid in diabetic ketoacidosis. N Engl J Med 284:283–290, 1971

27. Assal J-Ph, Aoki TT, Manzano FM, Kozak GP: Metabolic effects of sodium bicarbonate in management of diabetic ketoacidosis. Diabetes 23:405–411, 1974

28. King AJ, Cooke NJ, McCuish A, et al: Acid-base changes during treatment of diabetic ketoacidosis. Lancet 1:478-481, 1974

29. Beigelman PM: Severe diabetic ketoacidosis (diabetic 'coma'): 482 episodes in 257 patients; experience of three years. Diabetes 20:490-500, 1971

30. Clements RS Jr, Blumenthal SA, Morrison AD, Winegrad AI: Increased cerebrospinal-fluid pressure during treatment of diabetic ketosis. Lancet 2:671-675, 1971

31. Fein JA, Rackow EC, Waldroup LD, Tenner MS: Cerebral edema in the treatment of diabetic ketoacidosis (abstract). Clin Res 26:414, 1978

32. Arieff AI, Carroll HJ: Nonketotic hyperosmolar coma with hyperglycemia: clinical features, pathophysiology, renal function, acid-base balance, plasma-cerebrospinal fluid equilibria and the effects of therapy in 37 cases. Medicine 51:73-94, 1972

33. Maccario M: Neurological dysfunction associated with nonketotic hyperglycemia. Arch Neurol 19:525-534, 1968

34. Guisado R, Arieff AI: Neurologic manifestations of diabetic comas: correlation with biochemical alterations in the brain. Metabolism 24:665-679, 1975

Chapter 7

Office Management of the Diabetic Patient

It is unfortunate that most of the physician's training in the care of diabetic patients occurs in the hospital. The management of these patients belongs in an office setting. The weekly diabetes clinic experience that may last from one to several months that serves as the house officer's experience in office management is woefully inadequate. For more than with most diseases. diabetes care requires an ongoing dialogue between patient and physician, and, unlike patients with other diseases, diabetics themselves make many important decisions regarding their care. This requires appropriate education and guidance by the physician and other health professionals. With the proper interaction between patient and doctor, many hospitalizations can be avoided. As discussed in chapter 4, even insulin therapy can be initiated and stabilized outside of the hospital in motivated patients if an office routine is established for this purpose.

No matter how experienced and dedicated the physician is, both the patient's knowledge of diabetes and his or her appropriate judgments in soliciting help from the doctor are usually the critical factors that prevent minor problems from becoming major ones. The education of diabetic patients is considered in detail in chapter 8, which was written for the patient as well as for the personnel (often nurses) carrying out the teaching. Although most physicians have neither the time nor the inclination to teach patients themselves, it is crucial that diabetics understand the material appropriate to their disease, as summarized in this chapter. If other professionals are not available to teach the diabetic, I urge physicians to read chapter 8 before carrying out the instruction. Too often, medical jargon prevents effective communication between patient and physician, and patients often are too overwhelmed to ask questions. Appropriate dietary information for patients is described in chapter 3.

Initial Evaluation and General Follow-Up

In keeping with the philosophy set out in the preface—that is, to discuss only those aspects of patient care that are either unique or particularly pertinent to diabetic patients—I will highlight here only a few aspects of the initial workup. Because of the increased susceptibility of diabetics to macrovascular disease, it is important to carry out baseline recording of pulses and to check for the presence or absence of bruits. These pulses include the carotid, femoral, popliteal (more easily palpated if the leg is slightly bent), posterior tibialis, and dorsalis pedis. The arteries to be examined for bruits are those of the neck (carotid), abdomen (aorta), flanks (renal), and groin (iliac). Because neuropathy may develop, a baseline evaluation of the functioning of two components of the peripheral nervous system should be performed. Such an evaluation consists of the threshold for vibratory sensation (especially in the lower extremities) and the reflexes. Impairment of one or both of these components is the initial sign of peripheral neuropathy.

With regard to the laboratory evaluation, the initial workup should include a urinalysis for protein, blood urea nitrogen (BUN) or creatinine levels, fasting triglyceride concentration, cholesterol level, and electrocardiogram (ECG). Since diabetic glomerulosclerosis is invariably associated with proteinuria, routine repetition of BUN or creatinine measurements (assuming the initial value was normal) is not really necessary in the absence of proteinuria. Elevated cholesterol and triglyceride levels are risk factors for coronary artery disease, and both are increased in diabetics more commonly than in nondiabetics. Lowering of these lipid concentrations through dietary therapy seems to be associated with a decreased risk of vascular disease. Whether use of drug therapy is helpful in accomplishing this is controversial. (One exception, of course, is hypertriglyceridemia due to uncontrolled diabetes, which responds readily to insulin therapy.) If the initial cholesterol level is increased, a high-density lipoprotein (HDL) cholesterol concentration should be measured to ensure that the elevated total cholesterol level is due mainly to low-density lipoprotein (LDL) cholesterol. Low-density lipoprotein cholesterol is the cholesterol fraction associated with coronary artery disease, while elevated HDL cholesterol levels seem to protect against heart disease (1). The physician should not alarm the patient unduly or treat an increased total cholesterol value if it were due largely to HDL cholesterol. I measure HDL cholesterol initially only if the total cholesterol level is elevated. I do not measure it in every patient, since little is known at present about what factors affect it or the importance of increasing it. If the initial lipid values are normal, I routinely measure them once a year. If the patient is being treated for elevated values, I measure lipid levels at approximately 3-month intervals.

A baseline ECG is usually recommended, especially in patients over the age of 40 or in those who have had diabetes for more than 10 years. The rationale is that this information will be valuable if the patient is ever evaluated for chest pain due to possible coronary artery disease. This supposition has been challenged, however, by a study of patients with chest pain seen in an emergency room. The study showed that comparison of the emergency ECG to a previous ECG did not influence the decision to hospitalize the patient (2). In spite of this, I do order an ECG on patients who fulfill the above criteria. I do not repeat them routinely in asymptomatic patients, however, since the findings would not influence specific therapies.

Blood pressure should be monitored closely and treated vigorously if elevated. In addition to the well-known detrimental effects of hypertension on macrovascular diseases of the heart, brain, and kidneys, hypertension also is associated with accelerated microvascular damage to the eyes (3) and the kidneys (4).

Finally, diabetic patients should wear some form of identification. This is especially important for those taking insulin. If a patient is ever unable to give a history and a family member or friend is unavailable, he or she may accidentally be given inappropriate and perhaps dangerous therapy unless the medical personnel present are aware of the diabetes. Medic alert bracelets or necklaces are the best form of identification. The information necessary for ordering them is included in the appendix to chapter 8. If other forms of identification are utilized, they should be placed on the outside of the wallet or on the back of a watch. When a patient is unconscious, medical personnel may not go through a patient's wallet or pocketbook before they initiate treatment.

If a patient has no specific complaints and if treatment is through diet alone or diet supplemented with sulfonylurea agents, he or she is seen in the office at approximately 4- to 6-month intervals. Blood sugar levels are measured more frequently (see under *Monitoring Diabetic Control*), and patients are contacted with the results. If the values are satisfactory, office personnel can relay the information. However, the physician should communicate unsatisfactory results personally so that explanations may be sought and, if indicated, adjustments in therapy be made.

The patient should be evaluated at 4- to 6-month intervals for the following: blood pressure, retinopathy, vibratory sensation, pulses, proteinuria, and condition of the feet. It is especially important to assess these in patients over the age of 40 or in those who have had diabetes for more than 10 years. If evidence of background (or simple) retinopathy is found, the patient should be referred to an ophthalmologist. Fluoroscein angiography will usually reveal much more extensive damage than will the ophthalmoscope, and prophylactic photocoagulation has been helpful in preventing severe visual loss (5). In order to rule out an asymptomatic urinary tract infection, a urine culture should be ordered, or at least the presence of pyuria evaluated, in patients with new onset of proteinuria. Elevated blood pressure must be followed closely and treated if persistent. Decreased vibratory sensation can serve to motivate patients to control their diabetes better. Definite pulse changes require further evaluation.

Monitoring Diabetic Control

The importance of strict diabetic control was discussed in chapter 2. The attainment of this goal is critically dependent on the ability to monitor the degree of control achieved. At present, there are five general methods of assessing diabetic control, each of which will be discussed in detail: (a) semiquantitative testing of urine for glucose and ketone bodies; (b) quantitative measurements of urine glucose in timed samples; (c) fasting and/or postprandial whole-blood or plasma glucose determinations obtained sporadically at a chemistry laboratory or the doctor's office; (d) home glucose monitoring; and (e) measurement of glycosylated hemoglobin (Hgb) or Hgb A_{1c} levels.

Semiquantitative Urine Testing

Evaluation of the results of urine testing requires an understanding of the concept of the renal threshold for glucose (T_m). Glucose is filtered at the glomerulus and reabsorbed back into the circulation in the proximal tubule. When the capacity of the proximal tubule to reabsorb glucose is exceeded, glucose appears in the urine. The amount of glucose reabsorbed is related to its concentration in the filtrate and to the rate at which it is presented to the renal tubular cells. It also is linked to sodium reabsorption in the proximal tubule. Therefore, the classic concept that the proximal tubule has an intrinsic maximal capacity to reabsorb glucose is not accurate. However, the concept that there is a limit to glucose reabsorption in the proximal tubule (even if it depends on other variables) is useful clinically. Under normal conditions, glucose does not appear in the urine until the plasma glucose concentration exceeds ~180 mg/100 ml. That is, at plasma levels below this value, virtually all of the glucose is reabsorbed and does not reach the urine. Therefore, the normal renal threshold for glucose is ~180 mg/100 ml. This level is relatively variable among patients. It tends to be lower in younger patients and to increase with age. Pregnancy lowers plasma glucose levels considerably for reasons that are not entirely clear. Pregnant women can even manifest glucosuria with normal plasma glucose concentrations (100 to 120 mg/100 ml). Renal disease, including diabetic glomerulosclerosis, raises the T_m. This explains why some (usually older) patients may be aglucosuric at elevated glucose levels (250 to 350 mg/100 ml).

There are four different products available for urinary testing of glucose: (a) Clinitest tablets, (b) Clinistix, (c) Tes-Tape, and (d) Diastix. Clinitest tablets utilize a copper-reduction reaction and may also measure substances other than glucose. Either two or five drops of urine are added to 10 drops of water before testing. With the remaining three methods, a piece of paper or a cellulose strip is simply dipped into the urine. These methods rely on a reaction involving the enzyme glucose oxidase, which is specific for glucose. The product of the reaction, hydrogen peroxide, reacts with another enzyme impregnated on the strip to produce nascent oxygen, which oxidizes a dye and thus causes the color of the strip to change. Substances that interfere with the measurement of urinary glucose by methods utilizing glucose oxidase usually inhibit the oxidation of the dye, not the enzyme reactions (6).

These four methods have different ranges of sensitivity (Table 7-1). Because the relations between positive reactions expressed as the plus signs and the amount of urinary glucose vary considerably among the different tests, efforts are now being made to report the results only as percentages. If this approach is successful, Clinistix will no longer be suitable because each color change represents a range of glucose levels. Note that Tes-Tape is the most sensitive method, since it gives a definite color change at 0.1% urinary glucose; however, there is little change in color between 0.5% and 2%. The two-drop Clinitest method extends readings at higher levels of urinary glucose (between 2% and 5%). Diastix and the five-drop Clinitest method are the most comparable, with approximately equal changes in urinary glucose associated with discernible color changes between 0.25% and 2%.

In addition to the effect of the renal threshold on urinary glucose testing, certain constituents and properties of the urine itself have important effects on the results. Both falsely low and falsely high readings are common and differ among the 4 methods. In a study in which 500 urine samples from both diabetic and nondiabetic patients were tested, both as collected and after a precise amount of glucose was added, approximately 25% of the samples gave falsely low readings and almost half gave falsely high readings (7). Only Clinistix and Diastix gave falsely low readings. In half of the urines yielding falsely low results, ascorbic acid (vitamin C) and/or a breakdown product of salicylic acid (aspirin) were found. Both of these substances interfere with oxidation of the dye, as mentioned previously. Aspirin and vitamin C are so commonly ingested that patients often do not mention them to physicians. In addition, numerous other, unidentified compounds were found in the urines, probably representing the diverse medications that the patients were taking or the degradative products thereof.

The reason that falsely low readings were not observed with Tes-Tape is interesting and could be useful clinically. Tes-Tape is a paper tape; as the urine ascends the tape, the glucose separates from the interfering substances (6). Therefore, the color change at the upper end of the tape (i.e., the interface between the wet and dry parts of the tape) is a valid measure of the amount of glucose present. A similar situation would occur if only the tip of the test area of the Clinistix and Diastix strips were immersed in the urine sample. However, this is difficult because the chemicals are contained in such a small area.

Almost half of the urines gave falsely high values (7), and two thirds of these occurred with Clinitest tablets. Low urine osmolalities (usually <100 mOsm/kg) were associated consistently with falsely high readings. The effect of the usual procedure of collecting a second-voided urine specimen 30 minutes after the patient drinks 16 ounces of water was evaluated in nine additional patients (7). Falsely high readings were found in all nine samples tested with Clinitest tablets, four of nine tested with Tes-Tape, in five of nine tested with Clinistix, and in four of nine tested with Diastix. These results raise a serious question about the accuracy of second-voided urines, a subject that will be discussed in detail later.

Table 7-1. Comparison of Results Among Different Methods of Testing for Urinary Glucose[a]

Product	Glucose Concentration							
	0.1%	0.25%	0.5%	0.75%	1%	2%	3%	5%
Clinitest (5-drop)		Trace	+	++	+++	++++		
Clinitest (2-drop)[b]			c		c	c	c	c
Diastix	Trace	+	++		+++	++++		
Clinistix[d]		. . . Light . . . (+)		. . . Medium . . . (++)		. . . Dark . . . (+++)		
Tes-Tape	+	++	+++			++++		

Blank spaces indicate that there are no color blocks for those concentrations.

[a]Adapted with permission from *Home Urine Testing for the Diabetic*. Ames Co., Division Miles Laboratories, Inc., Elkhart, IA, 1976.
[b]The two-drop chart provides a "trace" color block without a percentage value; a trace result merely indicates glucosuria of < 0.5%.
[c]Measures percentage of glucosuria at these levels, but equivalent + values are not available.
[d]Estimates relative presence of glucose but cannot show percentage value.

In addition to vitamin C and aspirin derivatives, several other substances have been implicated to interfere with the results of urine testing for glucose. Ketone bodies in moderate to large amounts may depress Diastix readings. Protein in the urine may cause excessive foaming with Clinitest tablets and may cause difficulty in interpreting the final color development, thus leading to artificially low readings. Cephalosporins, non-glucose-reducing sugars, and aspirin (6) will cause false-positive reactions with Clinitest tablets. Although vitamin C added directly to urine samples also may cause a false-positive reaction with Clinitest tablets, this effect was not noted in urine collected from subjects who ingested 4 to 6 g of ascorbic acid (8). The same pertains to isoniazid and methyldopa (Aldomet). Both of these drugs caused falsely low readings with glucose oxidase methodology (by inhibiting dye development) when added directly to urine (6) but had no effect on urine samples from patients taking the medications (9, 10). On the other hand, urine samples collected from patients taking L-dopa gave falsely high readings with Clinitest tablets and falsely low readings with Clinistix (6). Presumably, all tests utilizing the oxidation of a dye would show the same effect (except perhaps at the leading edge of the Tes-Tape strip). Finally, large amounts of urinary 5-hydroxyindoleacetic acid (5-HIAA), often seen in patients with the carcinoid syndrome, also blocks oxidation of the dye and cause false-negative results with tests using glucose oxidase methodology (6). Table 7-2 summarizes the effects of substances that interfere with tests for urinary glucose.

A breakdown product of L-dopa also causes false-positive results for urinary ketone bodies when measured by Ketostix (11). The same method for measuring ketone bodies is used in both Keto-Diastix strips and Labstix, which presumably would react similarly. Acetest tablets are not affected and therefore should be used to test for ketonuria in diabetic patients taking L-dopa.

The timing of urine collections obviously affects the results, but the reasons for this are mainly physiologic. A specimen obtained before breakfast when the patient is in the fasting state is least likely to show glucosuria simply because the plasma glucose concentration is usually lowest at that time. Thus, the fasting urine test is the least sensitive—i.e., it is least likely to show altered metabolism. The next most sensitive urine test is that performed on a sample collected preprandially. In this case, 3 to 4 hours usually have elapsed since the last meal, and the height of the postprandial glucose surge is over. A second-voided urine sample taken at this time measures the efficiency with which the meal-derived carbohydrates have been cleared by 3 to 4 hours and is more likely to show glucosuria than is the fasting specimen. However, the first-voided, preprandial urine sample is even more sensitive since it reflects the entire period following the meal, during which time postprandial glucose concentrations have reached their maximum. A sample collected 1 to 2 hours postprandially will be most likely to show glucosuria, since it will not be diluted with urine that may be sugar-free after the plasma glucose level has reached it peak.

Table 7-2. Effect of Substances That Interfere with Results of Urine Tests for Glucose

Substance[a]	Method[b] Nonspecific[c]	Specific[d]
Ascorbic acid (Vitamin C)	↑[e]	↓
Salicylic acid (aspirin)	↑	↓
Decreased osmolality	↑	
Ketone bodies		↓
Protein	↓	
Cephalosporins	↑	
Non-glucose-reducing sugars	↑	
Isoniazid (INH)		↓[e]
Methyldopa (Aldomet)		↓[e]
L-Dopa	↑	↓
5-HIAA		↓

Abbreviations: 5-HIAA, 5-hydroxyindoleacetic acid.

[a]Effect may be due to degradative product of substance.

[b]↑, falsely high; ↓, falsely low.

[c]Refers to nonspecific reducing method using Clinitest tablets.

[d]Refers to glucose oxidase methodology using Tes-Tape, Clinistix, or Diastix. Although all of these products were not tested for each interfering substance, it is assumed that all would be affected. The leading edge of the Tes-Tape strip, however, may give a true reading, since glucose is separated from interfering substances in this area.

[e]Effect is noted only when the substance is added directly to the urine; no effect is seen when the patient ingests the substance.

Although most diabetologists usually recommend that patients routinely collect and test a second-voided urine specimen and discard the initial one without testing it, this approach is currently being challenged. The arguments on each side are as follows.

The results of the second-voided specimen reflect what is happening at the time the sample is collected. When these results are compared with the prevailing plasma glucose concentration, the T_m is evident. (However, the T_m is not an exact glucose level, and several comparisons are needed that result in a small range and yield an approximate value for the T_m.) Since this sample is not "contaminated" with glucose that may have been excreted several hours before, the results of the second-voided specimen reflect more accurately the effect of exogenous insulin acting at that particular moment. Depending on which preparation has been injected and when (chapter 4, Table 4-1), the preprandial urine tests take place at times of peak insulin action. Therefore, the results are helpful in adjusting the insulin dose.

On the other hand, the same facts can be used to support routine testing of first-voided specimens. Overlooking postprandial glucosuria by testing only the second-voided sample may delude both patient and physician into thinking that diabetic control is really better than it is. Since tight control is so important (chapter 2), significant postprandial glucosuria must be appreciated and adjustments must made to abolish it. A forceful argument against the routine testing of double-voided urine specimens is the impracticality of the method. Many patients do not have or will not take the time to urinate twice before meals. Indeed, a survey of almost 1,200 urine tests at the inpatient diabetic ward at Cedars-Sinai Medical Center, where testing of both first- and second-voided urines is allegedly part of the nursing routine, revealed that the second-voided urine was not tested 45% of the time! Perhaps the poor compliance with urine testing at home is related in part to the requirement that patients produce and test a second-voided specimen.

If second-voided urine were tested routinely, how often would it yield results different from those of the first-voided specimen? Several recent studies have attempted to answer this question (Table 7-3). The results were the same 60% to 80% of the time. As was expected, only a small number (5%) of second-voided urines gave higher readings than the initial sample. First-voided urines gave higher readings in only 14% to 33% of the comparisons. For reasons already discussed, more glucosuria might have been anticipated in the first-voided specimen more often than it was found. Perhaps falsely high readings caused by the formation of dilute urine in the process of collecting the second sample was responsible for this discrepancy.

In view of these considerations, I use the following approach to urine testing. In ketosis-resistant (type 2) patients, I prefer Diastix because they are simple to use and the color changes represent gradually increasing amounts of glucose (Table 7-1). Although the latter feature is also characteristic of Clinitest tablets, testing with them requires so much preparation and time as to profoundly limit patient compliance. Tes-Tape, although convenient, shows most of its color development at urinary glucose values of up to 0.5%, with the final change representing an increase from 0.5% to 2%. Clinistix has too broad a range of glucose concentrations for each color change.

Ketosis-prone (type 1) patients should not test with Diastix since moderate to large amounts of ketone bodies may depress the glucose readings. In this situation, a falsely low reading will not be appreciated because the patient will not be aware of ketonuria. If Keto-Diastix are used, results of <1% urinary glucose in the face of moderate or large ketone bodies requires retesting with Clinitest.

Table 7–3. Comparison of Test Results for Urine Glucose Using First- and Second-Voided Urine Samples

Study (Reference No.)	Method	No. of Comparisons	Same	Results (%)	
				First-Voided Higher	Second-Voided Higher
Guthrie and co-workers (12)	Clinitest (2-drop)	754[b]	62	33	5
McCarthy (13)	Tes-Tape	406	81	14	5
CSMC[a]	Keto-Diastix	646	72	23	5

[a]Unpublished study conducted on the Diabetes Ward at Cedars-Sinai Medical Center.

[b]Three comparisons in the published report were omitted from this table because the patients ate between the first- and second-voided urine collections.

This is important because uncontrolled diabetes with falsely low glucose readings must be distinguished from "starvation" ketosis (described later). Since ketosis-prone diabetics do not need to test routinely for ketone bodies, an alternative approach is use of Clinitest tablets and testing for ketone bodies when the results show a consistent glucosuria of 1% to 2%.

When diabetes is initially diagnosed and the patient is introduced to urine testing, it is important to know the T_m in order to interpret the results. Measuring the T_m was described in chapter 4 and requires, of course, routine testing of second-voided urine samples. However, once the T_m has been determined, I usually ask only patients on insulin to test a double-voided urine sample before breakfast. Since this is often the time of lowest glucose concentration during a 24-hour period, it is important not to be misled by glucosuria that has occurred during the early part of the night and thus does not represent the true metabolic situation before breakfast. Following the glucosuria of the first-voided specimen may result in inappropriate increases in insulin doses, whereas the results of the second-voided specimen would have dictated otherwise.

Although the same argument could be advanced for testing urine at other times of the day, there is an important difference. The length of time between completion of a meal and the preprandial urine test before the next meal is much shorter than the time between the bedtime snack and the before-breakfast test. Therefore, the difference between the postprandial glucose level (which peaks 1 to 2 hours after eating) and the glucose concentration before the next meal is much more likely to be smaller than the one between the bedtime snack and breakfast (8 to 12 hours later). For this reason, even if postprandial glucosuria is present in the next preprandial urine sample, adjustment of insulin doses on the basis of this test should not lead to overtreatment very often. In addition, tight control cannot be achieved if postprandial glucosuria is ignored. Therefore, during the day, my patients test only the first-voided urine. They are instructed to test both the first-voided sample (on arising) and the second-voided sample (before they take their insulin) before breakfast.

It should be obvious from this discussion that semiquantitative urine testing for glucose is at best only a crude index of diabetic control. A measure of the imprecise relation between urine tests and prevailing plasma glucose levels is shown in Table 7-4. Blood was sampled continuously for the 30-minute period between collection of first- and second-voided urine samples. The double-voided specimen was tested by the two-drop Clinitest method in 37 patients with insulin-dependent diabetes (14). Although the mean (30-minute integrated) glucose concentration is roughly proportional to the level of glucosuria, the wide range of associated plasma glucose values precludes an accurate assessment of diabetic control on the basis of urine testing.

In addition to the important effects of the renal threshold, interfering substances in the urine, and the osmolality, the interpretation of urine test results is also affected by whether the bladder is emptied completely. However, at present, urine testing still is the most practical and accurate way to judge day-to-day diabetic control for most patients. It is unfortunate that many diabetics refuse to test their urine routinely. This leaves both them and their physician uncertain about their control and therefore unable to improve it (which, in my experience, is necessary in a substantial proportion of the diabetic population).

Table 7-4. Relationship Between the Prevailing Plasma Glucose Concentration and Glucosuria in a Second-Voided Urine Specimen[a]

| Urine Glucose (g/100 ml or %) | Plasma Glucose (mg/100 ml) | | No. of Comparisons |
	Mean ± SD	Range	
Negative	116±49	31–214	25
0.5	165±41	105–214	7
1	205±4	201–208	3
2	234±37	201–294	5
3	236±30	189–297	24
5	314±67	193–506	43

Abbreviation: SD, standard deviation.

[a]Adapted with permission from Winter RJ, Traisman HS, Green OC: Glucosuria in children with diabetes: advantages of the 2-drop Clinitest method. Diabetes Care 2:349-352, 1979.

Quantitative Urine Testing

A more accurate assessment of diabetic control by means of testing urine is quantitative measurement by the chemistry laboratory of the amount of glucose excreted. The advantages of this method are as follows: (*a*) it eliminates the influence of substances that give falsely low or falsely high readings; (*b*) it eliminates the influence of urinary osmolality; (*c*) it measures the exact level of glucosuria; and (*d*) it allows assessment of diabetic control over longer periods.

There also are several disadvantages to the quantitative method. The major one is the inconvenience of accurate urine collection. The bladder must be emptied at both the beginning and end of the evaluation period, and *all* urine passed during that period must be brought to the laboratory. As with semiquantitative methods, the T_m for glucose has an important effect on the level of glucosuria. In addition, the amount of dietary carbohydrates may influence the interpretation of the results. A commonly accepted criterion for good control is excretion of less than 10% of the total dietary carbohydrate intake. Therefore, a patient who loses 22 g of urinary glucose over 24 hours would be considered well controlled if he or she ate 250 g of carbohydrates but only fairly controlled if the diet consisted of only 150 g of carbohydrates.

I use quantitative measurement of urine glucose only to help determine whether a patient is experiencing the Somogyi phenomenon (posthypoglycemia hyperglycemia). Although this usually is obvious (and will be discussed later), an occasional patient may have persistent fasting hyperglycemia even though they take increasing amounts of intermediate-acting insulin and show no evidence of nighttime hypoglycemia. In this situation, it can be helpful to compare the daytime level of glucosuria with the amount of glucose excreted overnight. If the 12-hour daytime urine (8 AM to 8 PM) contains much more glucose than does the 8 PM to 8 AM portion, it is likely that the patient is experiencing unrecognized nighttime hypoglycemia with rebound hyperglycemia. If the level of glucosuria in the overnight collection is approximately equal to or greater than that in the daytime collection, underinsulinization is the more likely explanation. Similarly, a quantitative measurement of urinary glucose from the beginning of one meal to the beginning of the next would reflect the effectiveness of a dose of preprandial regular insulin in limiting the rise in postprandial glucose. In my view, these are the two most useful applications of quantitative determinations of urinary glucose (although I do not use the latter one very often).

Plasma Glucose Measurements

The plasma glucose concentration obviously is the best available index of diabetic control. However, since it reflects the situation only at that particular moment, the results may not represent the patient's usual metabolic state. For instance, if the trip to the laboratory, clinic, or doctor's office is stressful for the patient, the resulting glucose value will be higher than usual. Alternatively, some patients (at least, some of mine) change their usual pattern of treatment just before testing, e.g., by adhering to their diet or even occasionally by taking extra insulin. Obviously, the glucose concentration will be lower than their usual level. Therefore, although I rely on plasma glucose concentrations for assessment of control, I usually do not change therapy on the basis of one (spurious?) value. Comparing the plasma glucose level to the pattern of urine test results and/or obtaining several additional plasma samples for glucose is very helpful in deciding both the validity of the first result and whether to alter the therapeutic regimen.

The timing of plasma glucose measurements also is important in evaluating control. A postprandial sample obtained 1 to 2 hours after the patient has eaten is the most sensitive index, since glucose levels are maximal at this time. The caloric and especially the simple-carbohydrate content of the meal will affect this result. The preprandial glucose concentration is the next most sensitive index of how efficiently meal-derived carbohydrates have been cleared from the plasma. Finally, the fasting glucose concentration is the least sensitive index of diabetic control, since it does not reflect a postprandial challenge to the pancreas. In diabetics, the glucose level is usually at its lowest in the fasting state, and, as carbohydrate metabolism deteriorates, this value is the last to rise. Recommendations concerning the timing of samples under different circumstances will be discussed later.

Glycosylated Hemoglobin

Measurements of glycosylated Hgb (15) or Hgb A_{1c} have been introduced recently into clinical practice as an index of long-term diabetic control. Some knowledge of the biochemistry of red blood cells is necessary to understanding the rationale for measuring and interpreting glycosylated Hgb or Hgb A_{1c} levels in diabetics.

In nondiabetics, 90% of hemoglobin consists of two alpha and two beta chains and is called Hgb A. Approximately 2% of hemoglobin contains two alpha and two delta chains (Hgb A_2, a normal variant), while 1% is fetal hemoglobin (Hgb F), which is composed of two alpha and two gamma chains. The remaining 7% of hemoglobin also consists of two alpha and two beta chains, with either glucose or a derivative of glucose attached to the beta chain. If glucose is attached, the resulting hemoglobin is called Hgb A_{1c}. Hgb A_{1c} is the major component of these hemoglobins and constitutes approximately 5% of total hemoglobins in nondiabetics. A number of hemoglobins with glucose derivatives attached have recently been isolated. The next two most common hemoglobins are Hgb A_{1a} and Hgb A_{1b}, each of which makes up approximately 1% of total hemoglobins in nondiabetics. Since all of these hemoglobins contain glucose or one of its derivatives, they are known collectively as glycosylated Hgbs. The entire glycosylated fraction is also called Hgb A_1.

These additions to the beta chain change the charge characteristics of Hgb A so that the molecules travel faster in chromatographic separation techniques. In older terminology, this fraction was called the fast, or minor, hemoglobins. In

1962, diabetic individuals were first noted to have a higher percentage of fast hemoglobins than did control subjects. Since the structure of these hemoglobins was not yet appreciated, investigators thought that the increase in minor hemoglobins was related in some way to the genetic composition of the diabetic population. Subsequent studies in both animals and humans showed clearly that this was not the case.

The reaction between glucose and the beta chain of hemoglobin is (*a*) slow, (*b*) mostly irreversible, (*c*) not mediated by an enzyme, (*d*) continuous over the life span of the red blood cell, and (*e*) proportional to the glucose concentration to which the red cell is exposed. Thus, the amount of glycosylated Hgb or its major component, Hgb A_{1c}, is a time-integrated measure of the prevailing glucose concentration to which the red cells have been exposed. As such (within certain limitations) it should be helpful in monitoring diabetic control. A number of studies have demonstrated that levels of either Hgb A_{1c} or glycosylated Hgb (depending on which was measured) are proportional to fasting plasma glucose concentrations, postprandial glucose levels, values obtained during a glucose tolerance test, amount of urinary glucose excreted, and clinical estimates of control. One such correlation is shown in Figure 7-1. In this study, the amount of both Hgb A_{1c} and glycosylated Hgb were measured in a group of children with a wide spectrum of diabetic control. Biochemical criteria (16) for the different degrees of control were as follows: (*a*) excellent—essentially normal postprandial glucose concentrations on periodic clinic visits, aglycosuria, no ketonuria; (*b*) good—same as in (*a*), except for occasional minimal transient glucosuria (trace to 2% in no more than one of three to four daily urine specimens); (*c*) good to fair—somewhat more frequent transient glucosuria, usually related to dietary indiscretions; (*d*) fair—varying amounts of glucosuria in approximately half of the samples tested, occasionally transient ketonuria, postprandial glucose concentrations usually between 150 and 300 mg/100 ml; and (*e*) poor—various degrees of glucosuria in most urine specimens tested. The relation between the degree of control and levels of Hgb A_{1c} or glycosylated Hgb in these cases is striking. The difference between the best controlled patients and the nondiabetic group is minimal. Note that Hgb A_{1a} and Hgb A_{1b} levels are similar in all groups and that the fraction that changes in diabetics is Hgb A_{1c}. Therefore, the differences in the amount of glycosylated Hgb among the groups are due to changes in Hgb A_{1c}. However, for most clinical laboratories, measurement of total glycosylated Hgb is usually easier and is just as helpful as long as the higher normal range is appreciated.

Longitudinal studies (17, 18) have revealed that levels of glycosylated Hgb correlate best with the degree of diabetic control obtained several months earlier. This would be expected because of the 120-day life span of the red blood cell and because the glycosylation reaction of hemoglobin is mostly irreversible. The lag period before an improvement in diabetic control is reflected in changes in Hgb A_{1c} levels is shown in Figure 7-2. Comparison of the relatively rapid drop in urinary glucose with the gradual decline of Hgb A_{1c} values shows that the latter did not reach a plateau until 6 weeks after tight control was achieved.

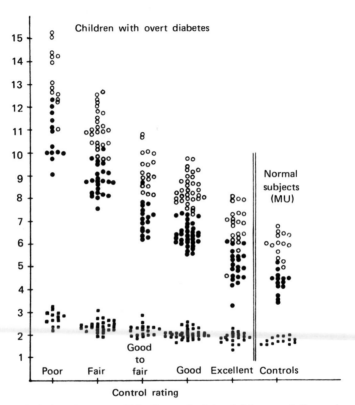

Figure 7-1. Relation between diabetic control in children and the various fractions of glycosylated Hgbs. ■, Hgb A_{1a+b}; ●, Hgb A_{1c}; ○, Hgb_{1a+b+c} or total glycosylated Hgb. (Reprinted with permission from Jackson RL, Hess RL, England JD: Hemoglobin A_{1c} values in children with overt diabetes maintained in varying degrees of control. Diabetes Care 2:391–395, 1979.)

There seems to be little doubt that levels of glycosylated Hgb are an excellent time-integrated measure of overall diabetic control. They are valuable in assessing control, both in diabetic populations and in individual patients. However, because of the lag period before this index reflects changes in diabetic control, it is not as helpful in deciding day-to-day therapy. For instance, the physician would not necessarily know exactly what change to make in the insulin prescription on the basis of a high level of glycosylated Hgb. On the other hand, this measure may be of value in patients whose office tests (or the record they bring to the office) do not coincide with other indices of diabetic control. In general, I do not routinely order glycosylated Hgb tests because they are expensive and they do not help to decide on specific changes in therapy. If the physician

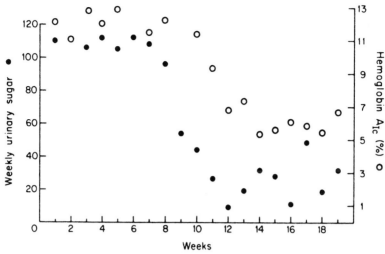

Figure 7-2. Temporal relation between weekly urinary glucose levels and Hgb A_{1c} in one patient. Urinary glucose was measured semiquantitatively with Clinitest tablets (on a scale of 0 to 4+) four times a day. The results were summed every 7 days to obtain a mean weekly index. (Reprinted with permission of the New England Journal of Medicine from Koenig RJ, Peterson CM, Jones RL, et al: Correlation of glucose regulation and hemoglobin A_{1c} in diabetes mellitus. N Engl J Med 295:417–420, 1976.)

decides to order these tests, he or she must remember several points. Since glycosylation occurs throughout the life span of the red cell, the presence of conditions that shorten this life span (hemolytic anemias, bleeding) will produce falsely low values. Conversely, if the life span is abnormally long (e.g., in patients with splenectomy, the values will be falsely high. Finally, Hgb F moves with the glycosylated Hgbs during chromatographic separation. Therefore, patients with the thalessemia syndromes (i.e., with increased amounts of Hgb F) will have artificially high levels of "glycosylated " Hgb.

Home Glucose Monitoring

Because there are many limitations to urine testing and because certain factors (discussed previously) influence occasional plasma glucose measurements obtained at the office or clinical laboratory, it is extremely helpful to monitor plasma glucose levels much more frequently in the patient's normal environment (19). The technology for this became available a number of years ago when the paper strip impregnated with glucose oxidase (Dextrostix) was adapted for use with whole blood. The results could be read visually, but the range of glucose concentrations that could be measured was limited and the delineation between successive glucose levels frequently was difficult to obtain. The results could be made more precise by reading the strip in a large, expensive ($\sim$\$600) machine (reflectance meter; Ames).

Several recent developments have made this approach to assessing diabetic control, termed *home glucose monitoring* (19), much more attractive. First, the importance of tight diabetic control has been substantiated by more and more animal and human data (chapter 2). Second, it is now possible to perform finger sticks to obtain capillary blood much less painfully than before with use of an automatic spring-loaded device called an Autolet (Ullster Scientific Inc.). Third, a new strip (Chemstrips; Bio-Dynamics/bmc) has been introduced on which the enzyme impregnates two adjacent areas, each of which is connected to a different dye system. Therefore, each glucose level produces two separate colors, which facilitates reading the results. Furthermore, the range of glucose values is extended at both the high and low end. A similar strip can be read in a less expensive ($\sim$\$350) machine (the Stat-Tek; Bio-Dynamics/bmc) for more precise results. Finally, a light, portable, less expensive (also $\sim$\$350) machine (Dextrometer; Ames) has been developed to read the Dextrostix. In spite of the fact that strips cost approximately \$ .50 each, many diabetologists are starting to monitor their patients with home glucose monitoring. Reasonably accurate blood sugar measurements are relatively simple to obtain, and, more important, the information makes it much easier to control the diabetes.

Home glucose monitoring is particularly useful when the patient is uncertain whether he or she is experiencing hypoglycemia. Patients taking insulin frequently have mild symptoms that they attribute to hypoglycemia; thus, they ingest simple carbohydrates to combat it. This leads to hyperglycemia that lasts for many hours; in some cases this episode is unnecessary because hypoglycemia was not present initially. This scenario can easily be avoided if the patient measures his or her capillary blood sugar before eating.

As long as glucosuria is consistently present, home glucose monitoring is unnecessary because virtually all plasma glucose values will exceed $\sim$180 mg/100 ml. An obvious exception is patients with a lowered T_m for glucose, the most common being pregnant patients. Since very strict diabetic control is extremely important for the well-being of the fetus and newborn, home glucose monitoring of pregnant diabetic patients is particularly valuable.

If most urine tests give negative results for glucose, home glucose monitoring is the only practical way to ascertain stricter degrees of control. I usually tell my patients who take insulin to start measuring capillary blood sugar at the times at which I would order them from a laboratory—i.e., before breakfast and supper, two or three days a week. If these concentrations are consistently >120 mg/100 ml, I gradually increase the appropriate insulin dose in order to lower glucose levels to this value or below (remember that a whole-blood glucose concentration of 120 mg/100 ml corresponds to a plasma glucose level of $\sim$140 mg/100 ml). If that can be achieved consistently, the patient then measures the capillary blood sugar approximately 1.5 hours after each meal. Again, the goal is to achieve postprandial glucose concentrations of 120 mg/100 ml or below (remember that, since capillary blood contains an arterial contribution, the postprandial glucose value will be somewhat higher than a concomitant venous sample). Judicious adjustment of the regular insulin doses in the morning and evening will affect the postprandial glucose concentrations after breakfast and after supper, respectively. The postprandial level after lunch is often more difficult to treat unless the patient is willing to take a small amount of insulin before the midday meal. Although it is not possible to achieve this level of control in all patients who take insulin, this pattern of home glucose monitoring is helpful at least in approaching this goal.

Home glucose monitoring is not as helpful in patients treated by diet alone or by diet supplemented with sulfonylurea agents. Glucose concentrations are more stable in such individuals, and changes in therapy usually result in a gradual overall lowering of glucose levels rather than in decrements at specific times of the day. In patients without glucosuria, blood sugar concentrations measured at home can substitute for those usually obtained in a clinical laboratory or doctor's office. However, high values with home glucose monitoring should be verified by a laboratory method before therapy is changed.

If the patient is going to read the strips visually, I recommend Chemstrips for two reasons. First, the differences in the colors for various glucose levels seem easier to appreciate with Chemstrips than with Dextrostix. Second, with Chemstrips, water is not required to wash off the blood, as it is with Dextrostix. This makes the procedure neater and slightly more convenient. On the other hand, if the strips are going to be read in a machine to obtain more precise values, the Dextrostix system offers several advantages. The Dextrometer is smaller and lighter than the Stat-Tek. Another important feature of the Dextrometer is that it can be run on batteries and therefore is more portable than the Stat-Tek. Finally, the Dextrometer is calibrated and utilized more conveniently than the Stat-Tek.

Monitoring Patients Who Take Insulin

As discussed in chapter 4 (Table 4-2), the results of urine tests performed both before each meal and before the bedtime snack reflect the maximal action of different components of the insulin prescription. Therefore, the patient must perform all four tests in order to ensure the maximal effectiveness of insulin therapy. The goal is to obtain negative results on urine tests throughout the day. If any results are positive, the test should be repeated on subsequent days to determine whether a consistent pattern is emerging. It is not widely appreciated that the inherent severity of the metabolic abnormality in diabetes can vary widely over time (20). That is, in the absence of a recognizable cause (e.g., infection, weight change, emotional stress), the metabolic abnormality becomes either more severe (and requires more treatment) or milder (and requires less treatment). This situation underscores the importance of the patient being able to adjust the insulin dose without constantly consulting with the physician.

If a urine test gives positive results for glucose at a level of $\geqslant 0.5\%$ for 3 consecutive days (assuming that diet and exercise remain relatively stable), the patient should increase the appropriate component of the insulin prescription. If the pattern of positive urine tests is such that both the short- and intermediate-acting insulins need to be increased, only the latter should be changed (see the discussion of insulin therapy in chapter 4). Once the results of urine tests reflecting the peak action of the intermediate-acting insulin revert to negative, the dosage of regular insulin should be increased, if still necessary. The intermediate-acting insulin should be increased by 4 units each time unless previous experience shows that the patient (who is almost always lean) is sensitive to insulin, in which case a 2-unit increase is in order. An observation period of several days (with continued testing) should elapse before further changes in insulin therapy are made. Since regular insulin acts over a much shorter period, I usually increase the dosage by only 2 units each time in order to decrease the likelihood of hypoglycemia. In obese patients, however, the regular insulin should be increased by 4 units instead of 2.

If the metabolic abnormality becomes milder in patients taking insulin, hypoglycemia will occur (again, assuming that diet and exercise remain relatively stable). An isolated episode of hypoglycemia usually does not necessitate a change in insulin dosage. If the episodes recur, however, an adjustment is necessary. In patients taking one injection of insulin per day, hypoglycemia that occurs in the afternoon, evening, or during the night requires a decrease in the dose of intermediate-acting insulin. If the individual is on a split-dose regimen, the morning dose should be decreased if hypoglycemia occurs during the afternoon, and the evening dose should be decreased if hypoglycemia occurs during the night. Morning hypoglycemia (after breakfast) requires a decrease in the before-breakfast dose of regular insulin.

Hypoglycemia that occurs in the evening presents more of a problem. If the patient takes regular insulin before supper, the hypoglycemia most likely is due to this component of the insulin prescription, especially if the hypoglycemia occurs early in the evening. Hypoglycemia that occurs just before or soon after bedtime can be due either to the before-supper dose of intermediate-acting insulin or to the regular component; most likely it is secondary to their combined actions. The regular insulin should be decreased first, because it is important that the intermediate-acting insulin control hepatic production of glucose throughout the night in order to avoid marked fasting hyperglycemia. The intermediate-acting insulin should be decreased by 4 units each time. I usually lower the dose of regular insulin by the same amount (4 units) in order to prevent the hypoglycemia from recurring; then I increase it slowly, if necessary.

I also attempt to measure glucose concentrations every 4 to 6 weeks. If possible, these values should be obtained as part of the patient's usual routine. Fasting and before-supper determinations are the most helpful because they help to assess the effectiveness of the intermediate-acting insulin, the most important component of the insulin prescription. Often it is more convenient for the patient to go directly to a clinical laboratory located near home or work rather than to travel to the physician's office. Fasting glucose concentrations, at least, tend to remain relatively stable in diabetics. Figure 7-3 depicts the relationship between two fasting blood sugar levels obtained within 1 week. Although the variation is wider in the higher values (where presumably patients on insulin would be), these differences are not clinically important. The physician should investigate persistent discrepancies between laboratory glucose values and the results of urine tests.

If urine test results are mostly negative, I ask well-motivated patients to consider home glucose monitoring in order to define the degree of control more precisely. Some patients whose compliance with urine testing is poor may elect to monitor their glucose levels at home. The approach outlined in the section on home glucose monitoring should then be followed.

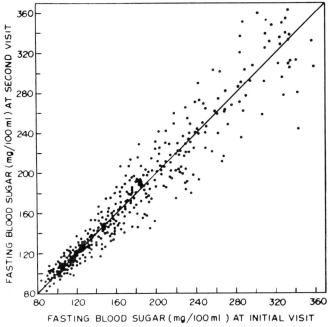

Figure 7-3. Relation between two fasting blood sugar concentrations in diabetic patients obtained within a 1-week interval. (Reprinted with permission from Kosaka K, Mizuno Y, Kuzuya T: Reproducibility of the oral glucose tolerance test and the rice-meal test in mild diabetes. Diabetes 15:901–904, 1966.)

Monitoring Patients Who Do Not Take Insulin

The main differences between monitoring patients who take insulin and monitoring those who do not are that the latter (*a*) return for office visits less frequently (discussed earlier), (*b*) follow a different pattern of testing to evaluate their control, and (*c*) have less difficulty managing their diabetes when they become ill (see section on sick-day rules). These distinctions are because the altered metabolic state is less labile and less abnormal in patients who do not take insulin than in those who require insulin. In the former group, urine tests performed before meals and before the bedtime snack are much more likely to yield negative results. If the results are negative, urine samples passed 1 to 2 hours after meals should be tested routinely, since urine tests are most likely to be abnormal at these times. The after-breakfast test is the most sensitive because (inexplicably) insulin is less effective in the morning than it is at other times of the day (21). If postprandial urine results are consistently negative, testing can be limited to 1 to 2 days a week. Positive results require further evaluation. Similarly, when plasma glucose is monitored in these patients, measurements should be taken 1 to 2 hours after the meal. Treatment of type 2 patients with both dietary therapy and sulfonylurea agents has been described in detail in chapter 5.

Goals of Therapy

Although the degrees of diabetic control described below may not be possible in many patients, these goals should be compromised only after diligent efforts to achieve them have been made. First, all urine test results should be negative. In patients with an increased T_m for glucose, this parameter obviously does not ensure very good control. Conversely, in the rare patient with a lowered T_m for glucose, negative urine test results may be associated with unacceptable hypoglycemia. In patients taking insulin, therapy should be adjusted so that the results of *preprandial* urine tests become negative. I do not recommend routine use of double-voided specimens. Consequently, in some patients, negative results of first-voided urine tests may be difficult to achieve without causing unacceptable hypoglycemic episodes. Therefore, under these circumstances, second-voided urine samples should be tested. If these results also are positive, further adjustments in therapy should be made; if the results are negative, the insulin dose should be maintained.

In patients who do not require insulin, the goal is to render the results of postprandial urine tests negative. Doses of sulfonylurea agents should be adjusted until this goal is achieved or until the maximal doses allowable are reached.

With regard to plasma glucose concentration, several levels of control theoretically are possible. The least stringent control, and one for which patient and physician should always strive, is a glucose value of <200 mg/100 ml, before both breakfast and supper. For patients taking intermediate-acting insulin, these are the times at which glucose concentrations usually are the lowest; therefore, higher glucose concentrations are present during most of the day and night. The next level of control is a glucose value of <150 mg/100 ml before breakfast and supper. Tighter control is achieved if the postprandial glucose concentrations can be kept below 200 mg/100 ml. Finally, the strictest criterion for control is a postprandial plasma value of <150 mg/100 ml. This usually is achieved only in patients who inject regular insulin before each meal or in those who use the new insulin infusion pumps, which provide a continuous basal supply of insulin and preprandial boluses.

Important factors in achieving control in insulin-dependent patients are a relatively inflexible pattern of eating and exercise and a stable emotional state. Under these circumstances, an insulin prescription can be ordered so that most patients can achieve the least stringent level of control (i.e., negative preprandial urine test results and plasma glucose values <200 mg/100 ml before breakfast and supper). Some patients (especially lean ones) can attain the next most stringent level (i.e., plasma glucose concentrations <150 mg/100 ml before breakfast and supper). More strict control in insulin-requiring patients is often not achieved. Obese patients usually have more difficulty in achieving control because the obesity interferes with the effectiveness of the insulin.

In controlling diabetes with use of insulin, a balance must always be achieved between attempting to return glucose concentrations toward normal and the risk of hypoglycemia. Under the present crude system of replacing endogenous insulin with exogenous insulin, some episodes of hypoglycemia are almost unavoidable if glucose concentrations are to approach normal most of the time. Since tight control has such important benefits (see chapter 2), I ask my patients to tolerate occasional (2 to 3 times per week) mild episodes of hypoglycemia. However, if these episodes occur more frequently than 2 to 3 times per week, are very distressing to the patient, and are not quickly aborted, I reduce the insulin dose and settle for less tight control.

Patients treated with diet and sulfonylurea agents usually achieve better diabetic control than do those who require insulin. The dose of the sulfonylurea agent is continually raised until either the postprandial glucose values are <150 mg/100 ml or until maximal doses of the agent are reached. As discussed in chapter 5, if the fasting plasma glucose concentration exceeds 200 mg/100 ml at the point of maximal dosage, the sulfonylurea agent should be discontinued and insulin therapy initiated.

"Honeymoon Phase" of Type 1 Diabetes

Shortly after the onset of type 1 diabetes, a *temporary* remission occurs in approximately 20% of patients (even in those who were in profound diabetic ketoacidosis). This is termed the *honeymoon phase*. The clinical manifestation of this remission varies from a slight reduction in insulin requirement to complete normalization of glucose tolerance without therapy. Secretion of endogenous insulin returns, at least in part, during the remission period (22). The duration of the honeymoon phase usually is short, lasting from a few weeks to several months, although an occasional patient has been in remission for many years. Although recent evidence suggests that the earlier and more intensive the initial treatment, the more likely and longer the remission will be, diabetes always returns. Thus, it is important to be aware of this phenomenon, in order both to anticipate the possible decrease in insulin requirement and not to offer the patient false hope that the diabetes has been cured.

Insulin Treatment of Grossly Obese Diabetics

Treatment of the obese diabetic patient who remains markedly out of control on maximal doses of potent sulfonylurea agents can be a difficult problem because these patients often do not respond to conventional doses of insulin. In general, the more obese the patient, the less responsive he or she is to insulin. Hospitalization to determine an appropriate insulin dose is useless, since the imposed ingestion of a suitable hypocaloric diet in the hospital improves their control considerably. Indeed, under these dietary conditions, obese diabetic patients often do not require insulin or even sulfonylurea agents. Thus, many physicians withhold insulin therapy from these patients, with the rationale that a weight-reducing diet is the appropriate treatment. Although this obviously is true, these patients are unable to adhere to such a diet, and their tissues remain exposed to greatly elevated levels of glucose. Therefore, I use insulin in obese diabetics even though it is usually only partially effective. I give two injections of intermediate-acting insulin per day in order to bring the diabetes under control. However, even the least stringent level of control usually is not attained, no matter how much insulin is administered subcutaneously. For practical reasons, I usually do not increase each injection to >100 U (which is equivalent to the contents of a 1-cc syringe) in order to limit the volume injected. Although 2-cc syringes are available, these patients respond so poorly to insulin that the additional amount often provides little extra benefit. With this approach, fasting glucose concentrations often can be reduced from 300 to 400 mg/100 ml to 200 to 300 mg/100 ml. Although this level of control is far from good, the reduction in the glucose concentration is healthier for the patient.

Brittle Diabetes

The pattern of diabetic control fluctuates extremely in a small minority of insulin-requiring patients. This situation has been variously termed *unstable, labile,* or *brittle* diabetes. Investigators disagree on the definition of this entity. Tattersall (23) suggests that a brittle diabetic is "any patient whose life is constantly being disrupted by episodes of hypo- or hyperglycemia whatever their cause." This is a good operational definition because this is exactly the situation with which the clinician must deal.

Several circumstances are associated with unstable diabetic control. First, individuals who do not secrete endogenous insulin are more likely to have labile diabetes than are those with some insulin secretion (24). However, this cannot be the entire explanation, because many patients devoid of their own insulin secretion do not have brittle diabetes.

Second, many brittle diabetics seem to have more severe emotional problems than those usually encountered in other patients. Although it is possible that this is the result of the labile course, the present consensus does not support this view (23). It is more likely that the hormonal responses to anxiety and anger in these patients lead to rapid rises in glucose concentration that cannot be counteracted by the slow absorption of subcutaneously injected insulin. Because the emotional state of these patients varies, increasing the insulin dose to improve diabetic control at one point may cause hypoglycemia at another. Thus, the identification and alleviation of emotional problems (see chapter 9) can be very helpful in treating brittle diabetes. This can be a difficult challenge, however.

In my experience, many patients with unstable diabetes are those who take relatively large amounts (>15 U per injection) of regular insulin. A rapid drop in glucose stimulates the release of contrainsulin hormones, the effects of which last for many hours (see chapter 10). Reduction or elimination of the dose of regular insulin is often helpful in improving control in brittle diabetics. (The Somogyi effect will be considered in greater detail in the next section.)

Finally, in a few labile patients neither emotional disturbances nor large amounts of regular insulin can be identified as a possible cause of the unstable course. Although endogenous insulin secretion probably is totally absent, this condition is not alterable at present. These patients respond best to two injections of intermediate-acting insulin per day; this dosage should be changed cautiously, if necessary, in small increments (usually by 2 units). Regular insulin should be avoided unless a relatively predictable pattern of diabetic control indicates its need. Then it is introduced into the regimen very slowly. Tight control in these patients is obviously much more difficult to achieve and probably is not a realistic goal.

Hypoglycemia

Although chapter 10 is devoted entirely to this subject, several issues concerning hypoglycemia in diabetic patients need emphasis here. The signs and symptoms of hypoglycemia that are caused by increased activity of the sympathetic nervous system (chapter 10, Table 10-3) can occur secondary to a rapid drop of an elevated glucose concentration to a lower (but still elevated) level. Therefore, a low glucose value may not be found in patients with suspected hypoglycemia.

Although episodes of hypoglycemia in insulin-requiring patients often occur inexplicably, decreased food intake or increased exercise should be explored as possible causes each time.

It is obvious that all patients who take insulin should carry with them a source of simple carbohydrates (e.g., candy, cookies, mints). What is not so obvious is that, after ingestion of these items and reversal of the hypoglycemic symptoms, the patient should eat something containing complex carbohydrates and/or protein within the next hour in order to avoid recurrence of this problem. The simple carbohydrate will be absorbed rapidly and will raise the plasma glucose concentration only temporarily. Glucose will be deposited in the tissues or lost in the urine if the plasma concentration exceeds the T_m and may not be available in the plasma long enough to buffer the continued effect of the insulin. Therefore, it is important to provide a source of more slowly absorbable carbohydrates. Amino acids from the ingested protein also will help to replenish stores of hepatic glycogen.

Home treatment of the unconscious hypoglycemic patient presents a difficult problem. Although preparations of "instant glucose" that are placed between the cheek and the teeth have been advocated in this situation, virtually no glucose is absorbed through the buccal mucosa with this technique (25). Since these preparations must be swallowed in order to be effective (25), they should not be given to an unconscious patient because of the danger of aspiration. Instead, glucagon should be available, and a responsible family member should be taught how to use it. The glucagon preparation consists of 1 mg of the powdered hormone in a sterile bottle and a vial containing 1 cc of sterile water. After the vial is broken, the diluent should be drawn into the patient's insulin syringe and injected through the rubber stopper of the bottle. The powder dissolves quickly, and the solution should be drawn back into the syringe and injected *intramuscularly*, rather than subcutaneously, to increase the rate of absorption. Within 5 to 10 minutes glucagon raises the blood sugar through stimulation of hepatic glycogenolysis. Although the effect is mild ($\sim$20 to 50 mg/100 ml increase), and transient (lasting $\sim$30 minutes), the patient often regains consciousness. At this point, the patient should immediately consume simple carbohydrates, followed by a substantial amount of complex carbohydrates.

Hypoglycemia secondary to the use of sulfonylurea agents usually lasts longer than insulin-induced hypoglycemia. Therefore, continued treatment for many hours may be necessary to prevent a recurrence. If the patient loses consciousness, hospitalization is advisable, since intravenous glucose therapy is indicated for several days (see chapter 10).

The final issue is the effect of unrecognized hypogl cemia or posthypoglycemia hyperglycemia. This is termed the Somogyi effect and is named after the person who first described this phenomenon. The clinical picture is one of worsening diabetic control in the presence of increasing insulin doses and is manifested especially by fasting hyperglycemia. The conventional explanation for this situation is that the hormonal response (catecholamines, glucagon, growth hormone, and cortisol) to unrecognized hypoglycemia (which usually occurs during the night) causes an insensitivity to insulin. Increasing the amount of insulin to treat the fasting hyperglycemia serves only to intensify the hypoglycemia; this in turn causes more insulin antagonism.

There are several clues to indicate the presence of the Somogyi effect in the uncontrolled diabetic (26): (*a*) rapid fluctuations in the results of urine tests for glucose and ketone bodies, sometimes changing from negative to maximal values within 4 hours; (*b*) wide swings in plasma glucose concentrations that are not related to meals; and (*c*) subtle clinical signs of hypoglycemia, such as mild nocturnal sweating, morning headaches, and hypothermia. Ketonuria often persists after glucosuria disappears; conversely, ketonuria may even precede the glucosuria.

Once the Somogyi phenomenon is suspected it must be documented. This can be accomplished only by assessing diabetic control at unusual times, usually during the night. Circulating glucose values can be measured by home glucose monitoring or, if the patient is hospitalized, by more conventional means. Split quantitative urinary glucose measurements are an effective way to measure glucose and have been discussed already. The simplest method is to compare results of semiquantitative tests of double-voided urine taken during the night with those taken before breakfast. If the results of the former are negative and those of the latter are markedly positive, the patient may be experiencing post-hypoglycemia hyperglycemia.

The ultimate criterion for diagnosis of the Somogyi phenomenon is improvement in diabetic control after a decrease in the insulin dose. This should be done gradually, since marked lowering (even to the same ultimate level) inexplicably worsens diabetic control (26).

In my experience, poor diabetic control is seldom due to the Somogyi phenomenon. The pattern of urine test results in most uncontrolled diabetics is one of unremitting glucosuria, and these patients invariably need more insulin. The lack of correlation between cortisol, glucagon, and growth hormone levels and a return to normal glucose concentrations after asymptomatic nocturnal hypoglycemia confirm this view (27). Instead, there is a close *inverse* correlation ($r = 0.99$) with free insulin levels, suggesting that the rapid rise in glucose values reflects a fall in circulating insulin concentrations (27).

"Starvation" Ketosis

The mechanism of "starvation" ketosis is similar to that of diabetic ketosis: increased breakdown of triglycerides in adipose tissue to free fatty acids, with their subsequent conversion to ketone bodies in the liver (see chapter 2). In diabetic ketosis, the absence of insulin causes overproduction of free fatty acids; in starvation ketosis, the signal is an underutilization of carbohydrates secondary to decreased carbohydrate intake. The utilization of ~80 to 100 g of exogenous carbohydrate per day is required to prevent ketosis. If much less than that amount is available, energy requirements in tissue must be met by increased fat metabolism, which leads to ketosis as described above. Although decreased carbohydrate intake usually is associated with diminished ingestion of total calories, ketosis also can occur with eucaloric diets that are low in carbohydrates. Thus, the term *starvation ketosis* is not entirely accurate.

There are two ways to distinguish between diabetic and starvation ketosis. The former almost always is associated with marked glucosuria, while the latter is not. However, ketonuria may interfere with the glucose reactions on Keto-Diastix, and type 1 patients thus may need an independent check of mild glucosuria occurring in the presence of moderate to large ketonuria by retesting with Clinitest. The most accurate way to distinguish between diabetic and starvation ketosis is to measure plasma ketone bodies. The degree of ketosis is much greater in uncontrolled diabetics as compared with that in patients whose ketosis is due primarily to inadequate carbohydrate intake. Therefore, in diabetic ketosis results of the nitroprusside test for plasma ketone bodies remain positive when the sample is diluted. In contrast, in starvation ketosis the results will almost invariably be negative after dilution.

There are two situations in which differentiation between diabetic and starvation ketosis is important. Occasionally, an obese type 2 patient will be given (and will actually follow) a hypocaloric diet whose carbohydrate content is low enough to lead to starvation ketosis. This usually is not difficult to distinguish from diabetic ketosis because the ketosis resistance of the patient will already have been established at the time of diagnosis. Furthermore, the urine tests should show little glucosuria. The other circumstance involves type 1 patients who become ill with gastrointestinal symptoms and are forced to limit their oral intake of food. This can be a difficult situation to resolve. On the one hand, gastrointestinal symptoms can be part of evolving ketoacidosis. Therefore, establishing the presence of diabetic ketosis and treating it vigorously is important in preventing hospitalization (see section on sick-day rules). On the other hand, if the situation is really one of viral gastroenteritis associated with starvation ketosis, overtreatment with insulin may cause hypoglycemia. Although a comparison of the degrees of glucosuria and ketonuria often help in making the decision, the patient may need to go to a laboratory facility for measurement of plasma ketone bodies.

Sick-Day Rules

In the presence of an infection of any kind, insulin action is impaired by unknown mechanisms. Therefore, in such circumstances diabetic control usually worsens, often quickly and profoundly. Because normal food intake is diminished, patients sometimes will decrease their insulin dose or omit it altogether. However, this is inadvisable. Rather, patients should take the prescribed amount and sometimes even additional amounts. The approach described below for adjusting insulin doses can also be used in patients whose diabetic control deteriorates in association with other kinds of stress (e.g., emotional upsets, trauma). Effective and frequent communication between patient and physician is an important component of care during these periods. Most hospitalizations can be avoided if adjustments in treatment are started early and continued appropriately.

Type 2 patients are less of a problem than type 1 diabetics. Most often their ketosis resistance persists and they very seldom become ketotic. The increasing hyperglycemia may need treatment, but their metabolic status will not deteriorate to the point where hospitalization is required. Since these episodes are self-limited, treatment regimens in patients on dietary therapy alone or dietary therapy supplemented with sulfonylurea agents usually are not altered. The dosage of the sulfonylurea agent can be increased temporarily if the patient becomes very symptomatic from uncontrolled diabetes. However, the benefits of starting either oral hypoglycemic therapy in those on diet alone or insulin are outweighed by inconvenience and by the short period for which these new therapies should be necessary. Furthermore, since most type 2 diabetics are obese, the decreased food intake usually associated with illness will tend to offset the worsening of control secondary to the infection in these patients.

The metabolism of type 2 diabetics receiving insulin, however, is more abnormal, and the deterioration of diabetic control is greater when these patients become infected. Therefore, insulin doses often have to be increased. If it is certain that the patient has an infection, urine tests should be carried out before each meal and before the bedtime snack, and the patient should receive 4 units of regular insulin for 1% or 2% glucosuria (≤0.5% glucosuria is not treated). Second-voided urine samples must be used because they permit determination of the patient's metabolic status at the time additional insulin may be needed. If regular insulin was given previously, the results of the first-voided specimen would not accurately reflect the effectiveness of the additional insulin; reliance on these results could lead to overtreatment.

If the patient has received additional amounts of regular insulin, the amount of intermediate-acting insulin must be increased the next day in order to prevent recurrence of similar poor control. For patients receiving two insulin injections, the morning dose is raised by 4 units if extra regular insulin was required before lunch or before supper. Even if supplemental insulin was given at both times, the morning dose of NPH insulin should be increased by only 4 units. The evening dose of intermediate-acting insulin should be increased by 4 units if additional regular insulin was required either that morning or before bedtime the previous evening. Again, the increase should be only 4 units, even if the patient received supplemental insulin at both times. For patients receiving one injection of intermediate-acting insulin in the morning, the dose of NPH insulin should be increased by 4 units the next day if one or two supplemental doses of regular insulin were required during the previous day and evening, and by 8 units if three or four doses were given.

As the infection improves, it is important to decrease the amount of insulin prescribed before hypoglycemia occurs. Thus, the dose of NPH insulin should gradually be lowered toward preinfection levels when results of the urine tests become negative. If the results remain negative, the decrease should be continued until basal levels are reached. If results of the urine tests generally remain at ≤0.5%, the new lowered level should be maintained in anticipation of further recovery from the infection and a quick return to the preinfection dosage of insulin. If 1% to 2% glucosuria reappears, the insulin dose should be raised again until the results of the urine tests improve.

This method of treating the infected insulin-dependent patient involves three basic principles: (a) that intermediate-acting insulin gradually be increased to prevent continued deterioration of diabetic control; (b) that regular insulin be administered only when needed; and (c) that NPH insulin be decreased gradually as the infection subsides and before hypoglycemia becomes a problem. Since this approach may not be entirely appropriate for all diabetics, it should serve only as a general guideline. Experience with individual patients will reveal to the physician that certain patients seem to be more sensitive to insulin and thus will require smaller increases, while others (especially obese individuals) are less sensitive and will require larger increases.

Insulin treatment in infected type 1 patients is similar to that in type 2 patients, with one important addition. Four additional units of regular insulin should be given if the urine test results also yield a moderate or large reaction for ketone bodies. Since infected type 1 diabetics can quickly slip into ketoacidosis, the extra amount of regular insulin is helpful in preventing this. In order to ensure that diabetic ketosis, not starvation ketosis, is being treated, 4 units of regular insulin are added to the 4 units that already were prescribed for the 1% or 2% glucosuria. If the test results for ketone bodies are moderate or large, ketonuria should not be treated unless significant glucosuria is present. Therefore, in patients with moderate or large ketonuria and <1% glucosuria with Keto-Diastix, it is important to ascertain whether the degree of glucosuria really is low or whether it represents a falsely low reading produced by the ketonuria, as discussed earlier. This problem is particularly vexing in infected patients with gastrointestinal symptoms, who could have either mild ketoacidosis (see chapter 6) or starvation ketosis secondary to diminished oral intake of food. Thus, an independent assessment of the amount of glucosuria with Clinitest is important in this situation.

The increase in the dose of intermediate-acting insulin the following day should be the same for infected type 1 patients as it is for infected type 2 patients. The governing factor is the number of times, not the amount, that additional regular insulin was prescribed; that is, if extra regular insulin were given once or twice, the increase in the dosage of NPH insulin the following day would be 4 U; if extra regular insulin were given three or four times, the increase would be 8 U. The principles of adjusting insulin doses in infected patients are illustrated in the following case.

Case 1

The patient is a 35-year-old woman who has had type 1 diabetes for 15 years. She takes 24 U of NPH insulin and 4 U of regular insulin before breakfast, and 8 U of NPH insulin before supper. On this regimen her urine test results usually are negative, except at times of dietary indiscretion. She smokes approximately one pack of cigarettes per day. On the evening of 10/22, she noticed the onset of a sore throat, nasal congestion, and myalgia. By the next morning the symptoms had progressed and her temperature was 100.2°F. Results of tests of double-voided urine and her regimen of insulin therapy are shown in Table 7-5. She called her physician on the afternoon of 10/22 and the approach discussed for treating infected type 1 diabetics was begun.

The patient's morning dose of NPH insulin on 10/23 was increased because she had required extra regular insulin the previous afternoon. In addition, she received more regular insulin before breakfast because of the results of the fasting urine test. These results before breakfast were also responsible for the increase in the before-supper dose of NPH insulin. She also required additional regular insulin that evening because of 1% glucosuria before bedtime.

On the morning of 10/24 the amount of NPH was not changed because additional regular insulin had not been necessary during the previous day (i.e., before lunch and supper). The evening dose of NPH insulin was increased because she had required additional regular insulin before bedtime the night before. On the evening of 10/24, her cough began to produce yellow sputum, which signals the onset of acute bronchitis in this heavy smoker.

The lower respiratory bacterial infection worsened her diabetic control further on 10/25 in spite of the increased amounts of insulin that she now was taking. Tetracycline was prescribed, and the amount of NPH insulin was raised by only 4 units even though she had required 4 units of extra regular insulin before both lunch and supper the previous day. Eight units of regular insulin also were added before breakfast on 10/25 because of the heavy glucosuria and ketonuria at that time. Additional short-acting insulin was not needed that day. The before-supper dose of NPH insulin was increased on the basis of the urine test results of the previous evening and that morning. (The increase was only 4 units even though a total of 12 units of regular insulin had been given at these times.)

The amount of NPH insulin was not changed on 10/26 because additional insulin was not required before lunch, supper, or bedtime the previous day or before breakfast that day. The final increase in insulin was made on the morning of 10/27 because she had required additional regular insulin the previous day. The results of the urine tests improved considerably as the therapy for her bronchitis took effect, and her insulin dose was reduced gradually to its usual levels. The advantage of increasing intermediate-acting insulin rather than short-acting insulin in anticipation of continued insulin antagonism was illustrated on 10/27. Both her bronchitis and her insulin sensitivity began to improve. If extra regular

Table 7-5. Insulin Treatment of an Infected Ketosis-Prone (Type 1) Diabetic Patient

Date	Before Breakfast				Before Lunch			Before Supper				Before Bed		
	Urine Tests		Insulin (U)		Urine Tests		Insulin (U)	Urine Tests		Insulin (U)		Urine Tests		Insulin (U)
	Glucose	KB	NPH	Reg	Glucose	KB	Reg	Glucose	KB	NPH	Reg	Glucose	KB	Reg
10/22	1%	N	24	4				1%	N	8	4	0.5%	N	
10/23	2%	N	28	8	0.25%	N		0.5%	N	12		1%	N	4
10/24	0.5%	N	28	4	1%	N	4	1%	1+	16	4	2%	1+	4
10/25[b]	2%	2+	32	12	0.25%	1+		0.5%	N	20		0.5%	N	
10/26	0.5%	N	32	4	2%	3+	8	0.5%	1+	20		0.5%	N	
10/27	0.1%	N	36	4	0.25%	N		N	N	20		N	N	
10/28	N	N	32	4	N	N		0.1%	N	16		N	N	
10/29	N	N	28	4	0.1%	N		N	N	12		N	N	
10/30	N	N	24	4	N	N		N	N	8		N	N	

Abbreviations: KB, ketone bodies; Reg, regular insulin; N, negative; 1+, small; 2+, moderate; 3+, large.
[b]Upper respiratory infection developed into acute bronchitis.

insulin had been prescribed, the likelihood of hypoglycemia occurring would have been greater, since the effect of the insulin would have been exerted over 4 to 6 hours rather than over 24 hours, as with NPH insulin.

In addition to adjusting insulin doses, three other modalities are important in treating infected diabetics; carbohydrate intake and, in patients with vomiting, diarrhea or marked polyuria, fluid (sodium) and potassium replacement. Since most of these patients receive insulin, some carbohydrate intake is important. A method for calculating the carbohydrate content in the diet and for obtaining that amount from more easily digestible foods is described in detail in chapter 3. In some patients this is not feasible because either they are not properly educated in this approach or their gastrointestinal symptoms may prevent them from eating the appropriate amounts of food. These patients should eat foods that they can tolerate from the milk, fruit, bread, and vegetable exchange lists. Liquids and soft foods are easier to digest, and patients often are able to consume 6 to 8 smaller meals rather than 3 to 4 larger ones. Soft drinks (not low-calorie ones) and fruit juices are good sources of carbohydrates.

Fluid losses from the kidney or gastrointestinal tract are high in sodium. In order to avoid marked depletion of the intravascular volume (dehydration), replacement must be with fluids that contain relatively large amounts of sodium. As long as enough insulin and fluids can be given, hospitalization can often be avoided. When the severity of the gastrointestinal symptoms precludes oral intake of fluid, patients usually must be hospitalized. Two good sources of sodium are bouillon (1 cup contains ~40 mEq) and tomato juice (1 cup contains ~20 mEq). Other foods high in sodium are canned soups, saltine crackers, and packaged custard pudding mixes. Salt can be added to other juices. Soft drinks contain little sodium.

Sources high in potassium include orange juice, tomato juice, and prune juice (1 cup ~15 mEq). Foods with a moderate potassium content (1 cup ~10 mEq) include milk, grapefruit juice, and pineapple juice. Apple juice, grape juice, and cranberry juice are low in potassium (1 cup ~5 mEq). A large banana contains ~10 mEq of potassium.

Exercise

Although exercise has been discussed in connection with dietary therapy (chapter 3) and insulin therapy (chapter 4), certain points will be repeated here because they are pertinent in the day-to-day management of insulin-dependent diabetics. Exercise increases the effectiveness of insulin, both by increasing its absorption from the injection site and by enhancing its intrinsic activity on insulin-sensitive tissues. Therefore, the insulin prescription should be matched to a relatively constant daily amount of exercise. If more exercise is planned, the patient should consume extra carbohydrate calories in order to offset the effect. A general approach for balancing the amount of extra food with the anticipated level of exercise is suggested in chapter 3. However, patients must determine for themselves whether these amounts are applicable to them or whether adjustments are needed. If the exercise period lasts longer than several hours, it sometimes is necessary to interrupt it briefly to ingest extra calories (in addition to eating before starting). Increasing calories is preferable to decreasing the amount of insulin for extra exercise. If the anticipated extra exercise is not performed, the patient will have taken too small a dose of insulin that day, and his or her control will suffer accordingly.

Foot Care

Infections of the feet are a major source of morbidity among diabetics and often lead to death. Even though many of these infections are preventable, foot ulcers and gangrene continue to exact a tremendous toll in the diabetic population. Thus, the physician must emphasize the importance of proper foot care (see chapter 8 for a detailed discussion of this topic). The feet of patients over the age of 40 and of those who have had diabetes for >10 years should be examined at every office visit. Patients with impairment of blood flow to the feet, secondary to either large- or small-vessel disease, should have their toenails cut by qualified medical personnel (i.e., podiatrist, nurse, or physician).

Calluses are an important sign of possible future trouble. They represent increased pressure on that area, and the patient often cannot feel them because of associated sensory neuropathy. Calluses should be shaved routinely (usually by a podiatrist, but other medical personnel can be taught how) and kept to a minimum. Unroofing an innocuous-looking callus will sometimes reveal an extensive ulcer, which could have been prevented by treating the callus when it first appeared. The source of the pressure (e.g., ill-fitting shoes, collapsed metatarsal arch, hammertoe) must be identified and corrective measures taken, if possible. Softer and better-fitting shoes usually are all that is needed, although persuading patients to forgo style simply to prevent calluses is not always easy. Prophylactic surgery to correct or remove a hammertoe is indicated in some patients with impaired circulation, since there is no orthopedic way to reduce the pressure on the offending digit.

In summary, *most foot ulcers and other infected lesions of the feet are preventable*. Although examination of the feet and instruction of patients in proper prophylactic foot care seem mundane, probably no other service that the physician performs offers as important a benefit for their diabetic patients, especially those who are older.

Travel

Insulin-requiring diabetics who travel should be advised about their insulin. Insulin is stable at room temperature, a feature that facilitates travel for these patients. Insulin vials and syringes should be taken along, especially if the patient is going to a foreign country. The timing, and occasionally the amount, of the insulin dose may need adjustment on the day of travel, especially if the patient is flying into a different time zone. The patient should find out from the airline what kind of meal will be served and at what time. The insulin dose is then adjusted to the meal pattern. Traveling from north to south, and vice versa, is the easiest change to accommodate, since the time does not change and the eating pattern usually is not too different from what the patient is accustomed to. Traveling from east to west, and vice versa, presents more of a problem because the change in time often disrupts both meal and sleeping patterns. A relatively smooth integration of the new eating and activity schedule with the insulin regimen can be accomplished by keeping both schedules geared to the patient's internal clock for the first 12 to 24 hours after arrival and by then shifting gradually to the changed external time.

For instance, for a patient taking two insulin injections per day, an afternoon flight from Los Angeles to New York City might be handled as follows. The flight leaves at 2 PM and a large meal is served 2 hours later. The patient would start his day ~1 hour earlier than usual. He would take the usual insulin dose and eat breakfast and lunch slightly earlier than normal. He would take his second injection of insulin on the plane just before the 4 PM meal (Los Angeles time) is served. The patient arrives in New York City at 11 PM local time (but at 8 PM according to his internal clock) and eats his bedtime snack shortly after arrival. This is necessary because he took his second injection of NPH insulin ~4 hours before. He goes to sleep at 1 to 2 AM New York time (9 to 10 PM Los Angeles time). On awakening the next day at 8 AM (5 AM Los Angeles time), his fasting glucose level should still be controlled by the NPH insulin, which was taken ~12 hours earlier. He now can follow his usual schedule. Although according to his internal clock he is taking his insulin 3 hours earlier than usual, his eating and activity patterns also have been shifted by 3 hours, and the relation between the two patterns have not been disrupted seriously.

Traveling from New York City back to Los Angeles requires more of an adjustment. A morning flight leaves the East Coast at 9 AM and arrives on the West Coast at noon (local time). The same patient would take his insulin and a small breakfast several hours before the flight. A large breakfast usually is served shortly after take off. The patient could either take a small amount of extra regular insulin to handle these calories or consume only a portion of them as a midmorning snack. Regardless of which he chooses, he needs to have some food available several hours before landing to serve as a small lunch. After arriving in Los Angeles at noon (3 PM by his internal clock), he should arrange to eat his major meal several hours later. Although this occurs in the middle of the afternoon on the West Coast, it is an appropriate time for his supper according to the peak action of his morning insulin injection. He should delay his second injection of NPH insulin for several more hours (5 PM Los Angeles time, 8 PM New York time). He would need to eat his bedtime snack at 8 to 9 PM (local time) to cover this injection, by which time he probably would wish to retire (approximately midnight by his internal clock). Although he might arise very early the next morning according to West Coast time, the hour would theoretically be appropriate for the East Coast, and he should delay taking his morning injection and eating until the appropriate Los Angeles time. This delay should not cause much of a problem because his last NPH injection was taken ~15 hours previously and should still be effective in controlling his fasting glucose concentration. His insulin regimen and eating patterns are now adjusted (with respect to time, at least) back to the West Coast schedule.

Although the disruptions encountered by patients taking longer plane trips are greater, the same general approach is used to treat them during the flight and to aid their adjustment after arrival. These examples do not take into account the stress effect of changing time zones ("jet lag"), which may impair diabetic control temporarily.

An alternative method is to give the patient the entire dose as short-acting insulin. Twenty-five per cent of the total daily dose should be taken as regular insulin before each meal during travel, starting the morning of departure. The normal amount of intermediate-acting insulin should be resumed with the first breakfast at the patient's destination. The disadvantage of this approach, however, is that the timing of the meals often is not evenly spaced during a 24-hour period. The patient may need a small dose of NPH insulin after arrival if he or she plans to sleep for 8 hours or longer before starting a more normal eating and activity schedule.

Dental Procedures

Dental infections, especially periodontal disease, are more common in diabetics than in nondiabetics. Therefore, diabetic patients are more likely to undergo dental procedures that impair food intake. This may be a problem for those taking insulin or sulfonylurea agents unless precautions are taken. Effective communication between the patient's physician and dentist is important so that the extent and timing of the diminished food intake and the severity of the operative stress can be judged.

If a patient taking sulfonylurea agents will miss more than one meal because of a dental procedure, the drugs should be omitted that morning and resumed when normal food intake occurs. Chlorpropamide (Diabinese) should be discontinued the previous day because of its long half-life.

Hypoglycemia is more likely to occur secondary to insulin therapy than to oral hypoglycemia agents. In these patients, dental procedures should be performed in the morning, if possible, because the effects of intermediate-acting insulins injected before breakfast peak late in the afternoon, and because an insulin reaction may occur if the supper calories are decreased. If the lunch calories are diminished, regular and Semilente insulin should be omitted from the morning dose. In addition, NPH insulin and breakfast might be taken a little later than usual to minimize the risk of early-afternoon hypoglycemia. If the amount of food intake at supper will be decreased, the dose of intermediate-acting insulin should be reduced. However, type 1 patients must have some insulin to avoid ketosis and possibly ketoacidosis. Therefore, a balance must be achieved between the decreased insulin requirements caused by decreased food intake and the need for insulin caused by the stress of the dental procedure and possibly by the infection that led to it. It is important that the patient monitor his or her control closely after the procedure and communicate with the physician. If extensive dental work that impairs food intake is necessary, in ketosis-prone diabetics, hospitalization sometimes is advisable.

Surgical and PostOperative Management

The goals of therapy during surgery in diabetic patients are threefold: to minimize fluid and electrolyte losses secondary to an osmotic diuresis by limiting hyperglycemia, to prevent diabetic ketosis in type 1 patients, and to avoid hypoglycemia while the patient is under anesthesia. Many different approaches have been recommended (28), and none has a clear-cut advantage over another. These include (a) withholding glucose and insulin until the postoperative period; (b) adding regular insulin to intravenous glucose infusions during surgery; (c) dividing the administration of intravenous glucose and subcutaneous regular insulin into equal periods, four intervals of equal duration; approximately one fourth of the previous total daily requirement of insulin is given each time, with additional amounts added as necessary according to the results of fractional urine tests; (d) giving insulin preoperatively and supplementing this amount postoperatively; and (e) giving the usual dose and type of insulin at the usual time.

Since intraoperative monitoring of glucose levels usually is not possible, many anesthesiologists fear that hypoglycemia will occur during surgery if insulin is given preoperatively. However, diabetologists state that such hypoglycemia rarely occurs (28). A recent prospective study done at UCLA (29) documents this observation. Glucose concentrations were measured hourly during surgery. Eighty-nine insulin-requiring patients were monitored. Insulin was withheld from 31 of them, 47 received one third of their total daily dose as NPH insulin on the morning of surgery, and 11 were given one half of theirs. In all 58 patients, glucose (6.25 g/h) was infused until the end of surgery.

Hypoglycemia occurred in only three of the 58 patients who received insulin. Two of the three experienced the hypoglycemia before their afternoon surgery was begun, and the third became hypoglycemic 30 minutes into surgery but 4.5 hours after the morning dose of intermediate-acting insulin.

The rise in glucose concentration during surgery was similar ($\sim$20 mg/100 ml per hour) in all 89 patients and thus seemed not to be related to whether or not the patient received insulin preoperative. Glucose concentrations during surgery exceeded 400 mg/100 ml in seven patients—four in the control group and three in the insulin-treated group. The apparent lack of effect of insulin on glucose concentration during surgery may be because most of the operations were performed in the morning during the lag phase of NPH insulin.

These results do not support the contention that preoperative insulin should be avoided because hypoglycemia may occur while the patient is under general anesthesia. Rather, they indicate that, in order to avoid hypoglycemia in insulin-requiring diabetics before surgery, operations should be performed in the morning.

Ideally, one would wish to administer rapid-acting insulin and monitor its effects frequently. Two recent studies (30, 31) have evaluated intraoperative intravenous insulin infusion with measurement of glucose concentrations every 2 hours. In general, small doses of regular insulin were effective in controlling glucose levels during surgery. However, unavailability of rapid glucose monitoring during surgery precludes the use of this method in most hospitals.

At Cedars-Sinai Medical Center, we are currently assessing this approach in the operating room with use of a Stat-Tek machine (see section on home glucose monitoring) to provide glucose values every hour. Patients do not receive insulin on the morning of surgery. An infusion of 5% dextrose in water at a rate of 125 cc/h is begun just before the administration of anesthesia. The glucose concentration is then measured, and an infusion of regular insulin is "piggybacked" onto the glucose infusion according to the protocol summarized in Table 7-6. The rate of insulin infusion is adjusted every hour on the basis of the results of the glucose measurement. (Note that this measurement is a whole-blood value, which is 15% less than the concomitant plasma concentration.) Other fluids required by the surgeon and the anesthesiologist are administered separately. Although the results of these investigations are not conclusive enough at present to advocate this exact approach, the rapidity and ease with which glucose concentrations can be measured in the operating room with the Stat-Tek machine should facilitate the general use of this method. If surgery is scheduled later in the day, the patient will require some insulin in the morning.

Table 7-6. Experimental Protocol for Treating Insulin-Requiring Patients During Surgery

Whole-Blood Glucose (mg/100 ml)	Insulin Infusion Rate (U/hr)
≤100	None
101–200	1
201–300	2
301–400	3
>400	4[a]

[a]Glucose infusion is discontinued.

Given the current limitations of monitoring glucose levels during surgery, the following approach is recommended for insulin-requiring diabetics. The patient should receive one half of his or her total daily insulin dose (i.e., one half of the entire amount of intermediate- and short-acting insulin taken normally) as NPH insulin on the morning of surgery. An infusion of 5% dextrose in water should be administered at a rate of 125 cc/h. If surgery must be delayed for ≥4 hours after the insulin is given, the fasting glucose concentration should be measured (ordered *stat*). If this value is <200 mg/100 ml, the rate of glucose infusion should be increased to 200 cc/h when the laboratory value is reported.

When the patient enters the recovery room after surgery, the patient should receive the second half of the NPH insulin, and the glucose level should be measured (ordered *stat*). If the glucose value is >350 mg/100 ml and/or moderate or large ketonuria is present, 8 to 10 U of regular insulin also should be given. If the patient requires only NPH insulin at this time, another glucose concentration should be obtained in ~8 hours; if he or she requires regular insulin as well, its effect should be monitored 2 to 4 hours later.

Patients undergoing minor surgical procedures should be able to eat the same day. If the glucose concentration obtained ~8 hours after the second injection of intermediate-acting insulin is high (>250 mg/100 ml), a small amount of NPH insulin may be required that evening to control the fasting glucose level the next morning. The patient should be back in his or her usual routine by the next day. Extra insulin may be necessary for several days to counteract the stress effects of postoperative discomfort. Insulin doses should be adjusted as described in chapter 4.

Patients undergoing major surgery, especially abdominal operations, will not be able to eat for various lengths of time postoperatively. Their parenteral nutrition should include at least 100 g of glucose (2 L of 5% dextrose in water) over each 24-hour period to avoid starvation ketosis. A convient way to administer insulin while the patient is not able to eat is to infuse the glucose continuously and give NPH insulin every 12 hours; this method provides continuous insulin coverage. The glucose concentration obtained before each administration of NPH insulin reflects the effectiveness of the previous injection (i.e., that given 12 hours before). Since that value will not be available from the laboratory until at least several hours after the most recent injection, it should be used to adjust the subsequent dose of insulin.

For instance, if the patient is receiving insulin at 0800 and 2000, the morning glucose concentration should be used to judge the evening dose and the glucose value at 2000 will help to determine what adjustments (if any) should be made the following morning. Lean patients are started on 10 U of NPH every 12 hours, and obese patients (i.e., those at >125% of ideal body weight; see chapter 3) are begun on 16 U of NPH insulin at both times. Each dose of NPH insulin is increased by 4 U if the appropriate glucose concentration is >250 mg/100 ml. If the glucose level is >350 mg/100 ml, 8 U of regular insulin is given when that value becomes known. As the patient begins to eat, increasing amounts of insulin can be added to the morning injection. When intravenous glucose is no longer infused overnight (which should occur after oral caloric intake improves considerably), some of the evening dose of NPH insulin also can be shifted to the morning. In this manner, the transition from total parenteral nutrition through partial oral supplementation to normal food intake can be accomplished smoothly without large fluctuations in diabetic control. The following case should serve to illustrate this approach.

Case 2

The patient is a 37-year-old woman who has had type 1 diabetes for 17 years. She is 5 feet 5 inches tall and weighs 142 pounds. Her insulin regimen consists of 28 U of NPH and 8 U of regular insulin in the morning, and 12 U of NPH insulin before supper. She was admitted to the hospital for an elective cholecystectomy after intermittent episodes of colicky pain in the right upper quadrant associated with mild postprandial nausea. On the morning of surgery, she received 24 U of NPH insulin; the appropriate glucose infusion was started, and she went to the operating room at 0900. Her postoperative course is summarized in Table 7-7.

The patient received the second half of her NPH insulin on entering the recovery room. The glucose concentration at that time was >350 mg/100 ml, for which 10 U of regular insulin was given when the laboratory reported the value. Her glucose level was measured 3 hours after she was given the short-acting insulin, and her response was satisfactory. Another sample was drawn at 2200 to monitor the effectiveness of the NPH insulin that was given 9 hours before, when she entered the recovery room. Since she is not obese, the evening dose (10 U) of NPH insulin was also given at 2200. Her morning glucose level on 7/24, the first day after surgery, revealed an inadequate response to the 2200 dose, and she was given 8 U of regular insulin when the value was reported. The response to the additional insulin was evaluated 4 hours after administration and was satisfactory. That evening, the amount of NPH insulin was increased to 14 U because the dose on the previous evening was inadequate. Because the glucose concentration that evening was 283 mg/100 ml, the morning dose of NPH insulin was increased the following day. Although the patient did not require any more regular insulin, the amounts of NPH insulin had to be increased gradually on 7/25 and 7/26 in order to maintain glucose concentrations of <250 mg/100 ml. Stricter control during the immediate postoperative period, when the patient is experiencing pain and receiving infusions of glucose, can be difficult to attain and is not necessary.

Although the patient began a liquid diet on 7/27, the insulin doses were not changed because the glucose infusions were maintained and the initial oral intake was limited. On 7/30, when she could tolerate a soft diet and the intravenous dextrose was discontinued, the effect of the morning dose of NPH insulin was evaluated before supper (at 1600 instead of 2000) and the evening dose of insulin was reduced. The pattern of adjusting her subsequent insulin requirements followed the guidelines discussed in chapter 4.

Table 7-7. Postoperative course of a Type 1 Diabetic Patient After Cholecystectomy

Date	Time	Plasma Glucose (mg/100 ml)	Amount (U) of Insulin (Type)	Remarks
7/23	1300	384	24 (NPH)	Enters recovery room;
	1430		10 (Reg)[a]	receives 5% dextrose
	1730	261		solution at 125 cc/hr
	2200	289	10 (NPH)	
7/24	0800	397	10 (NPH)	
	1000		8 (Reg)[a]	
	1400	241		
	2000	283	14 (NPH)	
7/25	0800	313	14 (NPH)	
	2000	275	18 (NPH)	
7/26	0800	225	18 (NPH)	Bowel sounds present
	2000	193	18 (NPH)	
7/27	0800	178	18 (NPH)	Liquid diet started
	2000	184	18 (NPH)	but patient vomited
7/28	0800	192	18 (NPH)	Liquid diet tolerated
	2000	210	18 (NPH)	
7/29	0800	163	18 (NPH)	Soft diet started
	2000	243	18 (NPH)	
7/30	0800	174	18 (NPH)	Glucose infusion
	1600	265	12 (NPH)	stopped; soft diet continued
7/31	0800	143	22 (NPH)	
	1600	225	12 (NPH)	
8/1	0800	158	26 (NPH)	Normal diet tolerated
	1600	179	12 (NPH)	
8/2	0800	138	26 (NPH)	Patient ambulatory
	1600	183	12 (NPH)	
8/3	0800	147	26 (NPH)	Regular insulin added
			4 (Reg)	because of persistent
	1600	163	12 (NPH)	glucosuria before lunch
8/4	0800	153	26 (NPH)	Patient discharged
			4 (Reg)	after breakfast

[a]Regular insulin given according to glucose values measured several hours previously.

The following approach is recommended for patients who do not require insulin. Those who are controlled by dietary therapy alone can be treated in the same way as nondiabetic patients. Monitoring of glucose concentrations is important, however, since hyperglycemia can occur secondary to the stress of surgery and postoperative discomfort. Although deterioration of diabetic control usually is temporary, glucose concentrations persistently elevated at >250 mg/100 ml should be treated with small doses of NPH insulin. Sulfonylurea agents should be discontinued on the day of surgery; chlorpropamide, however, should be discontinued the day before surgery because it has a long half-life. With minor surgery, oral medication should be resumed when the patient resumes eating. Major surgical procedures often cause marked elevations in glucose concentration in patients who require sulfonylurea agents. Therefore, lean individuals should receive 10 U of NPH insulin and obese individuals (>125% ideal body weight) should receive 16 U of NPH insulin on the morning of surgery. All patients should be monitored in the manner described for insulin-requiring diabetics. When the patient starts eating again, the insulin should be withdrawn gradually and the sulfonylurea agent resumed.

Some brief comments about two other methods of postoperative treatment for diabetic patients are in order. The sliding-scale method should *not* be used; the reasons for this are discussed in detail in chapter 4. Continuous intravenous administration of regular insulin can be used under the appropriate circumstances. There is no truth to the premise that the ratio of the amount of glucose given to the dose of insulin required is relatively stable. However, if the patient's actual response is monitored frequently, a constant infusion of insulin is an effective way to maintain acceptable glucose levels postoperatively.

The insulin solution (0.2 U/cc) is prepared by mixing 1.0 ml of U-100 insulin (100 U) in 500 cc of normal saline. Fifty milliliters are run through the tubing and then discarded in order to saturate the nonspecific adsorption sites for insulin and to ensure that the appropriate amount will be delivered. The initial dose is administered through a separate line at a rate of 2 U (10 cc) per hour. Glucose concentrations should be measured $\sim$2 hours after starting the infusion. If the glucose level is between 150 and 250 mg/100 ml, the infusion rate should not be changed, and the glucose concentrations should be measured routinely every 4 hours. Whenever the glucose concentration is >250 mg/100 ml, the rate should be increased by 1 U (5 cc) per hour; if it is <150 mg/100 ml, the rate should be decreased by 1 U per hour. Glucose levels should be measured 1 to 2 hours after each time the rate of infusion is changed. When the patient resumes eating, additional regular insulin (depending on the amount of caloric intake) should be given before each meal by temporarily increasing the infusion rate. When the glucose infusion is discontinued, insulin administration should be switched to subcutaneous NPH. Since this approach requires much closer laboratory and clinical monitoring of the patient, it may not be possible in all hospitals.

Practical Summary

Initial Evaluation and General Follow-up

In keeping with the basic philosophy of this book—i.e., discussing only material that is either unique or especially pertinent to the treatment of the diabetic patient—only a few aspects of the initial workup will be emphasized. This should include a baseline recording of the carotid, femoral, popliteal, posterior tibial and dorsalis pedis pulses; examination of the neck, abdomen, flank, and groin areas for bruits; and evaluation of vibratory sensation in the feet and of reflexes in all the extremities. In addition, in asymptomatic patients, the fundi should be examined thoroughly at least each year. Laboratory assessment should include a urinalysis for protein, blood urea nitrogen (BUN) or creatinine level, fasting triglyceride concentration, cholesterol level, and electrocardiogram (ECG). In the absence of proteinuria, routine measurements of BUN or creatinine concentrations are not really necessary. If the cholesterol concentration is elevated, high-density lipoprotein (HDL) cholesterol levels should be measured at least once to confirm that the increased total cholesterol level is due mainly to the low-density lipoprotein fraction and deserves treatment. If lipid levels are normal, they should be measured routinely each year. If the patient is being treated for elevated lipid concentrations, the lipids should be measured every 3 months. Electrocardiograms need not be repeated unless the patient complains of symptoms that may be related to the heart. Diabetic patients, especially those taking insulin, should carry or wear some form of identification that indicates they are diabetic (see appendix to chapter 8 for information on how to obtain a Medic Alert bracelet).

Patients who have no complaints should be seen every 3 months if they are taking insulin or every 4 to 6 months if their treatment consists of diet alone or diet supplemented with sulfonylurea agents. Blood sugar measurements should be ordered every 4 to 6 weeks, and the patient should be contacted with the results. Blood pressure, retinopathy, vibratory sensation, pulses, and proteinuria should be evaluated at ~6-month intervals. In patients over the age of 40 or with diabetes of ⩾10 years' duration, the feet should be examined at every visit. Elevated blood pressure must be vigorously treated because of its deleterious effects on diabetic retinopathy and glomerulosclerosis as well as on the heart. If any type of retinopathy (including the background variety) is found, the patient should be referred to an ophthalmologist. Fluorescein angiography probably will reveal much more extensive damage than is apparent on routine examination, and prophylactic photocoagulation is effective in preventing severe visual loss. A urine culture should be obtained, or at least pyuria should be evaluated, in patients with proteinuria of recent onset in order to rule out an asymptomatic urinary tract infection.

Monitoring Diabetic Control

There are five general methods for assessing diabetic control: (a) semiquantitative testing of urine for glucose and ketone bodies; (b) quantitative measurement of urinary glucose in timed samples; (c) laboratory measurement of plasma or whole-blood glucose concentrations; (d) measurement of capillary whole-blood glucose levels by the patient (home glucose monitoring); and (e) measurement of glycosylated hemoglobin (Hgb) or Hgb A_{1c} levels.

There are four different products available for semiquantitative measurement of urinary glucose: Clinitest tablets, Clinistix, Tes-Tape, and Diastix. Several factors can affect the results of these tests, including (a) the different ranges of sensitivity of each product (Table 7-1); (b) the patient's renal threshold for glucose (T_m); (c) certain properties and constituents of the urine that interfere with the chemical reactions involved in the tests (Table 7-2); and (d) the timing of the sample.

With regard to the last factor, specimens collected while the patient is in the fasting state are the least sensitive (i.e., least likely to show glucosuria); preprandial specimens are the next most sensitive; and samples collected 1 to 2 hours after the patient has eaten are the most sensitive. Another factor that influences sensitivity is whether a first- or second-voided urine specimen is tested. Second-voided samples give a more accurate reflection of the blood glucose concentration at the time the urine is excreted. Therefore, they must be used to determine the T_m. On the other hand, testing only first-voided samples is more convenient for the patient and thus compliance is much better. Additionally, the results of first-voided urine specimens reflect the postprandial surge of glucose and thus must be rendered negative to ensure strict diabetic control. Although the amount of glucosuria in second-voided urine samples is usually perceived to be less than that in first-voided samples, the results of both tests are the same 60% to 80% of the time (Table 7-3).

On the basis of these considerations, I recommend the following approach for semiquantitative urine testing of glucose. Ketosis-resistant (type 2) patients should use Diastix, and ketosis-prone (type 1) patients should use Keto-Diastix. Since in type 1 patients ketone bodies may falsely depress test results for glucosuria, in the presence of moderate or large ketonuria associated with <1% glucosuria, it is important to make an independent assessment of glucosuria with Clinitest tablets. Double-voided urine samples should be tested only for the initial diagnosis and for establishment of the T_m. First-voided specimens should be tested routinely except before breakfast, when second-voided samples should also be tested. Although semiquantitative testing of urinary glucose is at best only a crude index of the prevailing glucose concentration (Table 7-4), it is the only way to assess diabetic control routinely in most patients and thus should be encouraged.

Quantitative measurement of urinary glucose in timed samples gives a more accurate reflection of diabetic control. However, the results are influenced both by the T_m and by the carbohydrate content of the patient's diet. Because patients may find accurate collection of urine to be inconvenient, I use this method of assessing control only to determine whether the Somogyi phenomenon is present.

Plasma glucose concentrations obviously are the best index of diabetic control, but they reflect the metabolic situation at only a single point in time and thus may not represent the situation over an extended period. The fasting plasma glucose concentration is the least sensitive test; preprandial values taken during the day are of intermediate sensitivity, and measurements taken 1 to 2 hours postprandially are the most sensitive indices of control.

In the normal red blood cell, 90% of hemoglobin contains two alpha chains and two beta chains. This hemoglobin is called Hgb A. Approximately 7% of hemoglobin is composed of glycosylated Hgb (also called Hgb A_1), in which carbohydrate moieties are connected to the beta chains of Hgb A. These glycosylated Hgbs have a different mobility on ion-exchange chromatography and have been termed *fast Hgbs* because they precede the major peak of Hgb A when they are separated by this technique. There are five different glycosylated Hgbs: Hgb A_{1a}, Hgb A_{1b}, Hgb A_{1c}, Hgb A_{1d}, and Hgb A_{1e}, according to which specific carbohydrate moiety is attached to them. Hgb A_{1c} is the major hemoglobin and constitutes nearly 5% of the hemoglobin found in normal red cells.

The percentage of glycosylated Hgb is increased in diabetic patients, with Hgb A_{1c} showing the greatest change and the remaining glycosylated Hgbs remaining relatively stable. A number of experiments have demonstrated that the reaction between Hgb A and glucose (the major carbohydrate moiety) is slow, nonenzymatic, nearly irreversible, and continuous during the 120-day life span of the red cell. This means that the amount of glycosylated Hgb increases with the age of the red cell. The amount of glycosylated Hgb also depends importantly on the circulating glucose concentration to which the red cell is exposed. Therefore, the hyperglycemia of diabetes causes the increased percentage of glycosylated Hgb in diabetic patients. Since the life span of the red cell is 120 days, changes in the percentage of glycosylated Hgb are a time-integrated function of the glucose concentration prevailing during the preceding 2 to 8 weeks and do not reflect the glucose level at the time the sample is tested for glycosylated Hgb. Thus, when diabetic patients are brought under strict control, it is not surprising that changes in glycosylated Hgb lag (for weeks) behind other indices of control (Fig. 7-2). For this reason, measurement of glycosylated Hgb are not helpful in regulating the patient's day-to-day therapy.

Home glucose monitoring is the measurement of capillary whole-blood glucose concentrations by the patient. A drop of blood obtained by pricking the finger is placed on a specially treated plastic strip. The results are read either semiquantitatively, by comparing the resultant color change to a chart, or quantitatively, by placing the strip in a small, specially adapted machine. An automatic spring-loaded device for striking the finger has reduced considerably the pain involved in obtaining the sample. Although home glucose monitoring has been developed only recently, it is clear that this is the most efficient and accurate way to assess diabetic control. It is particularly helpful if the patient is uncertain whether hypoglycemia is present.

Home glucose monitoring is not useful in the presence of persistent glucosuria, since it already is obvious that glucose concentrations are elevated. In patients taking insulin who do not have glucosuria, glucose levels should be measured at least several times per day during 2 to 3 days per week. Initially samples should be taken before breakfast and supper. If these values are satisfactory (see below for criteria for control), measurements should then be obtained several hours after each meal. Home glucose monitoring is not as helpful in patients on dietary therapy alone or dietary therapy supplemented by sulfonylurea agents, since glucose levels in such patients are more stable. Changes in treatment usually result in a gradual overall decrease in glucose concentration rather than in decreases at specific times of the day.

Monitoring Patients Who Take Insulin

Since home glucose monitoring is not in widespread use, most patients evaluate their control by semiquantitative testing of fractional urines for glucose. The results of tests performed before each meal and at bedtime reflect the maximal action of different components of the insulin prescription (see chapter 4, Table 4-2). When glucosuria is present, tests should be repeated on subsequent days to determine whether a particular pattern is emerging. Since the metabolic severity of the diabetic state varies in the absence of a recognizable cause, such as emotional stress, infection, or weight change, insulin requirements will change. If glucosuria of $\geqslant 0.5\%$ occurs for 3 days (assuming that diet and exercise remain relatively stable), the appropriate component of the insulin prescription should be increased by 4 U (except in lean individuals taking regular insulin in whom the increment is 2 U). If the pattern of positive urine tests is such that the dose of both the short- and intermediate-acting insulins need to be increased, only increase the NPH insulin. Once the results of urine tests reflecting the peak action of the NPH insulin become negative again, the dose of regular insulin can be increased, if necessary. Several days should elapse (with continued testing) before further changes are made.

Isolated episodes of hypoglycemia do not require a decrease in the dose of insulin, especially if a precipitating cause, such as decreased food intake or increased exercise, can be identified. However, the intrinsic severity of the abnormal metabolic state also may diminish, and recurring hypoglycemia necessitates a reduction of insulin. The component of the insulin prescription that should be reduced (by 4 U) depends on when the hypoglycemia occurs. The same pattern of adjustment as that for counteracting excessive glucosuria should be followed, except that if recurrent hypoglycemia persists, the dose should be decreased more frequently than every 3 days.

Plasma glucose concentrations are also measured every 4 to 6 weeks. Fasting and before-supper values are the most helpful because they help to assess the effectiveness of NPH insulin, the most important component of the insulin prescription. Since these levels should be measured, if possible, as part of the patient's usual routine, samples should be obtained at clinical laboratories located near the patient's home or workplace. Persistent discrepancies between glucose values measured in the laboratory or doctor's office and results of the urine test at home require investigation.

Montoring Patients Who Do Not Take Insulin

The metabolic state in these patients is less abnormal and less labile than that in patients who require insulin. Therefore, results of preprandial urine tests are more likely to be negative. If this is the case, urine should be tested several hours after meals. If the postprandial results are consistently negative for glucose, testing can be limited to 1 to 2 days a week. Plasma glucose concentrations also should be monitored 1 to 2 hours after meals. Adjusting dietary and sulfonylurea therapy in these patients has been described in detail in chapter 5.

Goals of Therapy

In patients taking insulin, a balance must be achieved between the level of control and the occurrence of unacceptable hypoglycemia. Since tight control has such important therapeutic benefits (chapter 2), an occasional (2 to 3 times per week) mild hypoglycemic episode is acceptable in order to return glucose concentrations toward normal. The goals of insulin therapy,in order of increasing difficulty to achieve, are presented below.

Disappearance of the symptoms of uncontrolled diabetes should be achieved in all patients. In asymptomatic patients, the biochemical aspects of control should then be monitored. For semiquantitative urine tests, these aspects include (*a*) all negative results for glucose in preprandial second-voided urine samples; (*b*) all negative results for glucose in first-voided urine samples; and (*c*) all negative results for glucose in postprandial urine tests. For measurement of blood glucose concentrations the following should be achieved: (*a*) fasting and before-supper plasma glucose concentrations of <200 mg/100 ml, (*b*) fasting and before-supper plasma glucose concentrations of <150 mg/100 ml, (*c*) postprandial plasma glucose concentrations of <200 mg/100 ml, and (*d*) postprandial plasma glucose concentrations of <150 mg/100 ml.

Most insulin-requiring patients should be able to achieve negative results for glucose in preprandial double-voided urine samples and plasma glucose concentrations of <200 mg/100 ml before breakfast and supper. Continuous and strenuous efforts should be made to attain these goals. The next level of control to strive for is negative results for glucose in preprandial first-voided urine samples. This is possible in many patients. Negative results for glucose in postprandial urine samples and postprandial plasma glucose concentrations of <200 mg/100 ml comprises stricter levels of control. Many patients taking insulin may be unable to attain this degree of control without experiencing unacceptable hypoglycemia. However, many patients treated by dietary therapy alone or diet supplemented with sulfonylurea agents should be able to do so.

"Honeymoon Phase" of Type 1 Diabetes

Shortly after the onset of ketosis-prone (type 1) diabetes, approximately 20% of patients go into a *temporary* remission. This is true even in patients who have experienced severe diabetic ketoacidosis. Insulin requirements decrease dramatically and may not even be present in some patients. However, after a few weeks to several months, insulin-requiring diabetes almost invariably returns, although an occasional patient has remained in remission for several years.

Insulin Treatment of Grossly Obese Patients

Although hypocaloric diets are the most effective treatment for these individuals, many obese patients are not able to follow such diets and maintain fasting glucose concentrations of >300 mg/100 ml even while they take maximal doses of sulfonylurea agents. I treat such patients with two injections of NPH insulin per day. In order to limit the volume of insulin injected, the maximal dose given each time is 100 U. More than this amount usually has little extra benefit. Insulin therapy in these patients often lowers their glucose levels from 300 to 400 mg/100 ml to 200 to 300 mg/100 ml. Although this is far from good control, the reduction from the higher glucose concentrations probably is healthier for the patient.

Brittle Diabetes

A brittle (also called labile or unstable) diabetic is defined as "any patient whose life is constantly being disrupted by episodes of hypo- or hyperglycaemia whatever their cause." Fortunately, only a small proportion of insulin-requiring patients fall into this category. Many of them have more severe emotional problems than are usually encountered in other patients. Others take relatively large amounts (>15 U per injection) of regular insulin. Both of these factors may stimulate the release of hormones (glucagon, catecholamines, cortisol, growth hormone) that respond to stress or to rapid drops in glucose concentration. In the first instance, amelioration of the disturbed emotional pattern is helpful, although it is usually difficult to achieve. Patients with brittle diabetes respond best to two injections of NPH insulin a day. This dose then should be changed cautiously in small increments (usually by 2 U) when necessary. Regular insulin should be avoided unless a relatively predictable pattern of diabetic control indicates the need. It should be introduced into the regimen very slowly. Tight control is obviously much more difficult to achieve in patients with brittle diabetes.

Hypoglycemia

The adrenergic signs and symptoms of hypoglycemia (chapter 10, Table 10-3) may occur in response to a rapid fall in an elevated glucose concentration to a lower but still elevated level. Therefore, a low glucose value may not be found in patients in whom hypoglycemia is suspected. Although episodes of hypoglycemia in insulin-dependent diabetics often occur for no apparent reason, decreased food intake or increased exercise should be explored each time as possible causes. After treating the hypoglycemic symptoms with simple carbohydrates, the patient should ingest complex carbohydrates and/or protein within the hour to avoid a recurrence of the problem. Hypoglycemia associated with sulfonylurea therapy often is prolonged, and continued treatment is necessary for many hours to avoid a recurrence. A family member of diabetics receiving insulin should be instructed in the use of glucagon injections in the event that the patient experiences hypoglycemic coma.

Posthypoglycemic hyperglycemia is known as the Somogyi phenomenon. The hyperglycemia allegedly is secondary to the action of contrainsulin hormones stimulated by the hypoglycemia. Classically, the clinical picture is one of progressive hyperglycemia despite increasing doses of insulin. The hypoglycemia, which usually occurs when the patient is asleep but also may occur at other times, is unrecognized.

There are several clues to the presence of the Somogyi effect in uncontrolled diabetics, including (a) rapid fluctuations in urine tests for glucose and ketone bodies, sometimes changing from negative to maximal value within 4 hours; (b) wide swings in plasma glucose concentrations that are not related to meals; and (c) subtle clinical signs of hypoglycemia, such as mild nocturnal sweating, morning headaches, and hypothermia. Although ketonuria often persists after glucosuria disappears, it also may precede the appearance of glucosuria.

Once the Somogyi phenomenon is suspected, it must be documented. This can be accomplished only by assessing diabetic control at unusual times, usually during the night. Circulating glucose values can be measured by home glucose monitoring or, if the patient is hospitalized, by more conventional means. Split quantitative urinary glucose measurements also are effective. The simplest method is to compare results of semiquantitative tests on double-voided urine samples taken during the night and before breakfast. If the results of the former are negative but those of the latter are markedly positive, posthypoglycemic hyperglycemia may be occurring.

The ultimate proof that the diagnosis of the Somogyi phenomenon is correct is improvement in diabetic control after a decrease in the insulin dose. This decrease should be made gradually, since a marked lowering, even to the same ultimate level, inexplicably worsens diabetic control. In my experience, poor diabetic control is seldom due to the Somogyi phenomenon. The pattern of urine test results in most uncontrolled diabetics is one of unremitting glucosuria, and these patients invariably need more insulin.

Starvation Ketosis

If less than ~80 to 100 g of carbohydrates are utilized per day, increased amounts of adipose tissue triglyceride must be hydrolyzed to supply energy. The resulting increased plasma free fatty acids are converted to ketone bodies in the liver (see chapter 2). Although fasting is the ultimate way to decrease carbohydrate utilization, starvation ketosis also occurs in individuals who follow a low-carbohydrate diet regardless of the caloric intake.

There are two situations in which it is important to differentiate between diabetic and starvation ketosis. One occurs in type 2 patients on a hypocaloric diet in which the carbohydrate content is low enough to cause starvation ketosis. The other occurs in type 1 diabetics with gastrointestinal symptoms; the primary gastrointestinal problem impairs food intake, thus resulting in starvation ketosis. Alternatively, this could be diabetic ketosis with the gastrointestinal symptoms representing evolving ketoacidosis (see chapter 6).

There are two ways to distinguish between diabetic and starvation ketosis. Diabetic ketosis almost always is associated with marked glucosuria, while starvation ketosis should not. However, ketonuria may interfere with the glucose reactions on Keto-Diastix. Therefore, type 1 patients may need an independent confirmation of mild glucosuria in the presence of moderate or large ketonuria by retesting with Clinitest. The second, more accurate way to distinguish between the two conditions is to measure plasma ketone bodies. The degree of ketosis in uncontrolled diabetics is much greater than it is in patients whose ketosis is due primarily to inadequate carbohydrate intake. Therefore, in diabetic ketosis the nitroprusside test for plasma ketone bodies will give positive results on dilution of the sample, while in starvation ketosis the test will almost invariably give negative results after dilution.

Sick-Day Rules

Infection causes insulin antagonism. Therefore, infected diabetic patients should not decrease their insulin dose; in fact, additional amounts of insulin often are necessary. In ketosis-resistant (type 2) patients taking insulin, adjustments are made as follows. If it is certain that the patient has an infection, urine tests are carried out before each meal and before the bedtime snack. If the level of glucosuria is 1% or 2% ($\leq$0.5% glucosuria need not be treated), the patient should be given 4 U of regular insulin. Second-voided urine samples must be used because they reveal the metabolic status at the time the additional insulin may be needed. If the patient previously had received regular insulin, the test results with the first-voided specimen might not accurately reflect the effectiveness of this insulin, and the patient ultimately may be overtreated.

In order to prevent recurrence of a similar degree of poor control, the amount of intermediate-acting insulin must be increased the following day if additional regular insulin had been given. For patients taking two insulin injections, the morning dose should be raised by 4 U if extra regular insulin had been required before either lunch or supper. Even if supplemental insulin had been given at both times, the morning dose of NPH insulin should be increased by only 4 U. If additional regular insulin had been required that morning or before bedtime the previous evening, the evening dose of intermediate-acting insulin should be increased by 4 U. Again, the dose should be increased by only 4 U even if the patient had taken supplemental insulin at both times. For patients receiving one injection of intermediate-acting insulin in the morning, the NPH insulin should be increased by 4 U the following day if the patient required one or two supplemental doses of regular insulin the previous day and evening and by 8 U if he or she had required three or four doses.

As the infection improves, it is important to decrease the amount of insulin before hypoglycemia occurs. Thus, the dose of NPH insulin should be lowered gradually toward preinfection levels when the urine test results become negative. If the results remain negative, the decrease should continue until basal levels of insulin are reached. If the results of the urine tests generally remain at $\leqslant 0.5\%$, the new lowered dosage should be maintained in anticipation of further recovery from the infection and a quick return to the preinfection insulin dose. If 1% to 2% glucosuria reappears, the insulin dose should be raised again until the results of the urine tests improve.

Insulin treatment for infected ketosis-prone (type 1) patients is similar to that for ketosis-resistant (type 2) patients except that, in the former, an additional 4 U of regular insulin should be given if the urine test results also yield a moderate or large reaction for ketone bodies. In order to ensure that diabetic ketosis, not starvation ketosis, is being treated, the 4 U of regular insulin are added to the 4 U already prescribed for the 1% to 2% glucosuria. If the test results for ketone bodies are moderate or large, the ketonuria should not be treated if there is no significant glucosuria. Therefore, in patients with moderate or large ketonuria and $\leqslant 1\%$ glucosuria on testing with Keto-Diastix, it is important to ascertain whether the degree of glucosuria really is low or whether the value represents a falsely low reading caused by the presence of ketonuria. In infected type 1 patients, the increase in the dose of intermediate-acting insulin the following day should be the same as that for infected type 2 patients. The governing factor is the number of times additional regular insulin was prescribed, not the amount. The principles for adjusting insulin doses in infected type 1 patients are illustrated in Table 7-5.

This method of treating infected insulin-dependent patients provides that intermediate-acting insulin is increased gradually to prevent continued deterioration of diabetic control, that regular insulin is made available only when it is needed, and that, as the infection subsides, the dose of NPH insulin is decreased gradually before hypoglycemia becomes a problem. Since this approach may not be entirely appropriate for all diabetics, it should serve as a general guideline. Experience with particular patients will reveal to the physician that certain ones seem to be more sensitive to insulin and require smaller increases, while others (especially obese individuals) are less sensitive and require larger increases.

Patients who do not receive insulin usually do not require changes in therapy, since the episodes of infection usually are self-limited.

Other modalities of treatment are important in infected diabetics, including carbohydrate intake and, in patients with vomiting, diarrhea, or marked polyuria, fluid (sodium) and potassium replacement. Since most of these patients take insulin, some carbohydrate intake is important. A method for calculating the carbohydrate content of the diet and obtaining that amount from easily digestible foods is described in detail in chapter 3. This is not feasible in some patients because either they are not familiar with the fundamentals of this approach or their gastrointestinal symptoms may prevent them from eating the appropriate amounts of food. Such patients should eat foods that they can tolerate from the milk, fruit, bread, and vegetable exchange lists. Liquids and soft foods are easier to digest, and patients often are able to consume 6 to 8 small meals during the day than 3 to 4 large ones. Soft drinks (not low-calorie ones) and fruit juices are good sources of carbohydrates.

Fluids lost from the kidney or gastrointestinal tract contain large amounts of sodium. Therefore, in order to avoid marked depletion of intravascular volume, (dehydration), these fluids must be replaced with fluids that contain relatively large amounts of sodium. As long as the patient receives enough insulin and fluids, hospitalization can be avoided. If the severity of the gastrointestinal symptoms precludes oral intake of fluid, patients usually must be hospitalized. Two good sources of sodium are bouillon (1 cup ~40 mEq) and tomato juice (1 cup ~20 mEq). Other foods high in sodium are canned soups, saltine crackers, and packaged custard pudding mixes. Salt can be added to other jucies. Soft drinks contain little sodium.

Sources high in potassium include orange juice, tomato juice, and prune juice (1 cup ~15 mEq). Foods with moderate potassium content (1 cup ~10 mEq) include milk, grapefruit juice, and pineapple juice. Apple juice, grape juice, and cranberry juice are low in potassium (1 cup ~5 mEq). A large banana contains approximately 10 mEq of potassium.

Exercise

Exercise increases the effectiveness of insulin, both by increasing its absorption from the injection site and by enhancing its intrinsic activity on insulin-sensitive tissues. Therefore, the insulin prescription should be matched to a relatively constant daily amount of exercise. If more exercise is planned, the patient should consume extra carbohydrate caolories in order to offset the effect. A general approach to balancing the amount of extra food with the anticipated level of exercise is suggested in chapter 3. However, patients must determine for themselves whether these amounts are applicable to them or whether adjustments are needed. If the exercise period lasts more than several hours, it is sometimes necessary to interrupt it briefly to ingest extra calories (in addition to eating before starting to exercise). Consuming additional calories rather than decreasing the amount of insulin is preferable. If the anticipated extra exercise does not occur, the patient will have taken too small a dose of insulin that day, and his or her control will suffer accordingly.

Foot Care

Infections of the feet are a major source of the morbidity among diabetics and often lead to death. Although most foot ulcers and other infected lesions that lead to gangrene of the feet are preventable, they continue to exact a tremendous toll in the diabetic population. The physician must emphasize to the patient the importance of proper foot care. The feet of patients over the age of 40 or of those who have had diabetes for >10 years should be examined at every office visit. Patients with impaired blood flow to the feet secondary to either large- or small-vessel disease should have their toenails cut by qualified medical personnel.

Calluses are an important sign of possible future foot trouble. They represent increased pressure on that area and often cannot be felt by the patient because of associated sensory neuropathy. Calluses should be shaved routinely (usually by a podiatrist, but other medical personnel can be taught) and kept to a minimum. Unroofing an innocuous-looking callus sometimes reveals an extensive ulcer, which could have been prevented by treating the callus when it first appeared. The source of the pressure (e.g., ill-fitting shoes, collapsed metatarsal arch, hammertoe) must be identified and corrective measures taken, if possible. Softer and better-fitting shoes usually will suffice, although it can be difficult to persuade patients to forgo style simply to prevent calluses. In some patients with impaired circulation, prophylactic surgery to correct or remove a hammertoe is indicated if there is no orthopedic way to reduce the pressure on the offending digit.

Travel

Insulin-requiring diabetics who travel sometimes need advice concerning their insulin. Insulin is stable at room temperature, a characteristic that facilitates travel. Patients should take along insulin vials and syringes, especially if they are going to a foreign country. The timing and occasionally the amount of the insulin dose may need adjustment on the day of travel, especially if the patient is flying into a different time zone. The patient should find out from the airline what kind of meal will be served and when. The insulin dose should then be adjusted to the meal pattern. Traveling from north to south, and vice versa, is the easiest to accommodate, since the time does not change and the eating pattern usually is not too different from the patient's usual pattern. Traveling from east to west, and vice-versa, however, presents more of a problem because the change in time often disrupts both eating and sleeping patterns. A relatively smooth integration of the patient's new eating and activity schedule with the insulin regimen can be accomplished by making adjustments in the first 12 to 24 hours after arrival according to the patient's internal clock and then shifting gradually to the changed external time. An alternative approach is to give the entire dose as short-acting insulin (25% of the total daily amount as regular insulin before each meal starting on the morning of departure). The patient should resume the normal insulin schedule with the first breakfast at the patient's destination.

Dental Procedures

Dental infections, especially periodontal disease, are more common in diabetic than in nondiabetic individuals. Therefore, diabetic patients are more likely to undergo dental procedures that impair food intake. Unless precuations are taken, this can be a problem for patients who take insulin or sulfonylurea agents. Effective communication between the patient's physician and dentist is important in helping to judge the extent of the diminished food intake and the severity of the operative stress.

If a patient taking sulfonylurea agents will miss more than one meal because of a dental procedure, the drugs should be omitted that morning and reinstated when normal food intake resumes. Chlorpropamide (Diabinese) should be discontinued the day before the procedure because of its long half-life.

Hypoglycemia is more likely to occur secondary to insulin therapy than to oral hypoglycemia agents. In these patients, dental procedures should be performed in the morning, if possible, because the effects of intermediate-acting insulin injected before breakfast peak late in the afternoon, and an insulin reaction may occur if the supper calories are decreased. If the lunch calories are diminished, regular and Semilente insulin should be omitted from the morning dose. In addition, NPH insulin and breakfast can be taken a little later than usual to minimize the risk of early-afternoon hypoglycemia. If food intake at supper will be decreased, the dose of intermediate-acting insulin should be reduced. However, type 1 patients must have some insulin to avoid ketosis and possibly ketoacidosis. Therefore, a balance must be achieved between decreased insulin requirements due to impaired food intake and the need for insulin produced by the stress of the dental procedure and possibly by the infection that led to it. It is important that the patient monitor diabetic control closely after the procedure and that he or she communicate with the physician. Hospitalization of ketosis-prone diabetics sometimes is advisable if extensive dental work that impairs food intake is necessary.

Surgical and PostOperative Management

The goals of therapy during surgery in diabetic patients are to minimize fluid and electrolyte losses secondary to an osmotic diuresis by limiting hyperglycemia, to prevent diabetic ketosis in type 1 patients, and to avoid hypoglycemia while the patient is under anesthesia. The following approach is recommended for insulin-requiring diabetics. On the morning of surgery, the patient should be given one half of his or her total daily insulin dose (i.e., one half of the entire amount of intermediate- and short-acting insulin taken normally as NPH insulin. An infusion of 5% dextrose in water should be administered at a rate of 125 cc/hr. If surgery must be delayed for ≥4 hours after the insulin is given, the fasting glucose concentration should be measured (ordered *stat*). If this value is <200 mg/100 ml, the rate of glucose infusion should be increased to 200 cc/hr when the laboratory reports the value.

When the patient enters the recovery room after surgery, the patient should receive the second half of the NPH insulin, and the glucose level should be measured (ordered *stat*). If the glucose value is >350 mg/100 ml and/or moderate or large ketonuria is present, 8 to 10 U of regular insulin should also be given. If the patient requires only NPH insulin at this time, the glucose level should be determined again in ~8 hours. If he or she requires regular insulin as well, its effect should be monitored 2 to 4 hours later.

Patients undergoing minor surgical procedures should be able to eat the same day. If the glucose concentration obtained ~8 hours after the second injection of intermediate-acting insulin is high (>250 mg/100 ml), a small amount of NPH insulin may be required that evening to control the fasting glucose level the next morning. By the following day, the patient will be back in his or her usual routine. Extra insulin may be necessary for several days to counteract the stress effects of postoperative discomfort. Insulin doses should be adjusted as described in chapter 4.

Patients undergoing major surgery, especially abdominal operations, will not be able to eat for various lengths of time postoperatively. Their parenteral nutrition should include at least 100 g of glucose (2 L of 5% dextrose in water) over each 24-hour period to avoid starvation ketosis. A convenient way to administer insulin while the patient is not able to eat is to infuse glucose continuously and give NPH insulin every 12 hours; this method provides continuous insulin coverage. The glucose concentration obtained before each administration of NPH insulin reflects the effectiveness of the injection given 12 hours previously. Since the laboratory will not report that value until at least several hours after the most recent injection, it is used to adjust the subsequent dose of insulin.

For instance, if the patient is receiving insulin at 0800 and 2000, the morning glucose concentration should be used to judge the evening dose, and the glucose value at about 2000 will determine what adjustments (if any) should be made the following morning. Lean patients should be started with 10 U of NPH insulin every 12 hours, and obese patients (>125% of ideal body weight; see chapter 3) should be started with 16 U of NPH insulin at both times. Each dose of NPH insulin should be increased by 4 U if the appropriate glucose concentration is >250 mg/100 ml. If the glucose level is >350 mg/100 ml, 8 U of regular insulin should be given when that value becomes known. As the patient resumes eating, increasing amounts of insulin can be added to the morning injection. When intravenous glucose is no longer being infused overnight (which should occur after oral caloric intake improves considerably), some of the evening NPH insulin also can be shifted to the morning. In this manner, the transition from total parenteral nutrition through partial oral supplementation to normal food intake can be accomplished smoothly without large fluctuations in diabetic control. Table 7-7 illustrates this approach.

The following approach is recommended for patients who do not require insulin. Those who are controlled by dietary therapy alone can be treated in the same way as nondiabetic patients. Monitoring of glucose concentrations is important, however, since hyperglycemia can occur as a result of the stress of surgery and postoperative discomfort. Although deterioration of diabetic control is usually temporary, persistent elevation in glucose concentration of >250 mg/100 ml should be treated with small doses of NPH insulin. Sulfonylurea agents should be omitted on the day of surgery; chlorpropamide, should be discontinued the day before because of its long half-life. For minor surgery, medication should be restarted when the patient resumes eating. Major surgery often causes marked elevation in glucose concentrations in patients who require sulfonylurea agents to maintain diabetic control. Therefore, lean individuals should receive 10 U of NPH insulin and obese individuals (>125% ideal body weight) should receive 16 U of NPH insulin on the morning of surgery. These patients should be monitored in the same way as insulin-requiring diabetics. When the patient resumes eating, the insulin should be withdrawn gradually and the sulfonylurea agent reinstated.

There are two other methods of treating the diabetic patient during the postoperative period. The sliding-scale method should *not* be used. The reasons for this are discussed in detail in chapter 4. Continuous intravenous administration of regular insulin can be used if the patient's actual response is monitored frequently, and appropriate adjustments of the rate of insulin infusion can be made.

The insulin solution (0.2 U/cc) is prepared by mixing 1.0 ml of U-100 insulin (100 U) in 500 cc of normal saline. Fifty milliliters are run through the tubing and then discarded in order to saturate the nonspecific adsorption sites for insulin and to ensure that the appropriate amount will be delivered. The initial dose is administered through a separate line at an infusion rate of 2 U/hr (10 cc/hr). Glucose concentrations should be measured ~2 hours after starting the infusion. If the glucose level is between 150 and 250 mg/100 ml, the infusion rate should not be changed, and glucose concentrations should be measured routinely every 4 hours. Whenever the glucose concentration is >250 mg/100 ml, the rate should be increased by 1 U (5 cc) per hour; when it is <150 mg/100 ml, the rate should be decreased by 1 U/hr. Glucose levels should be measured 1 to 2 hours after the rate of infusion is changed. When the patient starts to eat again, additional regular insulin (depending on the amount of caloric intake) is given before each meal by increasing the infusion rate temporarily. When the glucose infusion is discontinued, insulin administration is switched to subcutaneous NPH. Obviously, this approach requires much closer laboratory and clinical monitoring of the patient and thus may not be suitable for all hospitals.

References

1. Rhoads GG, Gulbrandsen CL, Kagan A: Serum lipoproteins and coronary heart disease in a population study of Hawaii Japanese men. N Engl J Med 294:293-298, 1976

2. Rubenstein LZ, Greenfield S: Importance of the baseline ECG: an expensive myth? Clin Res 26:337A, 1978

3. Knowles WC, Bennett PH, Ballintine EJ: Increased incidence of retinopathy in diabetics with elevated blood pressure. A six-year follow-up study in Pima Indians. N Engl J Med 302:645-650, 1980.

4. Mogensen CE: Renal function changes in diabetes. Diabetes 25:872-879, 1976

5. The Diabetic Retinopathy Study Research Group: Preliminary report on effects of photocoagulation therapy. Am J Ophathalmol 81:383-396, 1976

6. Feldman JM, Kelley WN, Lebovitz HE: Inhibition of glucose oxidase paper tests by reducing metabolites. Diabetes 19:337-343, 1970

7. Feldman JM, Lebovitz FL: Tests for glucosuria. An analysis of factors that cause misleading results. Diabetes 22:115-121, 1973

8. Nahata MC, McLeod DC: Noneffect of oral urinary copper ascorbic acid on reduction glucose test. Diabetes Care 1:34-35, 1978

9. Self TH, Wester VL: Noneffect of isoniazid on urine glucose tests. Diabetes Care 3:44-45, 1980

10. Bowers CB, Self TH: Noneffect of methyldopa on urine glucose tests. Diabetes Care 1:36, 1978

11. Wolcott GJ, Hackett TN Jr: Levodopa and tests for ketonuria (letter). N Engl J Med 283:1522, 1970

12. Guthrie DW, Hinnen D, Guthrie RA: Single-voided vs. double-voided urine testing. Diabetes Care 2:269-271, 1979

13. McCarthy J: Double-voided dilemma. Am J Nurs 79:1249, 1979

14. Winter RJ, Traisman HS, Green OC: Glucosuria in children with diabetes: advantages of the 2-drop Clinitest method. Diabetes Care 2:349-352, 1979

15. Gonen B, Rubenstein AH: Haemoglobin A_1 and diabetes mellitus. Diabetologia 15:1-8, 1978

16. Jackson RL, Hess RL, England JD: Hemoglobin A_{1c} values in children with overt diabetes maintained in varying degrees of control. Diabetes Care 2:391-395, 1979

17. Koenig RJ, Peterson CM, Jones RL, et al: Correlation of glucose regulation and hemoglobin A_{1c} in diabetes mellitus. N Engl J Med 295:417-420, 1976

18. Gabbay KH, Hasty K, Breslow JL, et al: Glycosylated hemoglobins and long-term blood glucose control in diabetes mellitus. J Clin Endocrinol Metab 44:859-864, 1977

19. Bleicher SJ (editor): Symposium on home blood glucose monitoring. Diabetes Care 3:57–126, 1980

20. Pirart J: Diabetes mellitus and its degenerative complications: a prospective study of 4,400 patients observed between 1947 and 1973. Diabetes Care 1:168–188, 1978

21. Clarke WL, Haymond MW, Santiago JV: Overnight basal insulin requirements in fasting insulin-dependent diabetics. Diabetes 29:78–80, 1980

22. Park BN, Soeldner JS, Gleason RE: Diabetes in remission. Insulin secretory dynamics. Diabetes 23:616–623, 1974

23. Tattersall R: Brittle diabetes. Clin Endocrinol Metab 6:403–419, 1977

24. Yue DK, Baxter RC, Turtle JR: C-peptide secretion and insulin antibodies as determinants of stability in diabetes mellitus. Metabolism 27:35–44, 1978

25. Gunning RR, Garber AJ: Bioactivity of instant glucose. Failure of absorption through oral mucosa. JAMA 240:1611–1612, 1978

26. Bloom ME, Mintz DH, Field JB: Insulin-induced posthypoglycemia hyperglycemia as a cause of 'brittle' diabetes. Am J Med 47:891–903, 1969

27. Gale EA, Kurtz AB, Tattersall RB: In search of the Somogyi effect. Lancet 2:279–282, 1980

28. Stone DB: Surgery in the diabetic patient. In *Diabetes Mellitus: Diagnosis and Treatment*, vol 2. Edited by Hamwi GJ, Danowski TS. American Diabetes Association, New York, 1967, pp 167–170

29. Walts LF, Miller J, Davidson MB, Brown J: Perioperative management of diabetes mellitus. Anesthesiology (in press)

30. Taitelman U, Reece EA, Bessman AN: Insulin in the management of the diabetic surgical patient. Continuous intravenous infusion vs. subcutaneous administration. JAMA 237:558–560, 1977

31. Meyer EJ, Lorenzi M, Bohannon NV, et al: Diabetic management by insulin infusion during major surgery. Am J Surg 137:323–327, 1979

Chapter 8

Diabetes Education for the Nurse, Patient, and Family

Roz Morgan
Mary A. Pearce
Mayer B. Davidson

The diabetic patient is unique because diabetes is lifelong and requires involvement and concern 24 hours a day. Active participation is required of the patient in order to manage the diabetes successfully from day to day. This can be accomplished only if the patient is totally knowledgeable in all areas of diabetes management that are appropriate to his or her care. This knowledge may be a key motivating factor in the diabetic's compliance with a daily regimen. Our experience indicates that control of blood sugar is unattainable in individuals who either lack knowledge about the diabetic syndrome or who fail to apply the information.

Physicians often are too busy to spend enough time to educate their diabetic patients. Thus, the nurse becomes the major educator on the teaching team. The purpose of this chapter is to provide information that the nurse can utilize in educating diabetic individuals. Patients then can follow a program of self-management that the nurse can evaluate later.

Each section of this chapter (diabetic syndrome, monitoring, diabetic emergencies, exercise) is written as a separate unit according to the teaching/learning process. This process includes an assessment of the diabetic's knowledge and skills, an education record, behavioral objectives (outcome criteria) for the diabetic, goals for the nurse, content, and evaluation.

Teaching/Learning Process

Assessment

The first step in implementing an education program is to collect patient information (Fig. 8-1) that may influence the ability of the diabetic individual to manage his or her own disease. An example of this is the patient who has retinopathy.

Social History

Name _____ Age _____

Occupation _____ Retired _____

Lives with spouse _____ Family _____ Alone _____

Medical History

Chief complaint _____

Height _____ Weight _____

Type of diabetes: Type 1 _____ Type 2 _____ Duration _____

Frequent infections: _____ Skin _____ Bladder _____

                Vaginal _____

Other illnesses _____

Medications taken at home _____

Complications of Diabetes

1. Cardiovascular: MI _____ Angina _____ HTN _____ CHF _____

                      CABG _____ Pacemaker _____

2. Cerebrovascular: CVA _____ TIA _____

3. Peripheral vascular: Leg pain: On exercising _____

                           At rest _____

                           Bypass surgery _____ Amputations _____

4. Retinopathy: Yes _____ No _____ Vision affected _____

                  Laser treatment _____

5. Other eye problems: Cataracts _____ Glaucoma _____

                        Color blindness _____

6. Nephropathy: Protein in urine _____ Dialysis _____ Other _____

7. Neuropathy:

     a. Peripheral: Numbness _____ Burning sensations _____

                   Tingling _____ Pain _____

     b. Autonomic: Infrequent voiding _____

                   Not feeling empty after voiding _____

                   Voiding frequent small amounts _____

                   Intermittent diarrhea _____

                   Feeling full after eating small amounts _____

                   _____

                   Nausea after eating _____

                   Vomiting _____

                   Impotence _____

Figure 8-1. Patient Assessment Form. MI, myocardial infarction; HTN, Hypertension; CVA, cerebrovascular accident (stroke); TIA, transient ischemic attack (pre-stroke); CHF, congestive heart failure; CABG, coronary artery bypass graft.

The patient may encounter problems with insulin administration if he or she has visual problems. In such situations, special aids for the visually impaired will need investigation. For the patient with nephropathy, urine testing may not be meaningful, and home glucose monitoring may be the best method for evaluating diabetic control.

Certain information, such as frequent infections, or neuropathy, may indicate the need for greater attention to those aspects of the patient's illness. The Patient Assessment Form (Fig. 8-1) is designed to record such information in a simple and concise manner. On the initial visit, the nurse can obtain a social and medical history for the assessment form from either the physician's record or the patient.

The Knowledge Assessment and Education Record (Fig. 8-2) is designed to serve a dual purpose. First, it identifies the patient's knowledge and skills by asking questions about such skills as insulin administration and urine testing using the material presented in this chapter as a guideline for knowledge. If the nurse feels that the patient is competent, check the Yes column; if not, check the No column. The patient needs instruction in only the areas that have been checked No.

For the newly diagnosed diabetic, the assessment portion of Figure 8-2 is not pertinent. The area dealing with insulin administration can be omitted for the patient who does not require insulin. The second purpose of Figure 8-2 (second portion) is to document the instruction given and the patient's progress. When the patient has been instructed in a particular area, the letter "I," (i.e., instructed) is entered. When the patient is competent in that area, the letter "C" (i.e., competent) is entered. If the patient requires further assistance in a particular area, the letters "RA" (i.e., requires assistance) are entered. If the patient consistently requires assistance, such as in the area of insulin administration, intervention is needed by a family member or by an organization that provides nursing service in the home.

Behavioral Objectives for the Student

The second step in the teaching-learning process is identification of the skills and knowledge that the student (i.e., the patient and/or family) needs. Imparting this knowledge becomes the objective of the teaching plan. Objectives are statements that describe a desired outcome (results) on the level of knowledge, skill, or attitude. Behavioral objectives differ from other objectives in that they are student oriented rather than teacher oriented. That is, these objectives describe desired outcomes (results) that the student achieves on completion of the education. Action verbs, such as *demonstrate, identify,* or *state,* best describe the outcome in measurable terms. The advantage of using behavioral objectives in diabetes education is that the objectives give specific rules for measuring the results of teaching, including when and how the student will accomplish the objectives.

	Assessment		Teaching Done					
	Yes	No	Date					
Diabetic syndrome								
Patient can state								
1. Definition of diabetes and its effect on glucose metabolism								
2. Methods of control								
Urine testing								
Patient can state/demonstrate:								
1. Reasons for urine testing								
2. Correct urine testing procedure and record keeping								
3. Frequency of testing								
Insulin								
Patient can state/demonstrate:								
1. How insulin works								
2. Type of medication and dosage schedule								
3. Correct technique for preparing insulin								
a. Single dose								
b. Multiple dose								
4. Correct technique for insulin injection								
a. Rotation sites								
Oral hypoglycemia sulfonylurea agents								
Patient can state:								
1. Action of sulfonylurea agents								
2. Name of medication and schedule								
Hypoglycemia								
Patient can state:								
1. Definition and causes								
2. Symptoms/treatment/prevention								
3. Reason for carrying I.D. (Medic Alert identification card)								
4. Frequency of occurrence								
Foot care								
Patient can state:								
1. Reasons for daily foot care								
2. Dos and Don'ts of foot care								
Exercise								
Patient can state the effect of exercise on blood glucose control								

Figure 8-2. Knowledge Assessment and Education Record. Nurse records the appropriate responses (yes, no, I, C, RA), according to the patient's level of learning and/or ability in relation to the designated task.

Goals for the Teaching Nurse

The terms *goal* and *objective* frequently are used interchangeably in this chapter. Goals are teacher oriented, whereas behavioral objectives are student oriented. Our goal is to provide information that will educate the nurse on specific topics so that he or she will be able to educate the student.

Content

The technique of providing information separately for patient and nurse is used to differentiate the information essential to the diabetic from the detailed information that the nurse should know in order to educate the diabetic. The information for the patient is written simply and concisely, while that for the nurse is more detailed and technical. The more background knowledge the nurse has in the area being taught, the more effective will be the teaching. Also, intelligent patients often will want to know more than the bare essentials, and, unless the nurse understands the material, he or she will not be able to accommodate the patient.

Methods and Teaching Tools

In order to facilitate learning and self-management of diabetes, the teacher should utilize audio and visual teaching materials. The media available for diabetes education at present is prolific. Companies such as Becton-Dickinson and Monoject have provided slides and filmstrips on insulin injection and on other aspects of diabetes care. These materials are available from local and regional distributors at minimal cost. Printed literature for patient instruction also is widely available and can be supplied by companies such as Upjohn, Ames, and Lilly, which manufacture drugs and urine testing products for diabetics (see Appendix).

Evaluation

When behavioral objectives are used, evaluation becomes a process of assessing the student's behavior (i.e., knowledge) according to some acknowledged and defined criteria.

Each section of this chapter has an evaluation (test form) that should be given to the student when they complete the specific content in order to determine their level of knowledge. If the student cannot take a written test, an oral test can be given using the same questions. The questions given after each section are only examples for evaluating the objectives (answers are given at the end of the chapter). Others may be formulated by the nurse or physician. Some objectives are best evaluated by demonstrating a particular skill, such as insulin injection, testing urine, or capillary-blood glucose monitoring.

Example

Objective: Upon completion of the instructions, the student will be able to verbalize or write what effect insulin has on blood sugar.
Evauation: True or False
Insulin

a. lowers blood sugar
b. increases blood sugar
c. has no effect on blood sugar

THE DIABETIC SYNDROME

Diabetes mellitus is a chronic disease that requires lifelong management. In the past these features have frequently been misunderstood and sometimes taken lightly. Educating the diabetic patient is an attempt to correct this misunderstanding and, as a result, to allow the patient to attain control of glucose levels. This section will address both the differences between normal and abnormal metabolism (taking into consideration the definition, etiology, and new classification of diabetes) and the effect of diabetes on the vascular system over the long term.

Outcome Criteria (Student) and Goals (Nurse)

Objectives

STUDENT

Upon completion of the instruction, the student will be able to verbalize and/or write the following:

1. Definition of diabetes.
2. Causes of diabetes.
3. Two major types of diabetes and their differences.
4. Sources of body fuel.
5. Role of insulin in metabolism.
6. Signs, symptoms, and treatment of diabetes.
7. Body organs that may be affected by diabetes.

Goals

NURSE

To provide information on the following:

1. Normal and abnormal metabolism of carbohydrate, protein, and fat.
2. New classification of diabetes.

3. Etiology of diabetes.

4. Complications of diabetes.

What is Diabetes?

STUDENT

Diabetes mellitus is a chronic disease that can affect the entire body system and tends to run in families. In 1976, the National Commission on Diabetes reported that as many as 10 million people in the United States (about 5% of the population) have diabetes. The incidence appears to be increasing by 6% per year. At this rate, a person born in the United States today has a one-in-five chance of ultimately developing the disease.

There are two main disorders that occur in diabetes. One affects the ability of the body to use and store sugar (glucose). The use and storage of this fuel is controlled by a hormone called insulin. This hormone is made and stored in special cells in the pancreas. The pancreas (about the size of a fist) is located in the abdominal area near the stomach. Individuals with diabetes have problems with the production of insulin and/or the effectiveness of the insulin that is produced. The second general disorder that affects many systems in the body involves the structure, and therefore the function, of blood vessels and nerves.

NURSE

Diabetes mellitus is a disease that was first recognized almost 4,000 years ago. The term *diabetes mellitus* comes from a Greek word meaning "to pass through" and a Latin word meaning "honey." Diabetes actually is a syndrome that is manifested by abnormalities in both metabolism and the vascular system. Metabolically, diabetes is the result of a lack of insulin action on carbohydrate, protein, and fat metabolism. In some patients, this defect is caused by decreased or absent production of insulin and in others by impaired effectiveness of the insulin that is produced. Abnormalities in glucose metabolism have received the most attention.

Diabetes affects both the large (macrovascular) and small (microvascular) vessels in the body. The clinical expressions of macrovascular disease are heart attacks, strokes, and peripheral vascular disease; the last affects primarily the lower extremities, causing pain on walking and, possibly, gangrene. The microvascular disease affects the eyes (diabetic retinopathy) and the kidneys (diabetic nephropathy or glomerulosclerosis). The peripheral nerves also are affected, probably as a result of the altered metabolism.

Certain signs and symptoms of diabetes are related to the uncontrolled metabolism. These are discussed in the section on diabetic emergencies. Other signs and symptoms are caused by the vessel disease and depend on which vessels are involved. Vessel-related signs and symptoms are much different from those caused by uncontrolled metabolism.

Classification

STUDENT

There are two main types of diabetes: type 1 (formerly known as juvenile-onset) and type 2 (formerly known as maturity-onset). In type 1 diabetes, the insulin-producing cells in the pancreas no longer can make enough insulin to maintain normal levels of blood sugar. For this reason, type 1 diabetes requires lifelong injection of insulin. The onset of type 1 diabetes occurs primarily in young people but may occur in individuals of any age.

Type 2 diabetes is the most common type of diabetes. Most type 2 diabetics are middle-aged and overweight. These individuals usually produce substantial amounts of insulin but are not able to use this insulin effectively to control blood sugar. Type 2 diabetes usually can be controlled by diet and/or oral medications that lower blood sugar. However, some of type 2 diabetics require insulin for control as long as they are overweight. A small percentage of type 2 diabetics are not overweight and are more likely than obese patients to require insulin therapy.

NURSE

In 1978 an international work group convened at the National Institutes of Health (Bethesda, Maryland) to develop a new, uniform terminology and a functional classification of diabetes. This step was taken because (a) it was difficult to compare epidemiologic data from different research centers or from different countries, (b) the old criteria were thought to be inappropriately strict for diagnosing diabetes, and (c) new subtypes of diabetes had emerged that did not fit comfortably into the old classification. Measurement of the fasting blood glucose concentration and, if necessary, glucose levels during an oral glucose challenge remained the cornerstone of diagnosis. However, the work group modified the values that were considered to be abnormal and carefully defined an important classification termed *impaired glucose tolerance* (IGT).

Type 1 diabetes mellitus is also called *insulin-dependent diabetes mellitus* (IDDM). Patients with type 1 diabetes (a) are insulinopenic (lacking insulin production) and thus dependent on exogenous insulin for sustaining life; (b) are ketosis-prone unless treated appropriately; (c) experience onset primarily in youth but possibly at another age; (d) frequently have pancreatic islet-cell antibodies at diagnosis; and (e) show a genetic association between diabetes and certain histocompatibility antigen (HLA) types.

Type 2 diabetics mellitus is also called *non-insulin-dependent diabetes mellitus* (NIDDM). Patients with NIDDM fall into two categories, non obese and obese. The characteristics of both types include (a) high, low or normal insulin levels; (b) no ketosis, even without treatment; (c) onset primarily at more than 40 years of age but may occur at any age; (d) maturity-onset diabetes of the young (MODY; i.e., type 2 diabetes presenting in childhood or adolescence); (e) possible insulin requirement if hyperglycemia doesn't respond to sulfonylurea agents (i.e., oral drugs that lower blood sugar) and/or dietary therapy; (f) obesity in 60% to 90% of patients; and (g) family history of NIDDM.

Other types of diabetes formerly known as secondary diabetes include diabetes associated with (a) pancreatic disease (usually pancreatitis); (b) excess of certain hormones (glucocorticoids or steroids, growth hormone, adrenaline); (c) drug or chemical-induced diseases (e.g., thiazide diuretics, cortisone, estrogen); (d) abnormalities in insulin receptors; and (e) certain genetic syndromes.

Impaired glucose tolerance is a new category of diabetes. Previous terms for IGT included *asymptomatic diabetes mellitus, subclinical diabetes mellitus, chemical diabetes mellitus, borderline diabetes mellitus, latent diabetes mellitus,* and *prediabetes*. Patients with IGT may or may not be obese. Impaired glucose tolerance may be associated with other conditions and is characterized by (a) mild glucose intolerance, falling between normal and diabetic levels; (b) 1% to 5% of patients per year progressing to overt diabetes; (c) most patients either reverting to normal or continuing to experience IGT; (d) absence of renal and retinal complications; and (e) increased susceptibility to atherosclerotic disease.

The characteristics of gestational diabetes mellitus are (a) onset or recognition of glucose intolerance during pregnancy; (b) association of glucose intolerance with increased perinatal complications; (c) association of glucose intolerance with increased maternal risk of subsequent diabetes; and (d) need to reclassify the condition after pregnancy as previous abnormality of glucose tolerance, (PrevAGT) IGT, or diabetes mellitus.

There are two categories of diabetes that are characterized by normal glucose tolerance but an increased statistical risk of future abnormalities. Patients in these two categories previously were labeled *prediabetic*. The classification of PrevAGT is limited to persons who now have normal glucose tolerance but who at some time have had hyperglycemia or IGT, either spontaneously or in response to stress (e.g., pregnancy, obesity, trauma, injury). The classification of potential abnormality of glucose tolerance (PotAGT) includes persons who have never had an abnormal glucose tolerance test but who are at risk because of (a) a strong family history of diabetes, (b) delivery of a child weighing more than nine pounds, (c) obesity, (d) belonging to a particular racial or ethnic group (e.g., certain American Indian tribes) with a high incidence of diabetes (evidence for including these individuals in the PotAGT category is not well established).

Etiology

STUDENT

Most types of diabetes run in the family, although the exact inheritance pattern is not known. Some types are caused by a disease of or traumatic injury to the pancreas. Certain drugs (e.g., diuretics for high blood pressure, hormones such as cortisone or birth control pills) occasionally may bring out diabetes in a predisposed person.

The predisposition to diabetes is acquired through genes, the transmitters of all hereditary characteristics (e.g., eye, hair, and skin color). Although the parents may not have had diabetes, they have inherited the gene for diabetes from someone in the family. Although heredity plays a major role in who ultimately acquires diabetes, several environmental risk factors contribute to the onset of this condition. In adults these risk factors include obesity, pregnancy, trauma (i.e., accidents, major surgery, illnesses such as heart attacks and strokes), and psychological stress (e.g., divorce, death of a loved one, work-induced problems). These stresses require an increase in the amount of insulin the body needs, an amount that is too demanding for a hereditarily defective insulin-producing (pancreatic beta) cell. Therefore, blood glucose levels rise and remain high, leading to the onset of one of the types of diabetes. In children, environmental risk factors may include certain viruses that destroy pancreatic beta cells in susceptible individuals, thus causing diabetes.

NURSE

Type 1 Diabetes

The cause of type 1 diabetes is now being associated with a combination of genetic, immunologic, and viral factors. The interweaving of these factors comprises a fascinating story. It has long been suspected on clinical grounds that certain viral illnesses may precede the onset of type 1 diabetes by several weeks. Direct proof that a virus may help to destroy the pancreatic beta cell was furnished when a 10-year-old boy died in diabetic ketoacidosis and his pancreas was found to contain a Coxsackie B virus. Furthermore, this virus subsequently was isolated and injected into mice, who then developed diabetes.

It is clear, however, that the overwhelming majority of children who recover from a viral illness do not develop diabetes. This takes us to the genetic part of the story and also ties in with the role of the immune system. Antigens are substances against which antibodies are made. For example, foreign proteins are good antigens, and antibodies formed against these antigens when they are part of an invading virus or bacteria are responsible in large part for the ability to recover from an infection. If a cell were transplanted from one person to another, the cell would be rejected because the cell protein would be foreign to the patient receiving it, and antibodies would form against the proteins. These proteins are antigens (because they provoke antibody formation) and are located on the surface of the cell. Each person carries genes that determine which surface antigens his or her cells will produce. These antigens are called HLA (histocompatibility) antigens. The fact that different HLA antigens exist indicates that different genes are responsible for producing them. However, certain HLA types are very common in type 1 diabetes. This means that the genes responsible for these HLA types also are very common in these patients and provide the genetic background for a predisposition to type 1 diabetes.

Another aspect of the immune system that is related to type 1 diabetes involves a process called autoimmunity. Normally, antibodies are made only against foreign protein. The body's immune system somehow recognizes that its own proteins are not foreign and, therefore, that it should not form antibodies against them. This process fails in many patients with type 1 diabetes. Instead, these individuals make antibodies against their own tissues, especially against several endocrine glands. Antibodies against the islets of Langerhans (the pancreatic structure that contains the insulin-producing beta cell) are usually seen soon after the onset of type 1 diabetes and tend to disappear with time. Although the relations among anti-islet-cell antibodies, HLA types, and viral illnesses are not clear, an altered immune response to certain viruses in at least some predisposed individuals may play a role in causing type 1 diabetes.

In summary, diabetes mellitus does not appear to be a single disease with a simple etiology. Rather, the complex interaction between the genetic background of the individual and his or her environment in type 1 and type 2 diabetes still is not clear and needs further investigation.

Type 2 Diabetes

Until techniques were developed for measuring insulin concentrations in the blood, all types of diabetes were assumed to be caused by inadequate production of insulin by the pancreatic beta cell. However, when the assay for insulin was established, it became clear that type 2 diabetics did secrete insulin and that, in many of them, substantial amounts were released by the pancreas. Therefore, in a considerable number of type 2 patients, diabetes is related to impaired insulin action.

The effect of insulin on tissues that are sensitive to it is a very complicated process. The initial step involves the binding of insulin to a specific receptor located on the surface of the cell. This interaction generates a signal that causes a number of changes within the cell. Although little is known about this signal, the critical first step of insulin action (i.e., binding to its receptor) is being studied intensively. In many type 2 diabetics, insulin binding is decreased, and it has been postulated that this receptor defect may cause the decreased insulin action. Other type 2 diabetics seem to have normal insulin binding, indicating that their insulin antagonism must occur within the cell—i.e., by a "postreceptor" defect. Type 2 diabetes probably has several different causes, including decreased insulin binding, postreceptor defects, and, possibly, a primary abnormality of insulin secretion.

Metabolism

STUDENT

The metabolism of the tissues in the body involves three food components: carbohydrates, protein, and fat. After these substances are consumed, each is broken down in the intestine into their simpler building blocks; then they are absorbed into the blood stream and built back up into large particles for storage in different tissues. The building blocks of carbohydrates consist mostly of glucose; those of proteins, amino acids; and those of fat, mostly of fatty acids. Although abnormalities in the metabolism of all three components can occur in diabetes, changes in glucose metabolism usually are the most obvious and thus are used to monitor diabetic control.

There are two general kinds of carbohydrates found in food: the simple and the complex. Simple carbohydrates are composed of only a few building blocks and are broken down quickly by the intestine and rapidly absorbed into the blood stream. Some examples of simple carbohydrates are candy, table sugar, cookies, pies, cakes, and all fruits and juices. Normally, the body releases insulin immediately and prevents the blood sugar from rising very much. In diabetics, however, either the beta cell is unable to produce enough insulin to prevent the rise in blood sugar, or the insulin that is secreted is ineffective in lowering this rapid elevation of glucose levels in the circulation. For these reasons, diabetic patients should eliminate concentrated sources of simple carbohydrates (e.g., candy, table sugar) from their diet and should limit their intake of fruits and juices.

This is not the case with complex carbohydrates which contain many glucose particles that are linked together. Starch (e.g., rice, potatoes, cereals, beans, bread) is an example of complex carbohydrates in the diet. Complex carbohydrates are broken down slowly in the intestinal tract; as a result, glucose concentrations build up gradually in the blood stream. Therefore, not only can starches be included in the diabetic diet, but recent recommendations suggest that carbohydrates should constitute >50% of the diabetic's total daily calories as a way of reducing the fat content of the diet. (Low-fat diets are helpful in preventing some forms of vascular disease.)

After the glucose reaches the blood stream, it is stored in the tissues to be used as an emergency energy source. The form in which glucose is stored is called glycogen. Insulin is very important in storing glucose as glycogen. After a meal, ~80% of the carbohydrates ingested are deposited in the liver initially. Over the next several hours, the liver releases some glucose for use and storage by other tissues that also depend on insulin. In this way, insulin is responsible for clearing the blood stream of the glucose derived from dietary carbohydrates.

Most tissues in the body do not routinely use glucose for energy. Except for the period within several hours after a meal, when some glucose is used for energy, fats serve as the major energy source. There is one important exception to this, however. Under normal conditions the brain has an *absolute* requirement for glucose. Without glucose, brain function becomes impaired and symptoms of low blood sugar occur. In order to ensure that the brain always has sugar to use for energy, the liver produces glucose between meals and during the night to prevent blood sugar from dropping too low. In turn, insulin prevents the liver from making too much glucose. Therefore, after a meal insulin is important to help the liver store dietary carbohydrate. Between meals and during the night, insulin controls the amount of glucose released by the liver.

After a meal, insulin also is important in transferring the dietary protein and fat into tissue protein and fat (through complicated mechanisms). Since glucose can be stored as glycogen in limited amounts, insulin also changes excess dietary carbohydrates into fat and stores it as such. Between meals and during the night, insulin also prevents the breakdown of tissue protein and fat, as well as carbohydrates (glycogen).

In diabetes, either not enough insulin is produced by the pancreatic beta cell, or the insulin that is released is not entirely effective. In either case, postprandial blood sugar levels increase to abnormally high levels because insulin is not able to clear the circulation of glucose and store it in the tissues. Glucose levels also may be high between meals and during the night because the insulin does not control production of glucose by the liver. For this reason, the blood sugar sometimes is too high in the morning before breakfast.

A minority of patients (fortunately) produce so little insulin that, without treatment, the fat stored in tissue begins to break down. This leads to an accumulation of fatty acids (the building blocks of fat) in the circulation. Fatty acids are broken down further by the liver and changed into ketone bodies (also acids). If the ketone bodies build up too much, the patient can become very ill and coma may result. This situation will be discussed later in the section on diabetic emergencies.

NURSE

Insulin has many different effects on the three tissues that are sensitive to it (i.e., liver, muscle, and fat). For instance, in muscle and fat tissue, insulin not only stimulates the entrance of glucose into the cells but, once the glucose is inside the cell, also stores it as glycogen and fat. In the liver the situation is more complicated. Although insulin does not affect the entrance of glucose into the liver cell, it directly stimulates its storage as glycogen or fat, both of which are important after meals. In addition, between meals and during the night insulin both controls the breakdown of glycogen into glucose (a pathway called *glycogenolysis*) and regulates the synthesis or formation of new glucose from smaller molecules (a pathway called *gluconeogenesis*).

The liver is the most important of the three insulin-sensitive tissues. After the patient eats ~80% of the meal-derived carbohydrates are stored in the liver (at least initially). Therefore, if insulin does not act normally on the liver after a meal, an increased amount of glucose escapes storage in the liver. This raises the blood sugar level to abnormally high values. Since the liver is the only organ that produces glucose via glycogenolysis and gluconeogenesis, a diminished insulin effect when the patient is not eating results in increased production of glucose and causes fasting hyperglycemia.

In protein metabolism, insulin not only prevents the breakdown of stored tissue protein but increases the formation of new protein (protein synthesis). It accomplishes the latter not only by stimulating the entrance of amino acids (the building blocks of proteins) into cells, but also by directly increasing the formation of proteins from the amino acids inside the cell. The effect of insulin on fat metabolism is very complex. However, the net result of insulin action is enhancement of the formation of stored fat by an increase in fat synthesis and prevention of its breakdown.

Thus, the effects of insulin in all three areas of metabolism (carbohydrate, protein, and fat) is to increase the storage of their respective building blocks and to prevent the breakdown of the stored products. This building up of the tissues is called *anabolism*, as opposed to *catabolism*, or breakdown of tissue stores. Although a number of hormones are catabolic, insulin is the only one that is an anabolic hormone. Therefore, there is no backup system when insulin does not work effectively or is not available. Under such circumstances abnormal metabolism occurs, resulting in diabetes mellitus.

Abnormal Metabolism

STUDENT

In diabetes, either not enough insulin is produced by the pancreatic beta cell, or the insulin that is released is not entirely effective. In either case, postprandial blood sugar levels increase to abnormally high levels because insulin is not able to clear the circulation of glucose and store it in the tissues. Between meals and during the night, glucose levels also may be high because insulin does not control production of glucose by the liver. For this reason, the blood sugar sometimes is too high in the morning before breakfast.

The severity of the signs and symptoms of uncontrolled diabetes depend on the level of blood sugar. The cause and effect of hyperglycemia are described below.

Signs and Symptoms

1. *Increased urination.* Normally, all glucose in the blood passes through part of the kidney and then is reabsorbed into the blood stream before it can reach the urine (see under *Urine Testing*). In diabetes, as the blood sugar rises, the amount of glucose that enters the kidney is too great to be entirely reabsorbed into the circulation. The glucose that is not reabsorbed remains in the kidney and is passed into the urine. The glucose that stays in the kidney also prevents all fluid that entered with it from returning to the blood stream. This extra fluid becomes additional urine.

2. *Increased thirst.* When extra fluid is lost through the urine, the body becomes dehydrated. The brain responds by signaling thirst, and the resulting increased fluid intake is an attempt to correct this situation.

3. *Increased appetite.* Because the body lacks enough effective insulin, it is not able to utilize sufficient calories. The brain responds to this situation by signaling hunger. However, if the diabetes becomes very severe, ketone bodies (see under *Diabetic emergencies*) may form and will depress the appetite.

4. *Fatigue.* The cells in the body are not able to use carbohydrates, fat, and protein normally because effective insulin is lacking.

5. *Blurred vision.* High and fluctuating blood sugar levels increase the amount of fluid in the lens of the eye. This extra fluid changes the shape of the lens and vision becomes blurred. Normal vision may not return until weeks after the blood sugar has been treated.

6. *Frequent skin (boils, carbuncles) and vaginal (yeast) infections.* The body's ability to fight infection is reduced during periods of poor control (i.e., high sugar levels). In the well-controlled diabetic, defense mechanisms against invading bacteria and fungi operate normally.

NURSE

The lack of insulin inhibits the utilization of glucose by the three insulin-sensitive tissues (muscle, fat, and liver). Additionally, in the absence of effective insulin, glucose production by the liver is uncontrolled and excessive. Both of these conditions lead to elevated glucose concentrations in the blood, or hyperglycemia. Increased urination (polyuria) occurs because the kidney can not reabsorb all of the filtered glucose into the blood stream; thus, the excess sugar that is passed into the urine brings along extra fluid with it (see under *Monitoring Diabetic Control*). This loss of extra fluid results in dehydration, which in part may cause headache and fatigue. There is a center in the brain that responds to dehydration by signaling the patient to drink in order to restore the plasma volume. This increased thirst is called *polydipsia*. Unless ketosis occurs, diabetic patients in this condition often become very hungry. Although the mechanism for the increased appetite (or polyphagia) in uncontrolled diabetes is not clear, it probably is due to the decreased utilization of calories. Hyperglycemia causes blurred vision because the lens of the eye changes shape in the presence of high blood sugar levels. Patients with blurred vision should refrain from obtaining new glasses or changing their current prescription until the blood sugar has been lowered for 3 to 4 weeks.

Baterial infections due to *Staphylococcus aureus* (boils, carbuncles) and certain fungi (vaginal yeast infections) are more common in uncontrolled diabetics than in well-controlled patients. The ability of white blood cells to counteract these organisms effectively is impaired until control is attained. Prolonged poor control causes excess breakdown of proteins, leading to poor wound healing and further difficulty in combating infection. Ischemia or lack of tissue oxygenation due to impaired blood flow also may contribute to increased susceptibility to infection.

Treatment

STUDENT/NURSE

The treatment program for all diabetic patients should include a prescribed diet and exercise program. Some type 2 diabetics do not need further treatment, while others require either sulfonylurea agents or insulin. All type 1 patients require insulin therapy. The daily management of diabetes should include some form of glucose monitoring (e.g., urine testing, capillary-blood glucose evaluation) and personal hygiene (see sections on monitoring diabetic control and foot care.)

Goals of Treatment

1. To maintain a blood sugar level as close to normal as possible.
2. To maintain a normal body weight by following an individualized diet that includes adequate vitamins and minerals.
3. To engage in a planned exercise program.

Personal Hygiene

STUDENT/NURSE

The hygiene needs of diabetics do not differ from those of nondiabetics but must be attended to with more caution and diligence.

Eye Care

Chronic complications that may occur in the diabetic demand emphasis on frequent eye examinations. Cataracts, glaucoma, and retinopathy (hemorrhages in the eye) occur more frequently in diabetics than in nondiabetics. Yearly eye examinations by an ophthalmologist are recommended; examinations should be more frequent if eye pain or changes in vision occur.

Teeth

Diseases of the mouth, especially of the gums and surrounding tissue, are estimated to occur three times more frequently in diabetics than in nondiabetics. Poor oral hygiene is the main cause of periodontal (gum) disease.

Major signs and symptoms of periodontal disease include the following:

1. Inflammation of gum tissue (red and swollen gums).
2. Easily bleeding of gums on touching.
3. Dental plaque and calculus accumulation.

4. Spacing between teeth, receding gums, and loose teeth.
5. Early loss of teeth due to primary gum disease.

NURSE

Teaching Needs: Prevention

1. Achieve good control of blood sugar.
2. Clean teeth at least twice a day with a soft toothbrush and toothpaste; use dental floss.
3. Do not neglect toothaches, bleeding gums, poorly fitting dentures, or sores in the mouth.
4. Examine the gums by pulling the lips apart and looking for inflamed tissue.
5. When the patient is to undergo oral surgery, it is essential that the blood glucose be controlled, since stress and anesthesia raise the blood sugar.
6. Practice routine care of the mouth and take frequent prophylactic measures, since diabetics tend to have gum infections (gingivitis).
7. An insulin-dependent diabetic going to a dentist for general treatment should have breakfast before the appointment; however, special provisions for food need not be taken. The dental appointment should be scheduled so that it does not prevent the patient from having the usual meals and snacks.

STUDENT/NURSE

Candida albicans (Moniliasis)

Diabetic patients, especially those who are poorly controlled, frequently contract yeast infections. *Candida albicans* may affect the oral mucous membrane (causing thrush), axillary areas, under the breast, the groin, and tissue around nails. An infection of the last is termed a paronychia.

The most common disorder caused by *C. albicans* is vulvovaginitis. *Candida* is present normally in the vaginal mucosa. However, in diabetic individuals, the increased concentrations of glucose in the urine and surrounding tissues causes the organism to multiply rapidly. This problem is seen most commonly in the obese diabetic.

Signs and Symptoms

1. White, cheesy discharge with a peculiar yeasty odor.
2. Pruritus vulvae (itching).
3. Erythema (redness) and edema (swelling) of genitalia, perineal area, or inside of the thighs.

STUDENT/NURSE

Teaching Needs

1. Do not wear soiled underclothes.
2. Wear underclothing that will not promote or trap heat and moisture (e.g., cotton-crotch underwear, especially pantyhose with cotton crotch or cotton top).
3. After urination, cleanse perineal and vaginal area using a plastic squirt-type perineal bottle (can be purchased in stores) filled with tap water.
4. Always use front-to-back wiping (drying).
5. Although specific medicine is available to treat this fungus, the infection is difficult to clear up unless the diabetes is brought under control.

Long-Term Complications

STUDENT

Long-term complications of diabetes result from changes in the structure, and therefore the function, of blood vessels and nerves. Such complications do not necessarily affect all diabetics. Factors to consider in the development of complications are the type and duration of the diabetes and the degree of blood sugar control. Evidence now suggests that long-term complications, especially involvement of the eye, kidney, and nerves, can be delayed or prevented if the blood sugar is consistently maintained at nearly normal levels.

NURSE

Before the discovery of insulin, the major cause of death in diabetes was keto-acidosis. Today morbidity and mortality are due mainly to involvement of the vascular system, both of the small vessels (microangiopathy) and the large vessels (macroangiopathy). Diabetics have twice the prevalence of myocardial infarctions, a five times greater prevalence of gangrene and a 17 to 25 times greater risk of renal failure and blindness than do nondiabetics.

Retinopathy (eye disease), neuropathy (involvement of the nerves), nephropathy (kidney disease), and arterial calcification all increase in frequency and severity with the duration of diabetes. This is in contrast to the sequelae linked directly to atherosclerosis, which are related more to the age of the patient rather than to how long diabetes has been present.

Microangiopathy includes retinopathy and nephropathy. Pathologically, microangiopathy is characterized by an abnormal thickening of the capillary basement membrane, which is a structure that surrounds all capillaries and whose function is unclear. However, it is certain that all diabetics develop some thickening of this structure. The alteration is associated with the eye and kidney, dysfunction that is seen in some diabetic patients.

Macroangiopathy refers to arteriosclerotic vascular disease, which includes hypertension, myocardial infarction, cerebrovascular disease, and peripheral vascular disease. Pathologically, these changes are the same in diabetics as they are in nondiabetics. However, clinically these diseases occur much earlier and in a more severe form in diabetics.

Retinopathy

Retinopathy is classified as either nonproliferative (background or simple) or proliferative retinopathy. In background retinopathy, the veins on the retina become dilated, tiny outpocketings (microaneurysms) of the veins develop, and plasma or whole blood leaks from the veins, causing retinal exudates or small hemorrhages, respectively. This condition usually does not impair vision. However, ~5% of diabetics develop edema in the macular portion of the retina, causing a significant decrease in visual acuity.

Proliferative retinopathy is much more severe because vitreous hemorrhage, retinal detachment, and blindness often follow. In this type of retinopathy, formation of new vessels occurs. These new vessels are very friable and often break, causing large hemorrhages that create problems. Fortunately, background retinopathy progresses to proliferative retinopathy in only a minority of diabetics.

Control of hypertension is extremely important in preventing retinal bleeding. Avoidance of high altitudes (>12,000 feet), heavy lifting, and smoking also are good preventive measures. The patient should be referred to an ophthal mologist at the earliest sign of advancing background or the appearance of proliferative retinopathy.

Treatment. Photocoagulation is the use of concentrated light rays from an xenon arc (white light), argon laser (green light), or a ruby laser (red light). The argon laser is the newest form of treatment and can pinpoint and coagulate leaking blood vessels in the retina with great accuracy.

Vitrectomy is the surgical procedure of removing old blood and proteins from the vitreous cavity of the eye by using an instrument containing an extremely small drill and suction. The device enters the eyeball, removing the vitreous hemorrhage and replacing it with normal saline.

Nephropathy

Severe thickening of the capillary basement membrane of the kidney eventually impairs renal function. When this extra material is concentrated in one or several areas in the glomerulus it is termed *Kimmelstiel-Wilson's disease* or *nodular glomerulosclerosis*. The accumulation occurs most often throughout the glomerulus and causes diffuse glomerulosclerosis. It is the diffuse process that compromises renal function.

The first sign of nephropathy is leakage of protein into the urine (proteinuria). Initially this leakage is intermittent, but eventually it becomes constant. Many years can elapse between the beginning of proteinuria and evidence of impaired renal function. However, total kidney failure usually occurs within 5 years after renal insufficiency is evident.

Controlling both hypertension and blood sugar levels has been shown to delay the progression of renal disease. Treatment also consists of a diet restricted in protein, sodium, and potassium. When renal failure occurs, the patient must be treated with either peritoneal dialysis or hemodialysis. Recently, renal transplantation has been attempted more and more frequently in diabetic patients.

In renal disease, the renal threshold for glucose rises as function diminishes, making assessment of blood sugar control on the basis of urine test results very difficult. Capillary-blood glucose monitoring that can be done by the patient and/or family is the best way to assess control (see section on monitoring diabetic control). Once renal impairment occurs, the dose of insulin often needs to be decreased. This is because the kidney normally inactivates $\sim 40\%$ of the insulin injected. If this proportion of insulin cannot be broken down because the amount of functioning kidney tissue is decreased, then active insulin accumulates and causes hypoglycemia.

Neuropathy

Diabetic neuropathy probably is the most common long-term complication of diabetes and is the source of severe discomfort for many patients. There are two types of neuropathy: peripheral and autonomic. Peripheral neuropathy is much more common than autonomic. Symptoms consist of burning sensations, tingling, numbness, and pain in the lower extremities, especially starting in the feet. The pain can become very severe; it sometimes is relieved by walking and is often worse at night. Loss of feeling may occur eventually. This can be dangerous for the patient because he or she cannot appreciate any external trauma to the feet and thus take the appropriate measures to treat it. The upper extremities also can be involved. Patients may suffer burns, especially from cooking and smoking, because of the decreased sensation. Learning Braille (which sometimes is necessary when blindness secondary to diabetic retinopathy occurs) is more difficult. Muscle atrophy, which also can occur in the feet, leads to weakness and impairs the patient's ability to use his or her hands normally (e.g., for preparing insulin injections).

Autonomic neuropathy does not cause clinical symptoms unless peripheral neuropathy also is present. Autonomic neuropathy involves mainly the gastrointestinal and genitourinary tracts.

Gastrointestinal Tract

1. *Gastroparesis diabeticorum.* The neuropathy causes delay in the emptying of stomach (gastric) contents. This may lead to an unpredictable absorption of food and thus interfere with diabetic control. Symptoms include feeling full after eating only a small amount of food, nausea, and vomiting. It is common for the vomitus to contain food eaten many hours before. Although treatment is difficult, small frequent feedings are helpful.

2. *Diabetic enteropathy.* Involvement of the nerves that control the small intestine can cause diarrhea, which sometimes alternates with constipation. The diarrhea is more frequent at night and may get better or worse for no apparent reason. Occasionally, fecal incontinence also occurs (especially at night) because the anal sphincter does not function normally. Diabetic enteropathy does not appear to interfere with either diabetic control or the general health of the patient. Treatment includes antibiotics and antidiarrheal drugs.

Genitourinary Tract

1. *Neurogenic bladder.* When the bladder expands, autonomic nerves located in the muscle wall give the signal for the bladder to contract; this results in urination. If these nerves are affected by diabetic autonomic neuropathy, the urge to urinate is delayed until the bladder becomes very full. This process is slow and insidious, but the patient eventually may notice infrequent urination. In addition, the strength of contraction is weakened, causing incomplete emptying of the bladder. The urine that remains is a good source for bacterial growth. Therefore, patients with neurogenic bladder frequently have urinary tract infections that start in the bladder but, unfortunately, may ascend to the kidneys.

   Treatment involves drugs that promote bladder contraction, antibiotics and, in advanced cases, possibly surgery.
   Patients with neurogenic bladder should be instructed to:

   a. Void frequently (i.e., every 4 hours) on a scheduled basis; this may necessitate the use of a watch or clock with an alarm.
   b. Triple-void. This is a simple technique of voiding as much as possible, resting 1 minute and voiding again, and resting 1 more minute and then trying a third time.
   c. Perform Crede's maneuver. Press hands against the lower abdomen to increase the pressure and therefore empty the bladder.
   d. Increase fluid intake, as in any bladder infection.

2. *Impotence.* Impotence is estimated to be four or five times more common in male diabetics older than 30 years than in nondiabetics in the same age group.

Impotence is the inability to successfully complete the act of sexual intercourse because of failure to initiate or sustain an erection. An erection results from a reflex action that traps blood in the penile shaft. The reflex is transmitted through a group of autonomic nerves originating in the lower part of the pelvic area. As a result of autonomic neuropathy, these nerves are unable to respond to the appropriate stimuli and an erection cannot take place.

Other conditions that may cause impotence need to be ruled out before the diagnosis is made. These conditions include:

a. psychogenic (emotional) problems

b. poor control of blood sugar

c. drugs, such as alcohol, certain antihypertensive medications, tranquilizers, or antidepressants

d. organic causes, such as trauma, systemic disease, or hormone deficiency.

Treatment of impotence is as follows:

1. Obtain a urology consultation.

2. If poor control of blood sugar is the cause, proper management and control of diabetes may restore normal potency.

3. If emotional factors are the cause, psychological evaluation and counseling may produce good results.

4. If abuse of certain drugs, such as alochol, is the cause, eliminating them usually restores potency.

5. If impotence is due to medications given for hypertension or severe depression, other medications that do not cause this side effect should be substituted.

6. If impotence is due to autonomic neuropathy, counseling sessions with both partners on alternative techniques for sexual gratification may be of great benefit.

7. A penile prosthesis also should be considered for certain patients.

Other disorders that may occur secondary to autonomic neuropathy include orthostatic hypotension, unexplained tachycardia, and silent myocardial infarction.

Macroangiopathy

The main threat to the health of the type 2 diabetic patient is the increased prevalence of atherosclerotic disease in the major arterial systems. Macroangiopathy in the diabetic individual usually occurs at an earlier age and progresses more rapidly than in nondiabetic individual. It causes coronary artery, cerebrovascular, and peripheral vascular disease. Myocardial infarctions occur three to four times more frequently in the diabetic population than in the nondiabetic population. Myocardial infarction should be considered when symptoms such as chest pain, shortness of breath, or congestive heart failure occur. A heart attack (silent myocardial infarction) is much more likely to be painless in diabetics because associated neuropathy affects the pain fibers to the heart.

Cerebrovascular disease leading to stroke is approximately twice as common in the diabetic population as in the nondiabetic population. Symptoms may include intermittent dizziness, lightheadedness, weakness of an arm or leg, or slurring of speech. Noninvasive procedures (e.g., ultrasound, Doppler studies) and invasive procedures (e.g., angiography), for assessing the carotid arteries should be considered. Surgical procedures (e.g., endarterectomy) also may be performed. Medical treatment may include use of anticoagulant medications. Aspirin taken once or twice a day has recently been shown to help prevent a recurrence of symptoms in many patients.

Peripheral vascular disease should be suspected if the patient exhibits decreased pulses in the lower extremities and/or leg pain (usually in the calf) during exercise that is relieved with rest (intermittent claudication). If the pain persists during rest or if a foot infection results from impaired blood flow through the major leg arteries, surgery to bypass the diseased vessels may be indicated.

Medical treatment should aim to reduce the risk factors associated with macro-angiopathy. These factors include (a) hypertension, (b) smoking, (c) elevated levels of cholesterol and, possibly, triglycerides, and (d) hyperglycemia. Elimination of smoking (which causes constriction of the blood vessels) is particularly important. Although reduction of elevated glucose concentrations probably is helpful, the other risk factors have made it difficult to demonstrate conclusively that better diabetic control will be beneficial. Two other treatment modalities are very important. The feet must be protected and inspected regularly (see section on foot management). A planned program of walking, increasing the distance gradually, is helpful in increasing the patient's tolerance for exercise.

Evaluation

Select the correct answer or answers to each question.

1. Diabetes is a condition in which
    a. the liver produces too much glucose
    b. either the pancreas produces too little insulin or the body cannot properly respond to the insulin produced
    c. blood sugar is too low
2. Type 1 diabetes is seen more often in
    a. the young
    b. the middle-aged and older
    c. the obese
    d. the lean

3. In normal metabolism, the source(s) of body fuel is (are)
   a. protein
   b. carbohydrates
   c. fat
4. Insulin helps the body to use and store
   a. fat
   b. protein
   c. carbohydrates
5. Symptoms that may be seen when diabetes develops are
   a. frequent urination
   b. excessive hunger
   c. weight loss
   d. excessive thirst
6. Treatment of all diabetics includes
   a. diet
   b. pills or insulin
   c. exercise
7. Body organs that may be affected by diabetes are
   a. kidney
   b. eyes
   c. blood vessels
   d. nerves

INSULIN

Although control of diabetes depends on many factors, insulin administration (i.e., for patients who require it) is critical in attaining it. From an educational point of view, the need to take insulin increases considerably the amount of material the patient must master. It is not enough simply to teach patients how to fill a syringe and administer their injections. They should know what insulin is; where it comes from; something about its action in the body (especially on glucose levels); the onset, peak, and duration of different preparations; its possible side effects; and the body's response to too little or too much of it.

Outcome Criteria (Student) and Goals (Nurse)

Objectives

STUDENT

Upon completion of the instructions, the student will be able to verbalize, write, or demonstrate:

1. Where insulin is produced.
2. What effect insulin will have on the blood sugar level.
3. Type, strength, and time-course of the insulin prescribed for them.
4. Accurate preparation for the injection of one or two types of insulins.
5. Accurate selection of an injection site and injection technique using a pattern of rotation.
6. Storage and care of insulin and equipment.

Goals

NURSE

To provide information on:

1. The general structure, synthesis, storage, and release of endogenous insulin.
2. The source, types, strengths, administration, and associated complications of exogenous insulin.

DISCOVERY

STUDENT

In 1921, a young Canadian surgeon who had recently returned from service in World War I and a young Canadian graduate student performed one of the most notable experiments in medical history. The researchers injected into dogs dying of diabetes (induced by removal of the pancreas) an extract obtained from the pancreas of a normal dog. Not only did the dogs not die, but they regained their vitality. Further work on isolating the active part of the extract resulted in the discovery of insulin. In 1922 insulin was first given to a diabetic patient, who subsequently demonstrated rapid improvement. Since 1922, many improvements have been made in commercial insulin preparations.

NURSE

The story of the discovery of insulin can be said to have started as long ago as the end of the nineteenth century, when it was shown clearly that a relationship existed between the disease known long as diabetes and the pancreas, a gland lying directly below the stomach. But it remained for a young Canadian physician, the late Sir Frederick Grant Banting, to initiate the experiments that resulted in the discovery of insulin. In February 1922, Dr. Banting and Mr. Best published their work in the *Journal of Laboratory and Clinical Medicine.* Dr. Banting's first clinical studies were described in the March 1922 issue of the *Canadian Medical Association Journal.* The findings were summarized as follows:

Following the production of what appears to be a concentrated internal secretion of the pancreas and the demonstration of its physiological activity in animals, and under careful control, its relatively low toxicity, we are presenting a preliminary report on the pharmacological activity of this extract in human diabetes mellitus. Clinical observation at this juncture would appear to justify the following conclusions: 1) Blood sugar can be markedly reduced even to the normal values. 2) Glycosuria can be abolished. 3) The acetone bodies can be made to disappear from the urine. 4) The respiratory quotient shows evidence of increased utilization of carbohydrates. 5) A definite improvement is observed in the general condition of these patients and in addition the patients themselves report a subjective sense of well-being and increased vigor for a period following the administration of these preparations.

What is Insulin?

STUDENT

A hormone is a substance that is produced and released in one part of the body and travels to another part, where it exerts its effect. Insulin is a hormone produced and stored by special cells (beta cells) in the islets of Langerhans in the pancreas. This organ is about 6 inches long, or approximately the size of the hand, and is located behind the stomach. The name insulin comes from the term *islets,* or islands of cells where insulin is produced. (Langerhans is the name of the German physician who first described these cells.) After insulin is released from the pancreas, it travels in the blood stream to various parts of the body, where it has its effects.

NURSE

The islets of Langerhans contain three major types of cells. Alpha cells produce glucagon, a hormone whose main function is to raise levels of blood sugar by breaking down liver glycogen. Alpha cells comprise <1% of the islet cells. Delta cells secrete somatostatin, a hormone that inhibits the secretion of insulin and glucagon. Somatostatin also is present in other parts of the body and helps to regulate the secretion of other hormones.

The majority of islet cells are beta cells, which produce insulin through a complicated process. First, a long single chain of amino acids is formed; this chain curls back on itself so that it can be connected in two places by a bridge of sulfur atoms (Fig. 8-3). The entire structure is called *proinsulin.* Proinsulin is clipped in two places along the chain to form *insulin* (Fig. 8-3 closed circles) and the connecting peptide (or C-peptide) (Fig. 8-3 open circles). Insulin consists of 51 amino acids arranged in the A and B chains that are connected by two disulfide bonds (Fig. 8-3). All insulins isolated from mammals are very similar in structure and differ by only a few amino acids. The most common insulin preparation used to treat diabetics today is a combination of beef and pork

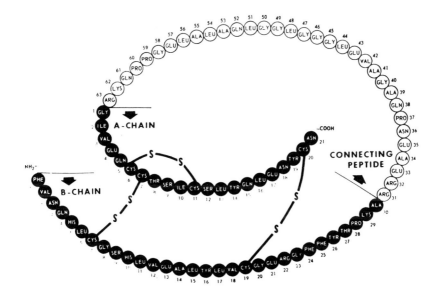

Figure 8-3. Structure of pork proinsulin, which is separated in the pancreas (at the thin straight lines) into insulin (dark circles) and the connecting peptide (open circles). (Reprinted with permission from Chance RE: Amino acid sequence of proinsulins and intermediates. Diabetes 21(Suppl 2):461-467, 1972.)

insulin. Pure pork and pure beef insulins also are available. Beef insulin has three amino acids that are different from those found in human insulin. Pork insulin has only one amino acid that is different from those in human insulin. Researchers recently have been able to "fool" certain bacteria into making synthetic human insulin, so that an unlimited supply of human insulin may be available for diabetics in the near future.

After proinsulin is broken down, insulin and the C-peptide are stored in the granules of the beta cell and are released together. Therefore, C-peptide concentrations in the circulation also reflect insulin secretion by the beta cell.

Measuring C-peptide levels has been helpful in two circumstances. When patients are treated with insulin, they form antibodies against it that interfere with the measurement of insulin concentrations. Therefore, C-peptide determinations can help to evaluate whether the beta cells of the insulin-requiring diabetic are still capable of producing insulin. Diabetics who can still secrete some of their own insulin usually are more stable and easier to control than those who cannot. Many times, an individual with juvenile-onset diabetes needs less and less insulin after the diagnosis is made and treatment is started. Sometimes insulin can be discontinued altogether. This is called the "honeymoon phase," and C-peptide measurements during this phase have documented that insulin secretion has returned. Unfortunately, this is a temporary situation, and, in virtually all cases, the beta cells fail again and insulin therapy must be either resumed or increased.

Second, in some patients (*not* diabetics) with hypoglycemia it is important to distinguish between those whose low glucose concentrations are caused by increased insulin secretion by a tumor of the beta cells (insulinoma) and those who may be surreptitiously injecting themselves with insulin. Since commercial insulin preparations do not contain C-peptide, the latter type of patient will have low glucose concentrations, high insulin levels, and low C-peptide values. However, if the hypoglycemia is caused by an insulinoma, the patient will show low glucose concentrations, high insulin levels, and high C-peptide values.

Why Insulin Cannot be Taken Orally

STUDENT/NURSE

Insulin is a hormone made up of many building blocks of protein arranged in a chain. If insulin were taken orally, this chain would be broken down and destroyed in the intestinal tract by the action of enzymes that help in the digestion of food. The pills that some diabetics take to lower blood sugar are not insulin and therefore can be taken orally (see under *Oral Hypoglycemic Sulfonylurea Agents*).

Commercial Insulin Preparations

STUDENT

Most insulin comes from the pancreas of cattle and pigs. The most common preparation of insulin is a combination of two thirds beef and one third pork insulin and can be purchased in 10-cc vials. Most medicines are measured in milligrams (e.g., Tylenol, 350 mg), grains (e.g., aspirin, 5 gr), or cubic centimeters (e.g., Maalox, 30 cc). Insulin, however, is measured in units (which appears on the label as "U"). The unit of insulin is the same amount in every preparation.

At present there are two different concentrations of insulin: U-40 and U-100. U-40 means that there are 40 U of insulin in every cubic centimeter; U-100 means that there are 100 U per cc. Thus, unit for unit the preparations are equal. For example, 10 U of U-40 insulin lowers the blood sugar to the same level as 10 U of U-100 insulin. The only difference is the amount of fluid that is injected.

One requirement is that the syringe must correspond to the concentration of insulin being used. Syringes are calibrated differently according to the concentration of insulin. A 1-cc U-100 syringe holds 100 U of insulin when filled completely, while a 1-cc U-40 syringe holds 40 U of insulin when filled completely. Therefore, in order to give 25 U of U-100 insulin, only one fourth (25/100) of the U-100 syringe would need to be filled. In order to give 25 U of U-40 insulin, five eighths (25/40) of the U-40 syringe would need to be filled. If by mistake a U-40 syringe were filled to 25 U with U-100 insulin, the patient would receive 2.5 times more insulin than was needed. This, of course, would be a serious error in dosage.

It is predicted that, before long, U-40 insulin will be discontinued and that U-100 insulin will be the only insulin used. Restriction of use to U-100 insulin has several advantages: (*a*) using one strength should reduce the errors in dosage; (*b*) the amount of insulin injected will be smaller, and (*c*) the U-100 syringe markings are easily adapted to the metric system. At the present time, 10% of the insulin sold in the United States is U-40 insulin.

NURSE

No further information is needed.

Characteristics of Insulin Preparations

STUDENT

The ingredients in the insulin preparation determine how quickly the insulin begins to work and how long the effects will last. For example, some cold medications (e.g., Contac) are time-released preparations (i.e., small amounts are continuously released), and their effects are noted for several hours or all day long. Other medications (e.g., Tylenol) are not time-released preparations, and their effects last for only a short time, perhaps 3 to 4 hours.

The same characteristics are true of insulin preparations. Clear insulin such as regular insulin does not have the time-release factor; therefore, it works quickly and is used up quickly. In contrast, the long-acting insulins have the time-release factor, which gives them a cloudy or white appearance.

Examples

Regular insulin given before breakfast will lower blood sugar mainly between breakfast and lunch.

Neutral protamine Hagedorn (NPH) or Lente insulin given before breakfast will lower blood sugar mainly between midafternoon and dinnertime.

A mixture of both regular and NPH/Lente insulins will have peak effects in lowering blood sugar twice during the day: between breakfast and lunch and between lunch and dinner.

NURSE

The patient must be informed about the onset, peak, and duration of action of the insulin preparations they use (Table 8-1 and Fig. 8-4). Protamine is used in NPH insulin and in Protamine zinc insulin (PZI) to retard the absorption of insulin from the injection site. In PZI there is an excess amount of protamine, which explains the long-acting characteristic of that preparation. The different sizes of the crystals in the Lente (Lente, Semilente, Ultralente) series explains the different time courses of these three insulins. The larger the crystal size, the slower the insulin is absorbed. Lente insulin itself is a mixture of three parts Semilente and seven parts Ultralente, and its time course is very similar to that of NPH insulin. Regular insulin can be mixed with any of the other insulin preparations. The combination of Regular and Semilente insulins is not helpful clinically since both are short-acting insulins. All insulin preparations are turbid or cloudy except for regular insulin, which is clear. Only Regular insulin can be given intravenously.

The patient should prepare a daily activity and eating schedule. Using the information in Table 8-1, the nurse should illustrate the onset, action, and duration of insulin as they relate to this schedule.

Table 8-1. Time-Course of Action of Insulin Preparations Available in the United States

Insulin Preparation	Type	Onset (hrs)	Action Maximal (hrs)	Duration (hrs)
Regular (crystalline)	Short-acting (rapid)	30 min–1 hr	2–4	4–6[a]
NPH (isophane)	Intermediate-acting (slow)	3–4	10–16	20–24
PZI	Prolonged-acting (very slow)	6–8	14–20	32+
Semilente	Short-acting (rapid)	1–2	3–6	8–12
Lente	Intermediate-acting (slow)	3–4	10–16	20–24
Ultralente	Prolonged-acting (very slow)	6–8	14–20	32+

Abbreviations: NPH, neutral protamine Hagedorn; PZI, protamine zinc insulin.
[a]In some patients, Regular insulin may peak between 4 and 8 hours after injection and last considerably longer.

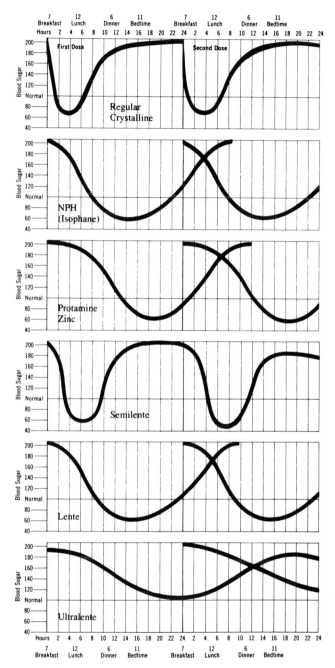

Figure 8-4. Time-course of action of various insulin preparations. (Reprinted with permission from Waife SO: *Diabetes Mellitus*, 7th ed. Lilly Research Laboratories, Indianapolis, 1973, pp. 42–43.)

Storage and Stability

STUDENT

Insulin is very stable and maintains its effectiveness in lowering blood sugar when stored at temperatures lower than 100°F. It should be remembered that your insulin can tolerate whatever temperature your body can. Therefore, insulin does not require refrigeration. Do not use insulin after the expiration date on the bottle.

NURSE

Changes in manufacturing methods have resulted in insulin of increased purity and with a neutral pH. The newer preparations also are more stable than the former, more acidic preparations. Neutral regular insulin maintains full potency when stored at room temperature (75°F) over a period of 24 months. Color changes and "clumping" of the liquid may be seen after 24 months. Both NPH and PZI insulins maintain their potency when stored at room temperature (75°F) for up to 36 months. After 36 months, the fine precipitate in NPH insulin forms clumps.

Summary

1. The potency of insulin is affected by extremes in temperature.
2. All insulins may deteriorate at temperatures over 100°F (37.6°C).
3. Freezing does not decrease insulin activity but may result in clumping of the suspension.
4. Although NPH and PZI are the most stable and regular insulin, the least all insulin preparations can be stored at room temperature or in the refrigerator for long periods. The expiration dates appear on the vials and should be observed.

New Insulins

STUDENT

Improvement in the purity of insulin has recently (1980) been achieved in all preparations manufactured by Eli Lilly & Company. As insulin is removed from the animal pancreas to begin the manufacturing process, certain impurities are also extracted. As many of these impurities as possible are removed during the purification processes, leaving a much purer form of injectable insulin. Labeling of the new insulins is the same as that of the old ones, except that the word "new" in red lettering appears on both the bottle and the box. The advantages of the new insulins have yet to be determined, but most authorities believe that the purer preparations will decrease the amount of certain (already uncommon) allergic reactions to insulin.

NURSE

Before 1972, all insulins manufactured in the United States contained various amounts of proinsulin and other higher-molecular-weight compounds, as well as glucagon and other pancreatic peptides. These impurities comprised ~10% of the insulin preparation; the remaining 90% was true insulin. Some of the complications of insulin therapy, such as localized skin reactions, insulin resistance, and lipoatrophy (see section on side effects of insulin), are thought to be related in part to the presence of impurities.

In 1972 insulin was purified further. The term *single-peak* was applied to these insulins, which were >95% pure insulin. In the spring of 1980, Lilly purified their insulin preparations even further to contain only a minuscule amount (<10 parts per million) of proinsulin. Lilly now manufactures two kinds of insulin—improved single peak (a combination of beef and pork) and Iletin II (a pure pork preparation). Two European pharmaceutical companies also manufacture insulin of this purity and market their products in the United States. Nordisk produces only pork insulin, while Nova manufactures pure pork, pure beef, or a combination of the two. As of fall 1980, E.R. Squibb & Sons, the other pharmaceutical company in the United States marketing insulin, is still routinely producing single-peak insulin. The clinical advantages of one or another of insulin preparation have not yet been established. (This information is intended as a guide to insulin preparations available from various pharmaceutical companies.)

Preparation and Administration

Preparation of One Type of Insulin

STUDENT

1. Wash hands.
2. Remove the cap from a new bottle of insulin. The cloudy sediment that collects at the bottom of the bottle contains most of the insulin. Therefore, roll the insulin bottle between the palms of the hands to mix the insulin. If the insulin is not mixed, the actual amount of insulin drawn up into the syringe will vary.
3. Wipe the rubber stopper and the top of the bottle with cotton moistened in alcohol or with an alcohol wipe.
4. Find the mark on the syringe that corresponds to the number of units of insulin to be given.

5. Pull the syringe plunger back to this mark using the portion of the plunger nearest to the needle to measure. (This step may be omitted in preparing only one kind of insulin if the patient encounters problems with it.)

6. The syringe is now filled with the volume of air that corresponds to the volume of insulin to be injected.

7. Keep the bottle in an upright position on the table and insert the needle through the center of the rubber stopper.

8. Push in the plunger to force air into bottle. This makes it easier to withdraw the insulin into the syringe.

9. Keep the needle in place.

10. Turn the bottle upside down.

11. Make sure that the needle is completely covered by the insulin solution.

12. Pull and push the plunger in and out three times to the prescribed mark to eliminate air bubbles in the syringe. Air bubbles will not cause harm but will interfere with drawing the correct amount of insulin into the syringe.

13. Pull back on the plunger *very slowly* until the prescribed mark is reached. The appropriate amount of insulin is now in the syringe.

14. Pull the needle out of the bottle.

15. Be careful not to touch the needle.

16. Prepare to give the injection.

Preparation of Two Types of Insulin in One Syringe

1. Wash hands.

2. Roll the insulin bottle containing the (cloudly) solution between the palms of the hands to mix the insulin. The insulin bottle containing the clear solution does not have to be mixed.

3. Wipe the rubber stoppers and tops of both bottles with cotton moistened with alcohol or with an alcohol wipe. When two insulins are to be mixed in one syringe, it is very important to increase the pressure within the bottles by pushing air into the bottles. The increased pressure in the bottle containing the long-acting insulin will prevent the Regular (clear) insulin from being sucked into the bottle.

4. Put an amount of air equal to the dose of the long-acting (cloudy) insulin into that bottle first.

5. Next push the appropriate amount of air into the bottle containing regular insulin.

6. Do not remove the needle from this bottle.

7. Turn the bottle upside down.

8. Pull and push the plunger in and out three times to the prescribed mark to eliminate air bubbles in the syringe.

9. Withdraw the prescribed amount of clear insulin into the syringe.
10. Pull the needle out of the bottle.
11. Insert the needle into the bottle containing the long-acting (cloudy) insulin.
12. Turn the bottle upside down.
13. Pull back on plunger *very slowly* to withdraw the prescribed amount of long-acting (cloudy) insulin. For example, if the prescribed dose is 40 U of NPH insulin and 10 U of regular insulin, there will be 10 U of clear insulin in the syringe at this point. Therefore, to obtain 40 U of the cloudy insulin, the plunger must be pulled back to 50 U. If more than the prescribed amount of insulin enters the syringe, pull the needle out of the bottle, discard the entire syringe, and *start over*. Do *not* put the mixture of insulin back into bottle or discard a portion of it by squirting some out of the syringe.

NURSE

Regular insulin manufactured today has a neutral pH and can be mixed with any other insulin preparation in any ratio. This is an advantage over old preparations of regular insulin, which had an acid pH and did not yield a stable solution when mixed with other insulins. The traditional practice of first drawing regular insulin into the syringe and then drawing the modified insulin was based on the instability of acidic regular insulin. In addition, the fast-acting property of regular insulin was diminished by contamination with modified insulin. This is no longer true. Since the advent of neutral pH insulins, stability no longer presents a problem, and the sequence of insulin withdrawal into the syringe does not matter. However, contamination of insulin bottles should be avoided because it prevents the patient from receiving the correct kind or amount of insulin. The magnitude of the error depends on both the amount of incorrect insulin introduced and the volume left in the bottle. Another potential problem is that only regular insulin can be given intravenously; and regular insulin contaminated with modified insulin may produce side effects when injected intravenously.

Dead Space

STUDENT

No information is needed.

NURSE

Another issue in mixing insulins is that of dead space. Dead space refers to the area at the tip of the syringe and in the hub of the needle where insulin remains after an injection is given. If the patient takes only one kind of insulin, dead space will not be a problem. For example, suppose 40 U of U-100 insulin must be given and the dead space is 0.1 cc (i.e., 10 U). When the 40 U is drawn into the syringe, the syringe and needle really are holding 50 U (40 units in the barrel of the syringe and 10 U in the dead space). After the injection is given, 10 U still remains in the dead space and the patient received 40 U of insulin, the correct amount. However, the dead space may cause problems if two kinds of insulin are given. For example, suppose the insulin dose is 40 U of NPH insulin and 10 U of regular insulin. Regular insulin is drawn into the syringe first. The barrel of the syringe and the dead space each will hold 10 U of regular insulin. When the NPH insulin is drawn, the 10 U of regular insulin in the dead space will enter the syringe. At this point, the syringe will contain 20 U of regular insulin and 30 U of NPH insulin, while the dead space will hold 10 U of NPH insulin. If the two insulins were not mixed, the appropriate amounts of each insulin would be given. That is, after the injection the dead space would contain 10 U of regular insulin, the kind and amount of insulin that was introduced into the syringe first. However, these proportions will be distorted if mixing of the two insulins occurs. The actual amounts of each that the patient receives depend on the degree of mixing. For this reason, the sequence in which two kinds of insulin are introduced into the syringe should always be the same. In this way, even if the exact proportions of the short- and intermediate-acting insulin prescribed are not given, the proportions delivered will be relatively constant and appropriate adjustments for controlling blood sugar still can be made. Of course, a better solution to the problem of dead space with administration of two kinds of insulin is simply to use syringes that do not have dead space, such as those manufactured by Becton-Dickinson or Monoject.

Administration of Insulin

STUDENT/NURSE

Insulin is injected into the subcutaneous tissue, which is a layer of fat that lies just beneath the skin. Insulin is absorbed from the subcutaneous tissue into the circulation at a certain rate. If it is injected into any other tissue, such as muscle, the rate of absorption changes. Injection into subcutaneous areas avoids large blood vessels, nerves, and bones. Changing the route of administration from subcutaneous to intramuscular will result in unpredictable onset, peak, and duration of insulin action. This would alter the control of blood sugar. Intramuscular injection not only increases the absorption rate of insulin, but also causes pain. Other factors that affect the absorption rate are exercise and the area used for injection.

Injection of insulin into an arm or a leg that is used in exercise (e.g., swimming, running) allows more rapid absorption into the system, thereby lowering blood sugar too soon and possibly causing an insulin reaction. If the rate of absorption is increased soon after injection, there may not be enough insulin available to last throughout its usual duration of action.

The rate of absorption varies also with area of injection. Studies have shown that insulin is absorbed most quickly from the abdominal area, next most quickly from the arm, and most slowly from the leg. However, the clinical importance of these various rates of absorption has not been established.

In order to find the initial injection site (Fig. 8-5):

1. *Legs.* Measure one hand width (fingers closed) down from the groin and one hand width up from the knee. Use the top and outer aspect of the leg to avoid the large blood vessels on the inner aspect of the thigh. Avoid areas where veins are visible.

2. *Abdomen.* Use the area beginning 2 in. from the belly button (umbilicus) and work sideways toward the hips.

3. *Arms.* Measure one hand width down from the shoulder and one hand width up from the elbow. Use the fleshy outer surface.

4. *Buttocks.* Use the *upper outer areas only*. This prevents injury to the large nerves and blood vessels located in the lower area of the buttocks.

Change the area for each injection daily for the following reasons:

1. To prevent changes in the skin covering the subcutaneous fat, such as pitting or dimpling (atrophy) or swollen and spongy areas (hypertrophy).

2. Repeated injections in the same site may lead to slow and incomplete absorption of insulin from the hypertrophied area. If injections are then introduced

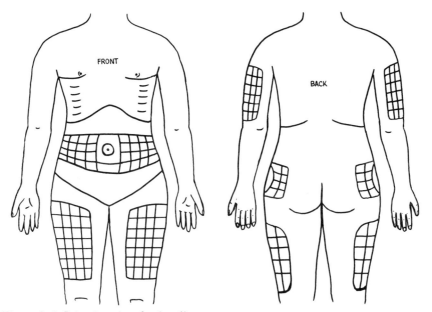

Figure 8-5. Injection sites for insulin.

into a new area, an insulin reaction may occur. This technique may cause uncontrolled blood sugar. If an injection site becomes numb or insensitive to touch, it may be a clue that the area is being used too frequently and indicates scarring of the tissues.

Rotation of injection sites is carried out by measuring two finger widths (~1 in.) away from the recent injection site. Do not use any injection site more than once in 4 to 6 weeks. Use one region, such as the abdomen, until *all of the area has been used.* Then proceed to another region, e.g., a leg, and then to the third site. A body map of injection sites in each region is shown in Figure 8-5.

The technique of injecting insulin is as follows:

1. Clean the area selected for injection with cotten moistened with alcohol or with an alcohol wipe.
2. Grasp ("bunch") the area with the entire hand so that the skin is firm.
3. Pick up syringe as you would a pencil.
4. Touch the needle to the skin at a 90° angle (i.e., straight up).
5. Insert the needle to its full length.
6. Inject the insulin at a medium rate.
7. Press an alcohol-moistened cotton or alcohol wipe firmly over the injected area and remove the needle.
8. Continue to press the area (do not rub) for a few seconds.
9. Dispose of the syringe and needle properly (i.e., do not reuse them).

NURSE (FURTHER INFORMATION)

Spreading versus Bunching. The choice depends on the amount of subcutaneous tissue at the injection site (i.e., thin versus fat).

1. If the patient has excess adipose tissue that is firm, the skin may be spread instead of bunched.
2. If the patient is of average weight or thin, the skin should be bunched in order to lift the fat from the muscle and thereby prevent injection into the muscle.

Angle of the Needle. For thin patients and most children, the needle should be positioned at a 60° to 90° angle. A 90° angle is desirable in most patients to ensure the delivery of insulin into the subcutaneous tissue instead of into the intradermal tissue. Intradermal injections may lead to reactions, such as itching, redness, lumps, and so on, and may result in an even slower rate of absorption.

Leakage of Insulin From the Injection Site. If this problem is encountered, the following possible causes should be investigated.

1. Is the insulin being injected too rapidly?
2. Is the skin being released before the needle is removed?
3. Is the injection being given intradermally?

Side Effects of Insulin

STUDENT

Insulin therapy can lead to several possible side effects. Low blood sugar is not considered a side effect because the action of insulin is expected to have this effect. Before purified insulin was available, many patients starting insulin therapy noted a burning or itching sensation at the injection site. Several hours later, an area about the size of a penny became red and slightly swollen. This lasted for 1 to 2 days and gradually disappeared. It occurred every time an insulin injection was given but gradually stopped after several months. It seemed to be related in some way to the impurities in the insulin preparations. Nowadays insulin is much more pure and such reactions are much less common.

Another possible side effect is gradual loss of the subcutaneous tissue at the sites of injection, causing large dimples in the skin. This seems to be most common in young women. It also seems to be related to the impurities in the insulin preparation, because, in most cases, when the new purified insulins are injected carefully into these areas over several months, the areas fill out again. However, an occasional patient may still experience dimpling. This is one reason why rotation of the injection site is so important.

The opposite effect also may occur. If a patient continues to inject insulin at the same site, a large buildup of fat may form. This is much less common than loss of fat tissue, which is only bad for cosmetic reasons. If insulin is injected into areas of increased fat deposition, absorption may be irregular and cause difficulties with controlling blood sugar.

The last two possible side effects are very uncommon and occur in <1 patient per 1,000 who take insulin. One is a condition called *insulin resistance*, in which a patient may require hundreds of units of insulin for a short period of time. The other is a generalized allergy to insulin that is characterized by a red, itchy rash that starts within minutes of injection at the injection site and spreads to other parts of the body. Although both of these rare side effects are troublesome, they can be handled relatively easily by experienced physicians.

NURSE

For skin reactions at injection sites that are characterized by itching, burning, redness or lumps, investigate the following possible causes:

1. Is injection being given intradermally instead of subcutaneously?

2. Has the alcohol evaporated from the skin before the needle is inserted?

3. Is the insulin at room temperature before injection?

If the patient is injecting correctly and the symptoms continue to occur, the patient may have an allergy to one of the impurities of the insulin preparation. The physician may elect to:

1. Take no action, since the symptoms will subside with time.
2. Give oral antihistamines.
3. Use cortisone preparations in the insulin syringe.
4. Use more purified insulin.

The loss of subcutaneous tissue at the injection site is known as lipoatrophy. Lipoatrophy is more common in children and adult females and is seen rarely in adult males. The mechanism is not known, but it may be related either to a low-grade inflamation caused directly by the impurities in the insulin preparation or to an immune response to these contaminants. Injection of highly purified insulin into the circumference of these lipoatrophied areas, with gradual working toward the center as the area fills in, often is successful in reversing the effect. The process may take months. The technique and results of this treatment are illustrated in chapter 4 (Figs. 4-6 and 4-7).

The buildup of subcutaneous fat tissue is known as lipohypertrophy (chapter 4, Fig. 4-8). Lipohypertrophy is not very common. It seems to be caused by the local effect of insulin on the production of extra fat. This explains its occurrence when insulin is injected repeatedly at the same spot (which the patient may elect to do because of decreased sensation in the lipohypertrophied areas). Treatment consists of simply not using this area for injections. However, since absorption from the lipohypertrophied area may have been irregular and slow, switching to a new site with the same dose of insulin may increase the possibility of an insulin reaction.

Although systemic allergy to insulin is rare, generalized skin manifestations may require a desensitizing process similar to that used for penicillin desensitization.

Insulin resistance is caused by the production of increased amounts of neutralizing antibodies against insulin. Every patient treated with insulin develops antibodies against insulin within several months after therapy begins. These antibodies are present in low titers (amounts) and do not cause problems. Occasionally the amount of these antibodies increases markedly and the patient requires hundreds (and sometimes thousands) of units of insulin. The antibodies usually decrease in several months and the patient's insulin requirement returns to normal. It is not known why these antibodies suddenly increase and then return to their normal levels.

Travel

U-100 insulin is not available in most foreign countries. For this reason, patients traveling abroad should plan so their trip includes the following:

1. Twice the amount of insulin and syringes that you will need for the length of the stay. *Do not put this equipment in luggage that is to be checked.* Pack it in the carry-on bag.
2. Two copies of (*a*) a statement verifying that the patient is an insulin-dependent diabetic and (*b*) prescriptions for insulin and syringes. Put one copy of each in the wallet or purse and one of each in the luggage.

In the event that the insulin, syringes, or prescriptions are lost or stolen and/or the patient is not able to purchase U-100 insulin and syringes, he or she should purchase U-40 or U-80 insulin *with matching syringes.* The same number of units as usual should be administered. The patient should not try to compute insulin dosages for an unmatched syringe (e.g., U-40 insulin for a U-100 syringe).

The patient should plan the trip by discussing with the physician any adjustments in insulin dosage that may be necessary. Such adjustments may be indicated if the patient must cross one or more time zones. The physician will need to know the schedule of meals served on the plane. If the patient is traveling alone, flight attendants should be informed that the patient takes insulin. The patient should carry a source of simple carbohydrates at all times, especially if a great deal of walking is anticipated.

It is essential that diabetics wear identification indicating their condition when traveling. Review the sick-day rules for food replacements if gastrointestinal upsets are experienced. The physician may prescribe antinausea or gastrointestinal medications for the trip.

When traveling in North America, the patient may contact local branches of the American Diabetes Association in the event that difficulties occur. When traveling outside North America, the patient should plan the trip by obtaining a list of physicians who specialize in diabetes from the American Diabetes Association, 2 Park Ave., New York, NY 10016; telephone, (212) 683-7444.

Evaluation

Demonstrate

1. The accurate preparation of one or two types of insulins (whichever is applicable).
2. The accurate selection of an injection site and injection technique using a pattern of rotation.

Select the correct answer or answers to each question.

1. Insulin is produced in the

   a. liver
   b. stomach
   c. pancreas

2. Insulin

    a. lowers blood sugar
    b. increases blood sugar
    c. has no effect on blood sugar

3. List or state the type, strength, and time course of action of the insulin(s) you take.

ORAL HYPOGLYCEMIC SULFONYLUREA AGENTS

Clinical experience has shown that, in general, patients who take oral hypoglycemic agents lack knowledge about diabetes and do not appreciate the importance of these medications in the control of blood glucose levels. Patients who start this therapy need to be informed (*a*) about what type of diabetes they have; (*b*) how to take the medications; (*c*) that they must be alert to any symptoms of hypoglycemia, especially with the long-acting chlorpropamide (Diabinese); (*d*) that these medications are not a substitute for a diabetic diet; and (*e*) that they must be monitored closely by their physician for control and side effects.

Outcome Criteria (Student) and Goals (Nurse)

Objectives

STUDENT

Upon completion of the instructions, the student will be able to verbalize and/or write the following:

1. Definition of oral hypoglycemic agents.
2. The side effects of oral hypoglycemic agents.
3. The portion of the diabetic population that can use oral hypoglycemic agents.

Goals

NURSE

To provide information about sulfonylurea agents currently in use. With this knowledge the nurse will be able to instruct the patient.

General Information

STUDENT

Oral medications that lower blood sugar but are not insulin were first used for the treatment of diabetes mellitus in the late 1950s. These medications are appropriate only for individuals (usually adults older than 40 years) who have no ketone bodies in their urine in the absence of treatment. This situation indicates that their pancreas is still producing insulin. Thus, their blood sugar is elevated because either not enough insulin is being made, or the insulin that is produced is not effective in lowering glucose levels.

NURSE

During the testing of the sulfonamide antibiotics during World War II, hypoglycemia was noted as a side effect of these drugs. By changing part of the structure of the drugs, the antibiotic properties were lost and the sugar-lowering properties increased. The result was the development of the oral hypoglycemic sulfonylurea agents. The clinical purpose of the sulfonylureas is to decrease glucose levels in diabetics. These new compounds are so different from sulfonamides that patients allergic to sulfonamides can still take sulfonylurea agents.

The sulfonylureas work only in patients whose pancreas can still secrete some insulin. For the first several weeks after the patient starts using the oral hypoglycemic agents, the amount of insulin produced by the pancreas is increased after the patient eats. Accordingly, the sulfonylurea compounds were thought to help control diabetes by increasing insulin secretion. However, after the patient takes sulfonylurea agents for ~1 month, the insulin concentrations return to pre-drug levels but diabetic control remains improved. This suggests (and other work proves directly) that the action of the sulfonylurea agents increases the effectiveness of insulin in metabolizing blood sugar. For this reason, the sulfonylureas work only in patients who can still make their own insulin.

Characteristics of Medications

STUDENT/NURSE

The four sulfonylurea agents currently used in the United States are listed in Table 8-2. Because of its short duration of action tolbutamide (Orinase) is usually given two to three times a day. Acetohexamide (Dymelor) and tolazamide (Tolinase) are given once or twice a day. Usually maximal amounts are split, while less-than-maximal amounts are taken only once a day. Because chlorpropamide (Diabinese) has a very long duration of action, it should be given only once a day.

Table 8-2. Sulfonylurea Agents Currently Used in the United States

Generic Name	Trade Name (Manufacturer)	Description	Duration of Action (hrs)
Tolbutamide	Orinase (Upjohn)	250 mg; white tablet 500 mg; white tablet	6 to 12
Acetohexamide	Dymelor (Lilly)	250 mg; white tablet 500 mg; yellow tablet	12 to 24
Tolazamide	Tolinase (Upjohn)	100 mg; white tablet 250 mg; white tablet 500 mg; white tablet	12 to 24
Chlorpropamide	Diabinese (Pfizer)	100 mg; blue tablet 250 mg; blue tablet	60

Tolbutamide is inactivated in the liver, which accounts for its short duration of action. Acetohexamide and tolazamide also are changed in the liver, but the resulting compounds continue to decrease blood sugar and are eliminated by the kidney. For all practical purposes, chlorpropamide remains unchanged in the body and is simply excreted in the urine. Therefore, all of these agents (with the possible exception of tolbutamide) should be used very cautiously in patients whose kidney function is impaired.

Adverse Effects

STUDENT/NURSE

Fewer than 5% of patients experience the adverse effects listed below. The first two are by far the most common.

1. Skin rashes.
2. Gastrointestinal symptoms (loss of appetite, nausea with occasional vomiting, heartburn, feelings of abdominal fullness, gas).
3. Dark urine, light-colored stools, yellowing of eyes or skin (rare).
4. Unusual bleeding (very rare).
5. Fever (very rare).

Use of these agents, especially chlorpropamide, may produce intolerance to alcohol. The unpleasant but usually harmless symptoms include sensation of warmth, flushed skin, headache, nausea, shortness of breath, rapid pulse, and giddiness. They begin 3 to 10 minutes after ingestion of alcohol, peak in about 20 minutes, and usually disappear after about an hour.

Hypoglycemia, although not really an adverse effect, may occur, since lowering blood sugar is the major function of the drugs. Hypoglycemia often occurs when patients (often older ones) eat irregularly and less food than they are supposed to. The condition seems more likely to occur with chlorpropamide (Diabinese) and least likely with tolbutamide (Orinase). However, hypoglycemia occurs much less frequently with sulfonylurea agents than with insulin. Because the former remain effective much longer than the latter, patients must be monitored carefully after they receive the initial treatment for the hypoglycemia. These individuals often are hospitalized, especially if chlorpropamide (Diabinese) is the culprit, with its very long duration of action.

A large study (the University Group Diabetes Program [UGDP] Study), begun in 1960, has raised questions regarding the possible harmful effects of sulfonylurea agents on the heart. In this study, tolbutamide (Orinase) and a placebo were compared in ketosis-resistant (type 2) diabetics. After 8 years, more patients taking the sulfonylurea agent apparently had died from vascular diseases (e.g., heart attacks, strokes) than had those taking the placebo. However, the design of this study had many problems, and the conclusions therefore are controversial. In addition, four other, similar investigations could not confirm that tolbutamide had a harmful effect on the heart. (This problem is discussed in detail in chapter 5.) Therefore, the majority of diabetes specialists continue to use sulfonylurea agents to treat patients who can use them.

Drug Interactions

STUDENT

No information is required.

NURSE

Certain drugs interact with the sulfonylurea agents and either interfere with or potentiate their ability to lower blood sugar. Some interactions are indirect; that is, the two drugs act on the same process but not on each other. Thus, potassium-losing diuretics, glucocorticoids (steroids), estrogen compounds, and diphenylhydantoin can interfere with the effects of sulfonylurea agents by indirect mechanisms. Conversely, salicylates, propranolol (Inderal), monoamine oxidase inhibitors, oxytetracycline, and ethanol (strictly speaking, the last is not a drug) potentiate indirectly the action of sulfonylurea agents.

The other way in which other drugs can affect the action of oral hypoglycemic agents is by interacting directly with the sulfonylurea. That is, the second drug influences the absorption, metabolism, or excretion of the sulfonylurea compounds. All drugs that interact directly with the sulfonylurea agents potentiate the effects of the latter. Such drugs are listed in chapter 5 (Table 5-2).

Evaluation

Answer true or false

1. Individuals with type 2 (adult-onset) diabetes often can be maintained by oral diabetic medications because the pancreas still makes some insulin.
2. Individuals with type 1 (juvenile-onset) diabetes cannot be maintained by oral diabetic medications because the pancreas usually does not make insulin.
3. Oral hypoglycemic medications are insulin.

  Select the correct answer or answers.

4. Which of the following adverse effects are produced by oral hypoglycemic agents?

   a. hypoglycemia
   b. skin rashes
   c. nausea and vomiting
   d. loss of hearing
   e. baldness
   f. intolerance to alcohol

MONITORING DIABETIC CONTROL

In most illnesses the physician controls the treatment, and the patient is the passive follower. In contrast, diabetics must assume responsibility for management and control of their illness. In order for the patient to assume an active role in treatment, a system of home monitoring is needed. Ideally, the monitoring system should be simple, economical, and provide information useful to both patient and physician. Currently there are two modes of home monitoring that fulfill these criteria: urine testing for sugar and ketones, and measuring capillary-blood glucose concentrations. In addition to home monitoring of blood glucose levels, the physician can assess blood glucose control using fasting, 2-hour postprandial or random venous-blood samples, 24-hour urine samples for glucose, and either glycosylated hemoglobin (Hgb) or hemoglobin A_{1c} determinations.

  This section will emphasize primarily home monitoring with urine testing and measurement of capillary-blood glucose. It will also briefly describe the quantitative measurement of urine glucose, glycosylated Hgb, and Hgb A_{1c}.

Outcome Criteria (Student) and Goals (Nurse)

Objectives

STUDENT

Upon completion of the section on urine testing, the student will be able to verbalize, write, and/or demonstrate:

1. Why and when urine tests are to be performed.
2. The meaning of urine test results.
3. What factors affect urine test results.
4. The ability to perform selected urine tests for sugar and ketones.
5. How to record the results of urine tests for sugar and ketones.

Goals

NURSE

To provide information about:

1. The mechanisms of glucosuria and ketonuria.
2. Factors that affect the renal threshold
3. The what, why, when, and how of urine testing.
4. The advantages and disadvantages of products for urine testing.
5. The quantitative measurement of urine glucose.
6. The significance of glycosylated Hgb and Hgb A_{1c} in diabetes.
7. The use of home monitoring of capillary-blood glucose levels.

Urine Testing (Semiquantitative)

Glucose (Renal Physiology)

STUDENT

Testing urine is one way of determining to some degree the level of sugar in the blood. Normally, all sugar in the blood passes through the kidney and is reabsorbed into the circulation. However, the amount of sugar that the kidney can reabsorb is limited. Usually, most sugar that is processed through the kidney is reabsorbed when the blood sugar level is <180 mg/100 ml. The concentration of blood sugar above which glucose starts to appear in the urine is called the renal threshold. That is, when the renal threshold is exceeded, the sugar from the blood spills over into the urine, much like water spills over a dam that has reached its storage capacity. The renal threshold varies among individuals and is affected by age, presence of renal disease, and pregnancy. Thus, some older people can have fairly high blood-sugar levels without much glucose appearing in the urine (high renal threshold). On the other hand, a child or a pregnant woman may have glucose in the urine if the blood sugar is normal or even low (low renal threshold).

NURSE

In order for the nurse to be able to explain the meaning of glucosuria and keto-nuria, he or she first must understand the principle of the renal threshold and the factors that determine the level at which glucose is spilled into the urine.

The excretion of glucose by the kidney depend on three factors:

1. The concentration of glucose in blood entering the glomerulus.
2. The glomerular filtration rate (GFR).
3. The maximal rate of tubular reabsorption (different for each person).

Blood circulates through the glomerular capillaries at a greater pressure than in other capillaries. This pressure causes the filtration of plasma constituents (which resemble blood plasma except that they lack an appreciable amount of protein and lipids) to pass from the glomerulus into the renal tubules. This process is known as glomerular filtration. Normally, the proximal tubules reabsorb 70% to 80% of the glomerular filtrate, which contains all of the glucose and protein and most of the sodium, while it rejects much of the urea and creatinine.

Glucosuria (glucose in the urine) occurs when the filtration of glucose through the glomerulus exceeds the capacity of the renal tubule to reabsorb the glucose into the circulation. The amount of glucose that is presented to the renal tubule depends on both the concentration of glucose and the rate at which the blood enters the glomerulus. The level of blood sugar at which glucose starts to appear in the urine is called the *renal threshold*. In most healthy individuals, the renal threshold is ~180 mg/100 ml. However, many factors affect the renal threshold, including age, presence of renal disease, and pregnancy.

The renal threshold tends to increase with age. Therefore, many older diabetics have negative results on urine tests for glucose in the presence of very high plasma glucose levels (occasionally as high as 350 to 400 mg/100 ml). Kidney disease also increases the renal threshold for glucose. Since renal insufficiency is not uncommon in older diabetics, it is another cause of negative urine test results in the presence of high blood sugar in these patients. On the other hand, children and young adults tend to have a somewhat lower renal threshold for glucose. This may lead to positive urine test results even when plasma glucose levels are only slightly high (e.g., 140 to 180 mg/100 ml). In pregnancy, blood flow to the kidney increases; this raises the GFR and lowers the renal threshold for glucose even further. The result is glucosuria in the presence of normal blood glucose concentrations, especially after meals.

Because there are so many variables, renal thresholds vary among individuals. Therefore, glucosuria is a useful but not always an accurate reflection of variations in blood glucose. Periodic blood glucose measurements with urine testing at the same time are necessary to monitor diabetic control. Not only does this approach provide information on the patient's control at a particular moment, but comparison of the two parameters provides a frame of reference for the interpretation of urine glucose test results on an ongoing basis.

Ketones

STUDENT

Two things happen when very little or no insulin is available. The blood sugar rises to very high levels because the insulin-sensitive tissues cannot use the available glucose and the liver makes too much. In addition, the fat stores in the body break down, and substances known as ketones or ketone bodies are produced as end products. Another term for these substances is acetone. Ketones are a sort of an acid "waste material" that can accumulate in excess in the blood of type 1 diabetics and then spill over into the urine. This condition is called *ketonuria* and is a sign of poor diabetic control. It is very important to reverse ketonuria because, if it worsens, diabetic ketoacidosis (one of the causes of diabetic coma) may result and the patient will become very sick.

Ketonuria occasionally can be seen in one other circumstance. If a patient east a diet very low in carbohydrates (the best example of this is starvation), the body has to break down increased amounts of fat for energy. This results in production of excess ketone bodies, as in uncontrolled diabetes. This condition is called *starvation ketosis* and occurs in both type 1 and type 2 diabetics and nondiabetics. There are two differences, however, between starvation ketosis and diabetic ketosis. First, in starvation ketosis glucose concentrations are not increased in nondiabetics and may not be too high in diabetics. This means that results of tests for urine glucose will be negative or only slightly positive in the presence of ketonuria secondary to starvation ketosis. Second, the amount of excess ketone bodies formed in starvation ketosis is much lower than in diabetic ketosis. Therefore, although ketonuria will be present in both situations, patients with starvation ketosis will not become very ill.

NURSE

Insulin deficiency is responsible for an accelerated lipolysis (fat breakdown), which causes overproduction of free fatty acids. The free fatty acids are then transported to the liver, where they are converted into ketone bodies. The two ketone bodies are β-hydroxybutyric acid and acetoacetic acid, which exist in equilibrium with each other. Acetoacetic acid is converted irreversibly to acetone, which is then excreted through the lungs. The abbreviation S&A (sugar and acetone) used in reference to urine testing should really be S&K (sugar and ketones). The chemical test for ketone bodies (nitroprusside reagent) measures only acetoacetic acid, not β-hydroxybutyric acid. Acetone also reacts with acetoacetic acid, but so weakly that there is not enough acetone in the urine to give a positive test results.

In general, starvation ketosis occurs when <80 to 100 g of carbohydrates are ingested per day. Thus, starvation ketosis is much more likely to be seen in ketosis-resistant (type 2) patients than in ketosis-prone (type 1) patients because the former follow hypocaloric diets. In one situation, however, diabetic ketosis in type 1 patients may be confused with starvation ketosis. One of the materials used for urine testing is Keto-Diastix. This strip contains two separate areas that are impregnated with chemicals: one area reacts to glucose and the other reacts to ketone bodies. Large amounts of ketone bodies may inhibit the chemical reaction for testing glucose. Therefore, if a patient spilling large amounts of both glucose and ketone bodies uses Keto-Diastix, the glucose results may be falsely low. This suggests starvation ketosis, and the patient must retest the urine specifically with Clinitest tablets. Usually, results of the urine test will be markedly positive for glucose, signifying the presence of diabetic ketosis. It is very important to educate type 1 diabetics about this possibility so that they will not be lulled into assuming they are experiencing starvation ketosis rather than diabetic ketosis.

Why Test?

STUDENT

Glucose

Urine testing for sugar is necessary in order to:

1. Provide information as to whether the body is utilizing the sugar in the blood.
2. Give a clue as to whether diet and insulin dosage are balanced.
3. Assist in adjusting the insulin dosage according to urine glucose levels when the physician specifically orders it.

Ketones

In ketosis-prone (type 1) patients it is not necessary to test the urine daily for ketones. It is important, however, to test for ketones as well as for sugar when:

1. Urine tests consistently yield $\geqslant 1\%$ to 2% glucosuria for two consecutive tests.
2. Acute illness occurs, especially when fever is present.
3. Episodes of nausea and vomiting are noted.
4. Surgery, injury, or other stress (including emotional problems) has occurred.

In ketosis-resistant (type 2) patients it is not necessary to test for ketones in the urine.

NURSE

Patients using Diastix should be warned that heavy ketonuria may depress the glucose reaction. Since patients will not know the ketones results (unless Keto-Diastix are used), they may not be aware that the glucose results are falsely low. Therefore, patients using Diastix alone for testing urine must be informed that, if the results are $<1\%$ glucosuria but either the conditions listed above pertain or they simply do not feel well, they should use another method of measuring glucose that is not influenced by ketonuria (e.g., Clinitest tablets) as an independent check. Although Keto-Diastix is slightly more expensive, if all type 1 patients routinely use it they will always be aware of the presence of ketonuria.

When to Test

STUDENT

When to test for urine glucose depends on what information is needed. Test as instructed. A minimum of two times a day is usually recommended, especially for insulin-dependent diabetics.

Insulin-Requiring Patients

In patients taking one injection of intermediate-acting insulin (NPH or Lente) per day, the before-breakfast urine test reflects the effect of the insulin taken ~24 hours previously on the fasting glucose concentration. In patients taking two injections of intermediate-acting insulin per day, the before-breakfast urine test best reflects the effectiveness of the before-supper dose. The before-supper urine test is most sensitive to the effects of the morning dose of NPH or Lente insulin. This is because the peak activity of these preparations occurs at about this time, and usually the major meal of the day has not yet been eaten and thus has not raised the blood sugar. The before-lunch urine test reflects how well the breakfast calories have been handled or how high the blood sugar was after breakfast. If the patient took Regular insulin with the morning dose of intermediate-acting insulin, the before-lunch urine test indicates its effectiveness. The bedtime urine test reflects how well the morning injection of intermediate-acting insulin has handled the supper calories of that day. If the patient took Regular insulin before supper, its effectiveness is best reflected by the bedtime urine test.

Patients Who Do Not Require Insulin

The timing of the urine test affects the sensitivity of the test. Blood sugar levels are the highest 1 to 2 hours postprandially. Therefore, results of the urine test are most likely to be positive at this time, making this test the most sensitive way to monitor diabetic control. The urine test performed just before lunch, dinner, or a snack is less likely to be positive because the blood sugar at those times is not as high as it is right after a meal. The before-breakfast urine test is least likely to be positive because the patient has not eaten for 10 to 16 hours and the blood sugar is usually at its lowest point of the day. Therefore, this test is the least sensitive way to monitor diabetic control. The physician should decide which urine tests to perform and how often. The patient should simply be aware that the before-breakfast test is the one least likely to give positive results. If it is positive, the fasting glucose level probably is >180 to 200 mg/100 ml, which most physicians feel is too high. A urine test taken soon after eating is most likely to be positive, and sometimes it is very difficult to lower the blood sugar enough after a meal to make these test results negative.

NURSE

The timing of the urine test usually depends on the degree of disordered metabolism and what information is being sought. In diabetic individuals, it takes approximately 4 to 5 hours for the carbohydrates in a meal to be completely absorbed from the gastrointestinal tract and stored in various tissues and the excess glucose to be excreted in the urine. Therefore, the more abnormal the carbohydrate metabolism, the more likely the urine test results will be positive soon after a meal. This is especially true for patients taking insulin. Therefore, urine testing is done routinely in these patients before each meal and the evening snack. If these test results are always negative, some physicians want the patient to test again 1 to 2 hours postprandially to determine whether better control is possible. Patients who do not require insulin are more likely to have negative urine tests before meals since their carbohydrate metabolism is less abnormal than that of diabetics taking insulin. In this situation, physicians will often require routine postprandial urine tests.

Another issue is whether testing only the first-voided urine specimen is sufficient or whether double-voided specimens also should be tested routinely. Again, this depends in large measure on the information that is desired. To collect a second specimen, the patient is instructed to drink 1 to 2 glasses of water after the first preprandial urine and to void a second time ~30 minutes later (still preprandially). The advantage of testing the second specimen is that its results reflect what has happened within the 30-minute interval. In addition, if a specimen for testing blood glucose is drawn during this period, the renal threshold can be evaluated. The second specimen is likely to show less glucosuria (for reasons discussed earlier). There are several disadvantages to routine testing of double-voided specimens. The most important is that patients often are unwilling or unable to take the time and effort to collect it properly. Since a second-voided specimens reflect only what is happening at the moment, the postprandial level of blood sugar is not reflected nearly as well in this sample as it is in the urine formed immediately after the meal.

Testing the first urine specimen is more convenient, a factor that increases the chances for patient compliance. Since the first-voided specimen reflects the level of blood sugar during the previous several hours, it serves as a better monitor to ensure tight control than does a double-voided specimen. For example, suppose the blood sugar of one patient had far exceeded the renal threshold after lunch but had returned to a level below the threshold before supper. In another patient, the blood sugar had remained below the renal threshold throughout the afternoon. In both patients, results of a second-voided before-supper urine test would be negative, and it would not be possible to tell which patient was better controlled. However, the results of the first-voided specimen would have revealed that the first patient had had higher glucose levels after lunch than the second patient (assuming that their renal thresholds were similar). The disadvantage of routine testing just the first urine sample, of course, is the difficulty both of establishing a renal threshold and of not knowing what the approximate level of blood sugar is at any particular time. However, several recent studies comparing both the first and second urine samples have demonstrated that the results are the same ~70% of the time, that results of the first are higher ~25% of the time, and that the results of the second are higher only 5% of the time. Thus, there are good arguments on both sides, and the controversy is still not resolved. We prefer to have our patients routinely test only the first-voided specimen, except before breakfast where the results of both are helpful in evaluating their control.

How to Test

STUDENT/NURSE

Test the first and/or second urine specimen as instructed. To test the first-voided specimen, simply obtain a urine sample. To test a second-voided specimen, empty the bladder 30 minutes to 1 hour before meals and bedtime and discard the urine (if a first-voided sample is not supposed to be tested). Drink a glass of water, and then urinate again within 30 minutes. Test this specimen for sugar and/or ketones.

There are many products used today for testing urine.

Clinitest, 5-drop method	Color	Record (% glucosuria)
a. 5 drops urine ⎱ Mix in a test tube b. 10 drops water ⎰	Blue	0
	Green	0.25
c. Add 1 Clinitest tablet	Light green	0.5
d. Wait 15 seconds *after boiling stops*	Olive green	0.75
e. Shake gently; compare with	Yellow to brown	1
color chart	Orange	2
	Orange to greenish brown	>2

Be alert to the "pass through" phenomenon. If the color goes through orange and back to brown or yellow, the concentration should be recorded as >2%. This means that you need to follow the color development closely and not simply look at the tube after 15 seconds. The Clinitest two-drop method measures glucose concentrations up to 5%. The "pass through" penomenon also occurs with the two-drop method. If it does, record >5% glucosuria.

Clinitest, 2-drop method (for >2% glucosuria)	Color	Record (% glucosuria)
a. 2 drops urine ⎫ Mix in a test tube	Blue	0
b. 10 drops water ⎭	Light green	0.5
c. Add 1 Clinitest tablet.	Olive green	1
d. Wait 15 seconds *after boiling stops*.	Greenish brown	2
e. Shake gently; compare with color	Yellowish brown	3
chart.	Orange	5

Tes-Tape	Color	Record (% glucosuria)
a. Withdraw approximately 1.5 in. of tape	Yellow	0
	Light green	0.1
b. Dip the end of the tape in the urine.	Dark green	0.25
Remove, and wait *exactly 1*	Dark green to blue	0.5
minute.	Dark blue	⩾2
c. Then immediately compare the color change next to the driest area of the tape with the color on the dispenser. Unchanged yellow color indicates urine is sugar free. If tape indicates ⩾0.5%, wait 1 additional minute and make the final comparison.		

Diastix	Color	Record (% glucosuria)
a. Dip the strip in the urine for	Blue	0
2 seconds.	Light green	0.1
b. Tap strip to remove excess urine.	Dark green	0.25
c. In exactly 30 seconds, compare	Olive green	0.5
the strip with the color chart.	Light brown	1
	Dark brown	2

Moderate or large amounts of ketones may depress the color development of Diastix. Ketosis-prone patients will probably use Keto-Diastix, which measures both glucose and ketone bodies. Therefore, if the results show large amounts of ketones and small amounts of glucose, another method of measuring glucose (e.g., Clinitest tablets) should be used in this specimen to determine more accurately the amount of glucose spillage.

Urine Tests for Ketones	Color	Record (amount)
Acetest		
a. Place white Acetest tablet on clean white paper or a paper towel.	No change Lavender	None Small
b. Put a drop or two of urine on the tablet.	Light purple	Moderate
c. Read color change at end of 30 seconds (no longer). (A color chart is supplied with each bottle of tablets.)	Dark purple	Large

Ketostix	Color	Record (amount)
a. Dip test end of strip in urine for 2 seconds.	No change	None
b. Tap strip to remove excess urine.	Light pink	Trace
c. Compare strip with color chart in exactly 15 seconds.	Rose	Small
	Medium rose	Moderate
	Dark rose	Large
	Purple	Large

Keto-Diastix strips are available for testing for both sugar and ketones.

Become familiar with and use the same method(s) each time. Reread the directions with the testing materials in hand. Since timing during the tests is very important, use a watch. Errors often occur when procedures become habits. Use a color chart that corresponds with the method of urine testing and record the results in a book. Also, check and observe the expiration date of the product. *Keep the bottles tightly closed and store them in a cool, dry place.*

How to Record Results

STUDENT

In the past, results of urine tests were recorded using plus signs (+). However, there are several urine testing products on the market whose plus signs indicate different concentrations of sugar in the urine (Table 8-3). Therefore, recording results as percentages avoids this problem, allowing a uniform interpretation of urine sugar results and helping to provide the physician with more meaningful information.

Table 8-3. Comparison of Results Among Different Methods of Testing for Urinary Glucose[a]

Product	Glucose Concentration							
	0.1%	0.25%	0.5%	0.75%	1%	2%	3%	5%
Clinitest (5-drop)		Trace	+	++	+++	++++		
Clinitest (2-drop)[b]			c		c	c	c	c
Diastix	Trace	+	++		+++	++++		
Clinistix[d]		...Light... (+)		...Medium... (++)	...Dark.... (+++)			
Tes-Tape	+	++	+++			++++		

Blank spaces indicate that there are no color blocks for those concentrations.

[a]Adapted with permission from *Home Urine Testing for the Diabetic*. Ames Co., Division Miles Laboratories, Inc., Elkhart, IA, 1976).

[b]The two-drop chart provides a "trace" color block without a percentage value; a trace result merely indicates glucosuria of <0.5%.

[c]Measures percentage of glucosuria at these levels, but equivalent + values are not available.

[d]Estimates relative presence of glucose but cannot show percentage value.

354

NURSE

Table 8-3 shows the differences between urine test results expressed as plus signs and those expressed as percentages. For example, a 3+ (1%) result with Diastix or Clinitest (five-drop method) signifies the presence of twice as much glucose as does a 3+ (0.5%) result with Tes-Tape. Thus, routine use of percentages alone avoids both confusion and potential errors in adjusting treatment.

Factors That Affect Urine Test Results

STUDENT

The following factors may decrease the accuracy of urine test results:

1. Touching the testing tablets or reagent paper may cause an adverse chemical reaction and therefore change the test results. Touching the tablets may also cause a burn to the skin.
2. Heat, sunlight, and moisture may hasten deterioration of the product. Do not store testing materials in a bathroom that becomes steamy and humid. Keep the lid tight.
3. Improper timing during the test.
4. Insufficient lighting for reading the test results.
5. Wrong proportions of urine and water (Clinitest).
6. Use of dirty equipment (Clinitest).
7. Use of outdated testing materials.
8. Incomplete emptying of the bladder for collection of the first specimen.
9. Incorrect interpretation of color changes.

NURSE

Several substances excreted in the urine can interfere with the results of urine testing for glucose. In some instances the same substances can have opposite effects, depending on which urine testing product is used. Table 8-4 summarizes some of the more common substances that interfere with testing for glucose. These substances often are degradation products of medication that the patient is taking and not the medication itself. L=Dopa may also induce a false-positive reaction for ketone bodies if Ketostix is used. Acetest gives true readings.

Quantitative Measurement of Urine Glucose

STUDENT

No information is required.

Table 8–4. Substances That Interfere with Results of Tests for Urine Glucose[a]

Substance in Urine	Product[b]	Effect on Readings[c]
Aspirin		
Usual dosage	Clinitest	None
	Clinistix	None
High dosage	Clinitest	High readings
	Clinistix, Diastix	Low readings
Vitamin C (ascorbic acid)		
Usual amounts (≤ 500 mg/day)	Clinitest	None
	Clinistix	Low readings
	Diastix	None
Large amounts (> 500 mg/day)	Clinitest	High or false-positive readings
	Clinistix	Low or false-negative readings
	Diastix	Little or none
Ketones		
Small amounts	Diastix	None
Moderate to large	Diastix	Low readings
Protein (albumin)	Clinitest	Low readings
Cephalosporins		
Reducing sugars	Clinitest	False-positive readings
other than glucose	Clinistix	None
(e.g. lactose during lactation)	Diastix	None
L-Dopa	Clinitest	False-positive readings
	Clinistix	False-negative readings

[a]Adapted with permission from *Home Urine Testing for the Diabetic*. Ames Co., Division of Miles Laboratories, Inc., Eckhart, IN, 1976.

[b]Tes-Tape is not included in this table because it is not distributed by Ames. In general, Tes-Tape is much less likely to give false-negative reactions if the patient reads the color change at the top of the strip (near the dry part). The glucose becomes separated from the inhibitor as the urine goes up the paper strip.

NURSE

Occasionally the physician may wish to measure accurately the actual amount of glucose excreted in the urine over a certain period. For instance, measuring how much glucose is lost during 24 hours gives an assessment of overall diabetic control during that day and night. If a patient consistently has high fasting glucose levels that the physician suspects are a reaction to nighttime hypoglycemia, the physician might order two 12-hour urine collections. If the amount of glucose lost in the urine during the night is low as compared with the daytime loss, then it is likely that the patient's blood sugar is relatively low during the night; thus, he or she requires less insulin at that time. On the other hand, if the night-time urine glucose excretion is as high or higher than the daytime values, the patient needs more insulin to work overnight. A 4-hour urine collection between breakfast and lunch will reflect how well the before-breakfast regular insulin handles the breakfast calories. Since the results depend critically on the total volume of urine passed during that time, it is essential that the bladder be emptied both before and at the end of the designated period and that the entire amount of urine be submitted to the laboratory for determination of glucose level.

There are several disadvantages to monitoring diabetic control with quantitative measurements of urine glucose. First, collections are very inconvenient for the patient and thus are often incomplete. Second, the results depend on the patient's renal threshold for glucose. Finally, the amount of carbohydrates consumed during the period under evaluation also influence the results.

Glycosylated Hgb and Hgb A_{1c}

STUDENT

No information is required.

NURSE

Monitoring diabetic control by measuring glycosylated Hgb or Hgb A_{1c} is a recent development in diabetes management. Approximately 90% of the hemoglobin in the red blood cell is Hgb A. This hemoglobin consists of four chains of amino acids, two alpha chains, and two beta chains. An additional 5% to 7% of the hemoglobin in the cell also consists of the same four chains, but glucose or a compound made from glucose is attached to the beta chains. When glucose is the extra substance, the resultant hemoglobin is called Hgb A_{1c}. If a related compound is attached, the hemoglobin is called Hgb A_{1a} or Hgb A_{1b}, depending on which compound is present. Normally, Hgb A_{1c} comprises about 5% of the hemoglobin in the red cell, while Hgb A_{1a} and Hgb A_{1b} account for only a few per cent.

The general chemical reaction that attaches glucose to proteins (in this case to hemoglobin) is called *glycosylation*. Therefore, these three hemoglobins are glycosylated Hgbs. Glycosylated Hgbs can be separated from Hgb A and measured. Some laboratories measure all three at the same time and report the results as a percentage of glycosylated Hgb. Other laboratories separate the three glycosylated Hgbs from each other and measure only Hgb A_{1c}. Hgb A_{1c} changes in diabetes, while Hgb A_{1a} and Hgb A_{1b} remain relatively stable.

The glycosylation reaction between glucose and hemoglobin proceeds slowly and depends, for the most part, on the glucose concentration during the period in which the red blood cells are exposed to them. Since the reaction is mostly irreversible, the amount of glycosylated Hgb is a time-integrated measure of the glucose levels. That is, the red cell "remembers" the level of blood sugar, and once the glycosylated Hgb is formed, it doesn't disappear.

As would be expected, the percentage of glycosylated Hgb correlates well with other measures of diabetic control. The value is higher than normal in diabetics and is very high in poorly controlled patients. However, since the life span of the red cell is $\sim$120 days, the level of glycosylated Hgb is correlated best with parameters of control measured 6 to 8 weeks previously. This is to be expected, since red cells exposed to the glucose concentration at that time are still present and can be measured. However, this limits the usefulness of glycosylated Hgb as an aid in adjusting treatment because it reflects mainly what the situation was several months ago. On the other hand, as a time-integrated measure of blood sugar, levels of glycosylated Hgb are an excellent way to assess overall diabetic control.

Home Monitoring of Capillary-Blood Glucose

STUDENT

No information is required unless the patient uses home glucose monitoring. Patients who monitor glucose at home should be taught how to use the techniques and how to interpret the results.

NURSE

Recent evidence strongly indicates that certain complications of diabetes, such as retinopathy (eye disease), nephropathy (kidney disease), and neuropathy (involvement of the nervous system), can be delayed and perhaps even prevented if strict control of the diabetes can be maintained. Since the normal renal threshold for glucose is 180 mg/100 ml, monitoring diabetic control with urine tests is somewhat inexact. Negative urine test results may mean a blood sugar ranging from normal ($<$100 mg/100 ml) to $\sim$180 mg/100 ml; if the renal threshold is elevated, the blood sugar may be as high as 300 mg/100 ml. Therefore, many patients (especially pregnant women, in whom strict control is essential to the health of the baby) are being introduced to a system of home glucose monitoring. With this method of monitoring diabetic control, the patient measures capillary-blood sugar levels obtained from finger sticks at appropriate times throughout the day. Recent developments have made the technique relatively painless and fairly accurate. In addition, patients are more involved in their treatment because they receive instant feedback concerning their level of control. Finally, multiple pre- and postprandial glucose values make it easier for the physician to adjust the treatment regimen.

Several methods can be used to measure capillary-blood sugar at home. The basic ingredient common to all systems is a paper strip impregnated at one end with the enzyme glucose oxidase. This enzyme reacts with glucose in the drop of blood that is placed on the appropriate part of the strip. The strip also contains other chemicals, which turn color when glucose reacts with the enzyme. The patient either matches the colors on the strip to those on a chart, or places the strips in a small machine that "reads" the glucose concentration.

Two systems of home glucose monitoring are available in the United States. The Ames Company produces a paper strip called Dextrostix, which can be read visually or be measured in one of two instruments. The older, larger, and more expensive model is called a reflectance meter; the newer, lighter, portable machine is the Dextrometer. The second system of home glucose monitoring is manufactured by Bio-Dynamics/bmc. The paper strips (Chemstrips) used for a visual reading are different from those used for machine (Stat-Tek) reading. Both the Ames and the Bio-Dynamics/bmc systems are expensive. At present, the reflectance meter and Stat-Tek costs ~$600, while the Dextrometer and Stat-Tek cost ~$350. Both Dextrostix and Chemstrips cost ~$.50 each. However, the degree of control obtained with home glucose monitoring (usually with just visual readings) usually is much better with these systems than it is with testing only urine. Admittedly, the better results may be explained by the fact that only well-motivated patients choose to do home glucose monitoring.

In order to obtain capillary blood relatively painlessly, the patient should use a blood glucose monitoring kit. This kit, manufactured by Ullster Scientific Inc., includes an *autolet* (an automatic spring-triggered device that drives a small lancet into the finger very rapidly when activated by pressing a button), *platforms* (inserted into the Autolet and pressed on the finger), and *monolet lancets* (small lances inserted into the autolet to prick the finger). The Autolet alone costs ~$30, a package of 200 lancets costs ~$8, and a package of 200 platforms costs ~$7.50. Local branches of the American Diabetes Association should be able to provide information on where to obtain the reagent strips and equipment.

Capillary blood from a finger puncture can be obtained in good quantity and relatively painlessly in the following way:

1. Before puncture, free flow of blood can be enhanced, especially in cold weather, by holding the hand under warm, running tap water for about 20 seconds. Avoid using hot water, particularly if neuropathy is present.
2. Although any finger may be selected as a source of blood, the thumb seems to serve this function better than the other digits because it has a greater surface area and superior blood supply. If tough skin on the thumb makes obtaining a good sample difficult, the ring finger has a better blood supply than the others and should be the second choice.
3. The ball of the finger tip usually is a more painful puncture site than the lateral aspects of the distal phalanx because the nerves are concentrated in this area. The less painful surface is U shaped and begins just above the distal joint and continues around the periphery of the tip and back toward

the same joint on the opposite side of the finger. The blood supply to the finger runs along the lateral aspect, so a puncture made in that area minimizes pain and maximizes blood flow.

4. Pain can be reduced if the patient presses the target digit with an opposing digit of the same hand while the puncture is being made. Pressure should be applied to the palmar surface immediately below the distal joint and should be great enough to cause marked erythema of the distal phalanx.

5. The finger must be dry before puncture, since moisture will cause the blood to spread over the skin surface rather than accumulate in a compact drop that can be transferred easily to the reagent strip.

6. It is not necessary to wipe off the first drop of blood, as some clinical laboratory manuals recommend. Results do not appear to be affected by this extra step.

7. A proper wound rapidly produces a drop of blood at least 5 mm in diameter without prolonged "milking" of the finger. If the blood does not flow freely, wipe off the finger and puncture again. This will prevent dilution of the specimen with tissue fluid.

8. Place a large drop of blood on the appropriate area of the reagent strip by inverting the finger, allowing the drop to fall on the appropriate area. Simultaneously begin timing.

9. The exact technique for measuring glucose concentration depends on the system of monitoring being used. Specific instructions (e.g., timing, how to remove the blood from the strip) are included with each system and should be followed exactly.

Evaluation

Select the correct answer or answers.

1. Testing urine for sugar is necessary in order to

   a. see how well the body is utilizing the sugar in the blood
   b. give an overall picture of control for both the patient and the physician
   c. adjust the amount and/or kind of insulin according to the urine sugar levels.

2. In insulin-requiring diabetics, the before-breakfast urine test tells

   a. whether regular (clear) insulin is effective in lowering blood sugar
   b. whether the dose of NPH or Lente insulin has reached its peak
   c. whether NPH or Lente insulin has been effective in lowering the fasting blood sugar (assuming insulin is given only once per day)

3. Large amounts of sugar in the urine of a diabetic may mean

   a. too much insulin
   b. too little insulin

c. too much food intake

d. too little food intake

4. In diabetes there sometimes is an excess of ketone bodies in the blood. This
   is caused by

   a. breakdown of stored protein

   b. breakdown of stored fats

   c. breakdown of stored sugar

5. Factors that affect urine test results are

   a. incorrect timing when performing the test

   b. exposure of the testing products to moisture

   c. old testing products

Demonstrate

   a. how to test

   b. how to record results

   c. urine record kept at home

DIABETIC EMERGENCIES

Diabetic emergencies are caused by the effects of too much or too little insulin.
The first situation leads to hypoglycemia, or low blood sugar. It also can be
caused by inappropriate use of sulfonylurea agents. Too little insulin leads first
to hyperglycemia, or high blood sugar. As less and less effective insulin is available, the glucose levels become higher and higher. In type 2 diabetes the pancreas is able to secrete enough insulin to prevent ketosis. However, the patient
may still go into coma as a result of the very high glucose concentrations. This
condition is called *hyperosmolar nonketotic coma*. In type 1 diabetes the pancreas
fails almost completely, and ketone bodies start to accumulate. If this situation
is not treated, diabetic ketoacidosis may result, which also can cause coma.

Outcome Criteria (Student) and Goals (Nurse)

Objectives

STUDENT

Upon completion of the instructions, the student will know the causes, signs and
symptoms, treatment, and prevention of hypoglycemia, ketoacidosis, and hyperosmolar nonketotic coma, and the reasons for purchasing Medic Alert identification.

Goals

NURSE

To provide information on:

1. Hypoglycemia

   a. The causes of insulin reactions.
   b. The effect of counterregulatory hormones.
   c. The Somogyi effect.
   d. Assessment for prevention.

2. Ketoacidosis and hyperosmolar nonketotic coma

   a. Pathophysiological events leading to diabetic ketoacidosis and hyperosmolar nonketotic coma.
   b. Current management techniques.

Definition

STUDENT

Hypoglycemia means:

$$Hypo \rightarrow low$$
$$gly \rightarrow sugar$$
$$cemia \rightarrow blood$$

In hypoglycemia, the blood sugar is <50 to 60 mg/100 ml. However, signs and symptoms of hypoglycemia may occur in some diabetics with a rapid drop from a high blood sugar level to a lower one that still is elevated.

NURSE

Blood glucose levels for hypoglycemia (50 to 60 mg/100 ml) vary depending on the sample measured. Plasma or serum values are 15% (not 15 mg/100 ml) higher than whole-blood values. The reason for this is that $\sim$30% of the red cell in whole blood is composed of solid material that cannot dissolve glucose. Therefore, when whole blood is used, glucose is distributed in only 85% of the total volume. However, the results are expressed as concentration per milliliter, which lowers the value by $\sim$15%.

Causes

STUDENT

A common cause of low blood sugar is an imbalance among the amount of insulin administered, activity, and food eaten. For example, the usual dose of insulin is given in the morning, and one or more of the following occurs: (*a*) the patient eats lunch several hours late; (*b*) the patient omits lunch altogether; (*c*) the patient eats only a small portion (especially of the carbohydrate content), or (*d*) the patient indulges in excessive or unusual exercise without eating extra food. Sulfonylurea agents can also cause hypoglycemia but are much less likely to do so than insulin.

NURSE

Hypoglycemia occurs when the rate of glucose entering the circulation (either from the gastrointestinal tract after eating or produced by the liver between meals and during the night) does not keep pace with the utilization of glucose by the peripheral tissues. Most tissues can use fat as a source of energy if glucose is not available. However, under normal circumstances, brain tissue cannot use any other substance except glucose. Therefore, when the brain is deprived of an adequate supply of glucose, brain cells are affected.

The most common causes of hypoglycemia are insulin, inadequate food intake, exercise, drugs, and age.

Insulin

1. Excessive dose
   a. Visual impairment causing inability to measure accurately.
   b. Use of syringes not calibrated for the type of insulin used.
   c. Deliberate manipulation by the patient.
   d. Reduced need for insulin due to either diminished caloric intake (illness and dieting) or termination of pregnancy.
   e. Approximately 40% of insulin is inactivated by the kidneys. After the kidneys fail, the effect of the injected insulin is increased because it is not broken down as rapidly. Unfortunately, since diabetics are prone to renal disease, this problem arises frequently.

2. Injection site
   a. Injecting into thighs and then exercising (e.g., running, swimming). Exercise increases blood flow, which causes insulin to be more rapidly absorbed from the site of injection and carried to the blood stream.

    b. Changing the injection site from hypertrophied to healthy tissue.

    c. Injecting into muscle instead of subcutaneous tissue.

Inadequate Food Intake

The procedure usually used for determining the insulin dose is first to ascertain the appropriate diet and then to match the insulin dose to that diet. Therefore, if the patient's food intake decreases, the usual insulin dose may be excessive. This occurs when the patient misses a meal. This also would occur if the patient voluntarily decreases his or her food intake by going on a diet. It also may occur if the patient becomes ill and cannot eat normally. However, infection tends to interfere with the action of insulin, and this leads to higher insulin requirements. Therefore, sick patients who have decreased their food intake do not necessarily need less insulin; in fact, some may even need more.

Exercise

In addition to increasing the rate of insulin absorption from the injection site, exercise also increases utilization of glucose by muscle. Both of these responses to exercise may lead to hypoglycemia in the insulin-requiring diabetic unless the patient eats extra food.

Drugs

Alcohol. Normal blood sugar is maintained either by the breakdown of glycogen or by the formation of new sugar by the process known as gluconeogenesis. Alcohol inhibits gluconeogenesis. A patient with poorly regulated juvenile-onset diabetes has less glycogen stored in the liver than well-regulated diabetics or nondiabetics. If a diabetic is taking insulin (which also can inhibit gluconeogenesis) has not eaten for a while (which depletes glycogen stores), and then drinks alcohol, severe hypoglycemia may occur.

Propranolol (Inderal). This drug blocks part of the effects of epinephrine (adrenaline). Therefore, it may mask or reduce the adrenergic symptoms that are the first to appear in hypoglycemia (sweating, nervousness, tachycardia). In addition because epinephrine is unable to stimulate glucagon secretion, glycogenolysis may be impaired. Finally, propranolol directly increases the utilization of glucose by muscle. All of these factors can lead to hypoglycemia that may not be appreciated by the patient. Therefore, the patient may not take the appropriate steps to combat it; this situation may eventually lead to loss of consciousness.

Age

In the elderly, cerebral arteriosclerosis affects the cerebral circulation, which in turn may interfere with the patient's ability to recognize a hypoglycemic reaction.

Hormonal Response

STUDENT

The body has a back-up system that responds to an emergency of low blood sugar. This system consists of several hormones that will supply the circulation with the sugar needed. The system also is responsible for some of the signs and symptoms that indicate low blood sugar.

NURSE

The hormones responsible for the body's attempt to correct a rapidly falling blood glucose are: epinephrine glucagon, cortisol, and growth hormone. Receptors for glucose are located at the base of the brain in the hypothalamus. When the glucose concentration falls, signals from this area activate the sympathetic part of the autonomic nervous system. This causes nerve endings to release norepinephrine and the adrenal medulla to release epinephrine. In addition, the pituitary gland releases growth hormone and the adrenal cortex releases cortisol. Finally, the sympathetic nervous system and epinephrine stimulate the release of glucagon from the pancreas. The secretion and action of these hormones are summarized in Table 8-5.

Signs and Symptoms

STUDENT

The alarm system that indicates the need for sugar includes sudden symptoms such as nervousness, anxiety, fast heartbeat, shaking, sweating, tingling of the tongue or lips, dizziness, headache, and extreme hunger. The patient may experience any combination of these symptoms. If sugar is not administered soon, the patient may experience some of the following symptoms: faintness, blurry or double vision, lack of concentration, irritability, personality changes, drowsiness, disorientation, or unconsciousness.

NURSE

The signs and symptoms of hypoglycemia are caused by activation of the autonomic nervous system and depression of the central nervous system. When the blood glucose level falls, the increase in activity of the autonomic nervous system causes signs and symptoms such as weakness, tachycardia, anxiety, tremor, irritability, hunger, palpitations, nervousness, and sweating. These signs and symptoms can be secondary to a *rapid* drop in glucose concentration (e.g., from 300 to 225 mg/100 ml), and hypoglycemia per se may not be present. Signs and symptoms due to depressed activity of the central nervous system require an absolutely low glucose level and may include headache, visual disturbances,

Table 8–5. Hormonal Responses to Hypoglycemia

Gland	Hormone	Response	Rate of Action	Mechanisms
Adrenal medulla	Epinephrine	Rapid	Rapid	Stimulates secretion of glucagon
				Inhibits insulin secretion by pancreatic beta cell and glucose utilization by muscle
				Increases hepatic gluconeogenesis (production of new glucose from noncarbohydrate sources)
Pancreatic alpha cells	Glucagon	Rapid	Rapid	Stimulates hepatic glycogenolysis (breakdown of glycogen into glucose)
Adrenal cortex	Cortisol	Delayed	Probably immediate	Increases hepatic gluconeogenesis; inhibits glucose utilization by muscle(?)
Pituitary	Growth hormone	Delayed	Delayed	Inhibits glucose utilization by muscle; increases hepatic gluconeogenesis(?)

mental dullness, confusion, amnesia, seizures, or coma. Such symptoms depend on the amount of glucose supplying the brain. The lower the blood glucose level, the greater the chance that the patient will become unconscious.

Treatment (Patient Conscious)

STUDENT

1. Liquids will be absorbed from the gastrointestinal tract much more quickly than solids.
2. Sweetened fluids should not be too concentrated because they will slow absorption and may cause nausea and vomiting.
3. 10 g of glucose (one fruit exchange) will relieve most reactions.
4. It should take 10 to 15 minutes for the sugar to become effective. If there is no improvement, repeat the treatment every 10 minutes.

Each of the following foods will provide $\sim$10 g of carbohydrate (one fruit exchange). Take only one of the following immediately.

1. $\frac{1}{2}$ cup (4 oz.) orange juice
2. $\frac{1}{2}$ cup nondiet carbonated beverage (cola, 7-Up, ginger ale).
3. $2\frac{1}{2}$ teaspoons sugar in $\frac{1}{2}$ cup water.
4. $\frac{1}{4}$ cup grape juice.
5. 2 teaspoons honey.
6. 2 packets sugar.
7. 4 sugar cubes.
8. 1 tablespoon jelly.
9. $\frac{1}{3}$ cup sweetened gelatin (Jello).
10. 5 to 6 Lifesavers (chew them).

The following items are easy to carry and can be wrapped in aluminum foil for traveling:

1. 5 sugar cubes.
2. 2 sugar packets.
3. 2 tablespoons raisins.
4. 2 large marshmallows.
5. 6 Lifesavers.
6. 7 jelly beans.

After you take sugar for an insulin reaction and your next meal is >30 to 45 minutes away, take small amounts of starch and protein (1 to 2 oz. protein + one bread exchange) to prevent recurrence of the reaction. To expedite treatment, always carry some form of sugar and always wear and carry some form of identification with you (see appendix).

You should attempt to determine the reason for the fall in blood sugar and correct the situation. Persons recovering from an episode of hypoglycemia may feel somewhat weak for a while and need to rest.

NURSE

There are several commercial products available for treating the conscious patient:

Glutose: 2 oz. (32 g of glucose; lemon-flavor red gel).

Insta-Glucose: 30.8 g (40% dextrose).

Cake Mate Gel: one tube = 12 g (61%) of carbohydrate.

Cake Mate Icing: $\frac{1}{2}$ oz. = 10 g (78%) of carbohydrate.

The primary advantages of these products are that they can be carried easily and may be less tempting to eat than candy. *These products are effective only when swallowed. Therefore, they should not be used if the patient is unconscious.*

Treatment (Patient Unconscious or Unwilling to Eat)

FAMILY MEMBER OR FRIEND/NURSE

An injection of glucagon should be given to the person who becomes unconscious from a severe reaction or who is stubborn about taking sugar by mouth (the irrational behavior can be the result of the hypoglycemia). Glucagon is a hormone that is made by the pancreas and raises the blood sugar. It is sold as a prescription drug for emergencies and comes in powdered form. Mix according to the package directions. Give the glucagon injection with the same syringe and needle used for insulin injection. After the glucagon injection, when the patient regains consciousness, give the same amount of carbohydrate and protein by mouth as recommended for the oral treatment of hypoglycemia.

Prevention

STUDENT

Many insulin reactions are caused by changes in the normal balance among insulin, food, and exercise. In general, first a diet is ordered, and then insulin is given in the appropriate dose and at the correct time to handle the food intake. After insulin is injected, the rate of absorption depends on the kind and amount of insulin given. In a sense, the food intake is a buffer for the insulin and must be eaten at specific times to counteract the glucose-lowering effects of insulin. Thus, if the usual relationship between insulin and food is altered, the insulin absorbed may be highly active at a time when there is no glucose from a meal to counteract its effects. The same is true for exercise. If patients exercise strenuously without taking extra food, the increased effectiveness of insulin (see section on exercise) may cause hypoglycemia because there is no extra glucose to buffer the increased action of insulin.

The following guidelines will assist in preventing an insulin reaction:

1. Correct technique of injection and rotation of sites (see section on insulin).
2. Regular mealtimes and snacks as ordered.
3. Understanding the meaning of urine test results.
4. When the patient is sick and normal intake of food is decreased, food must be replaced by carbohydrates.
5. The patient should eat a snack before engaging in some forms of exercise (see section on exercise).
6. Adjust insulin dosage only according to physician's guidelines.
7. Give correct amount of insulin.

NURSE

No further information is required.

Hazards of Hypoglycemia

STUDENT/NURSE

1. *Brain damage.* Although personality changes and mental dullness occasionally have been reported secondary to hypoglycemia, it should be stressed that only repeated and profound hypoglycemia can cause permanent changes. Stimulation of the adrenergic nervous system, although unpleasant, does no permanent damage. Even patients who lose consciousness due to low blood sugar seldom suffer any long-term effects. Permanent brain damage may develop only if the hypoglycemic coma lasts for a long time (i.e., many hours).
2. *Physical injury.* Dizziness or loss of balance may precipitate a fall, which in turn can cause contusions, fractures, or head injuries. Disorientation may cause self-injury, such as cigarette burns or automobile accidents. In addition, any of the hazards of unconsciousness may occur (e.g., aspiration).
3. *Socioeconomic factors.* Irritability may precipitate difficulty in personal relations on the job and with family members. Medical treatment for hypoglycemia (i.e., physician's, and emergency room services, hospitalization) is expensive, not only because of medical costs, but also because of loss of employment time.

4. *Uncontrolled diabetes.* Counterregulatory hormones produced during hypoglycemia (Table 8–7) cause glucose levels to increase. Care must be taken not to overtreat a reaction (e.g., with double or triple portions of sugar), because blood sugar levels will rise dramatically. This rise may in turn lead to further overtreatment with more insulin, which may cause yet another hypoglycemic reaction. This leads to a roller-coaster situation. The counterregulatory effects of the hormones will subside in time (usually within 1 day).

NURSE (FURTHER INFORMATION)

When a patient receives too much insulin, a rebound effect may occur, resulting in high levels of blood sugar. This is caused by the effects of the counterregulatory hormones. It was first described by Somogyi and is called the Somogyi effect. The patient may exhibit the following clues:

1. Marked fluctuations in urine glucose from negative to marked glycosuria.
2. Wide swings in ketonuria without glycosuria.
3. Nocturnal hypoglycemia, characterized by diaphoresis (sweating) and hypothermia (low body temperature), early-morning headache, or nightmares.
4. Increase in blood glucose with increasing insulin doses.

The nurse plays an important role in both assessing the situation and alerting the physician.

Diabetic Ketoacidosis

STUDENT

Ketoacidosis means

Keto → ketones in the blood
Acid → acid in the blood in addition to high blood sugar

Another term used for diabetic ketoacidosis (DKA) is diabetic coma. However, this term is not entirely accurate, since coma can also be seen in type 2 diabetics who become unconscious secondary to extremely high glucose levels without any accumulation of ketone bodies in the blood. This state is called hyperosmolar nonketotic coma (HNKC).

NURSE

The correct diagnosis of DKA is contingent on a blood pH <7.3, PCO_2 <40 mm Hg, HCO_3 <15 mEq/L, and strongly positive results for serum ketone bodies (nitroprusside test) in an undiluted serum or plasma sample. Severe hyperglycemia may be seen in DKA, but evidence for acidosis is necessary to make the diagnosis. Extremely high glucose concentrations ($>$1,000 mg/100 ml) are characteristic of HNKC (the two conditions will be contrasted later).

Causes

STUDENT/NURSE

Diabetic ketoacidosis is caused by a lack of effective insulin and is seen in the following circumstances:

1. Decreased amount or lack of insulin.
2. As an initial manifestation of diabetes. The patient goes into DKA without knowing that he or she has diabetes.
3. Infection.

Each of these factors is responsible for $\sim$25% of cases of DKA. No precipitating cause can be found for the remaining 25%. It should be mentioned, however, that stress can contribute to DKA because it interferes with the action of insulin. That is, the usual amount of insulin may be less effective because of the effects of stress. This includes both physical (e.g., illness, trauma, surgery) and psychological (e.g., emotional upset) stress.

Symptoms

STUDENT

The signs and symptoms of DKA are mainly those of uncontrolled diabetes. These include fatigue, weakness, headache, blurred vision, increased thirst, and increased urination. In addition, loss of appetite, nausea, vomiting, and, occasionally, stomach pain often are present. Finally, difficulty in catching one's breath and rapid or deep breathing are characteristic of DKA. Occasionally, others will be able to detect a sweet smell (acetone) on the patient's breath.

NURSE

The mechanisms leading to the signs and symptoms of DKA are illustrated in Figure 8-6. The lack of insulin inhibits the utilization of glucose by the three insulin-sensitive tissues (muscle, fat, and liver). Additionally, in the absence of effective insulin, glucose production by the liver is uncontrolled and excessive. Both of these situations lead to elevated glucose concentrations in the blood (hyperglycemia). Hyperglycemia causes blurred vision because the lens of the eye changes shape in the presence of high levels of blood sugar. Increased

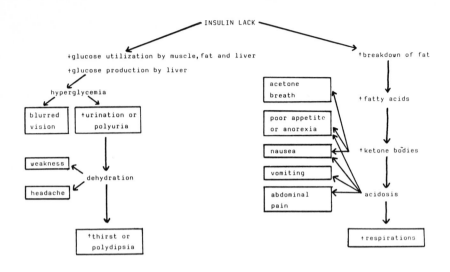

Figure 8-6. Abnormal metabolism that cause signs and symptoms of diabetic ketoacidosis. ↑, increased; ↓, decreased.

urination occurs because the kidney can not reabsorb all of the filtered glucose into the blood stream, and the excess sugar that ends up in the urine brings along extra fluid with it. This loss of fluid results in dehydration, which is responsible for headache and weakness. There is a center in the brain that responds to the dehydration by signaling the patient to drink in order to restore the plasma volume. This increased thirst is termed *polydipsia.*

Insulin lack also causes the stored fat to break down into fatty acids. Fatty acids are metabolized into ketone bodies in the liver and are released into the blood stream. Ketone bodies (acetoacetate and β-hydroxybutyrate) are changed into acetone, which is eliminated through the lungs. Acetone has a sweet or fruity smell and sometimes can be detected on the breath. The ketone bodies may be responsible for decreased appetite and may even cause mild nausea. Acetoacetate and β-hydroxybutyrate are weak acids, and when they accumulate the body becomes too acid (or an acidosis occurs). The acidosis probably is responsible (through unknown mechanisms) for the gastrointestinal symptoms of pain and vomiting and certainly contributes to the anorexia and nausea. In addition, the brain responds to the acidosis by increasing the patient's respirations, especially the depth of breathing. This is called Kussmaul respirations and is named after the physician who first described this overbreathing in DKA. Kussmaul respirations cause the body to become somewhat alkaline (which is the opposite of acidic) and thus is useful in counteracting the acidosis.

It should be stressed that the gastrointestinal signs (detected on physical examination) and symptoms may be so severe as to suggest the presence of an intra-abdominal emergency that requires immediate surgery. However, in almost all cases, this simply is a result of the DKA and appropriate treatment will alleviate the problem.

Treatment

STUDENT

In the early stages of ketoacidosis, treatment includes adjustment or initiation of insulin therapy and drinking lots of salt-containing fluids. For more advanced cases, especially if nausea and vomiting prevent oral intake of fluids, hospitalization is necessary to institute treatment.

NURSE

Although treatment of DKA is beyond the scope of this chapter, one should be aware that the three basic objectives of treatment are

1. Restoration of normal carbohydrate and fat metabolism by the use of insulin.
2. Replacement of lost fluids and electrolytes.
3. Identification of the precipitating factor(s). If an infection was the cause, isolate the organism and treat appropriately. If the patient failed to take insulin, determine the reason.

   In discussing DKA with the patient, the main emphasis should be on prevention, since most episodes of DKA can be avoided.

Prevention

STUDENT/NURSE

Since infections are responsible for ~25% of all cases of DKA, it is very important that the patient be aware of what to do in the event of illness. This will prevent the development of DKA. The most important element of prevention is communication with the physician before the symptoms become very severe. Certain sick-day rules are also helpful in preventing DKA.

1. Know how the illness affects diabetic control. Check urine for ketones and sugar at least four times a day. *Notify the physician* if sugar levels are consistently 1% to 2% and if any amount of ketones are seen. If you use Diastix or Keto-Diastix to measure urine glucose, be aware that moderate or large amounts of ketone bodies interfere with the test results. (See section on monitoring diabetic control for a full discussion.)

2. Do not omit the daily dose of insulin. The physician may need to change the amount and timing. Because infection and stress interfere with insulin action, insulin requirements may be even greater than usual at this time.

3. If you cannot follow your normal meal pattern, replace the food you do not eat with liquids or soft foods. Inability to keep down liquids because of nausea and vomiting is serious, and you should report this promptly to the physician. Pay particular attention to the replacement of carbohydrates, salts, and minerals. This can be accomplished with orange juice, carbonated beverages, popsicles, broth, or saltine crackers. (See chapter 3 for detailed information on food replacement.)

4. Although illness tends to increase blood sugar levels and thus you may require more insulin than usual, taking insulin without proper food replacement may lead to hypoglycemia. Negative results on tests for urine glucose should alert the patient to this possibility.

5. *Keep the physician informed*! You may be able to prevent ketoacidosis and avoid hospitalization.

6. Be alert to signs and symptoms that indicate possible DKA. These include increasing ketone bodies in the urine, nausea, vomiting, abdominal pain, fruity breath, or inability to catch your breath.

Hyperosmolar Nonketotic Coma

STUDENT

Little or no excess acid is present in HNKC. Therefore, patients do not feel as sick as quickly as they do in DKA, and thus they usually delay seeking medical help. This allows more time for the blood sugar to reach extremely high levels. Hyperosmolar nonketotic coma occurs in type 2 diabetes and sometimes is the first manifestation of diabetes in older patients. The symptoms are similar to those seen in DKA except that overbreathing and a fruity odor on the breath do not occur. Usually the gastrointestinal symptoms (nausea, vomiting, abdominal pain) are less severe. Increased urination and thirst are very prominent. Most patients, especially older ones, have decreased mental function as they go into HNKC. Urine tests will reveal minimal or no ketone bodies. The treatment and prevention of DKA also apply to HNKC.

NURSE

The differences between the signs and symptoms of DKA and those of HNKC is attributable to the relatively normal breakdown of fat in HNKC (Fig. 8-6). Therefore, signs and symptoms related to increased breakdown of fat in HNKC are either absent or minimal. Another difference is that many patients, especially older ones, have local neurologic changes that mimic stroke (e.g., slurred speech, weakness of an arm or leg). These changes usually disappear when the HNKC is treated. In addition, many patients experiencing HNKC do not need insulin after they leave the hospital, whereas virtually all diabetics in DKA need maintenance insulin therapy. Finally, almost all patients survive DKA. Unfortunately, a large number (30% to 50%) do not survive an episode of HNKC. This is due in part to the older age of the patients, the greater severity of their complicating illnesses, and the delay in making the diagnosis.

Evaluation

Select the correct answer or answers to each question.

1. Insulin reactions leading to hypoglycemia may be caused by

   a. delaying supper for several hours
   b. too much food and not enough insulin
   c. too little exercise without additional food
   d. too much exercise without additional food

2. Which of the following symptoms occur with low blood sugar?

   a. increased urination
   b. headache
   c. a nervous or shaky feeling
   d. dry tongue and mouth
   e. hunger
   f. fast heartbeat

3. In treating an insulin reaction, which of the following foods can be eaten?

   a. sugar cubes
   b. hard candy
   c. peanuts
   d. cola

4. When a diabetic increases his or her usual amount of daily activity, he or she will require

   a. the same amount of insulin with additional food
   b. more insulin with less food
   c. no insulin

5. The main cause of DKA is

   a. drinking too much water
   b. eating too much sugar

    c. lack of insulin

    d. excessive exercise

6. Which of the following may be associated with DKA?

    a. dry mouth

    b. increased thirst and urination

    c. increased sugar and ketones in the urine

    d. drowsiness and fatigue

    e. nausea and vomiting

7. When you are ill, which of the following steps should you follow?

    a. notify your physician

    b. check urine for sugar and ketones at least four times a day

    c. increase oral intake of fluids

    d. if vomiting, stop taking insulin

FOOT CARE

The number and seriousness of foot lesions that occur in diabetic patients is overwhelming. Assessment of the diabetic patient's foot reveals that trauma due to burns, injury to skin in cutting toenails, "home surgery" of corns and calluses, and blisters from new shoes are common occurrences.

Foot lesions in diabetics are related to three factors. First, neuropathy (nerve damage), which often is present, decreases the patient's ability to perceive pressure and pain. Therefore, the diabetic patient is unaware of repeated trauma. Second, circulation to the feet may be impaired, which slows down healing (sometimes considerably). Finally, poorly controlled diabetes compromises the patient's ability to deal with infection. The last factor is compounded by the effects of poor circulation. Foot lesions can be very serious and can lead to amputation. However, most such lesions are preventable. This section will emphasize how to educate the patient so that he or she can prevent trauma-induced foot lesions.

Outcome Criteria (Student) and Goals (Nurse)

Objectives

STUDENT

Upon completion of the instructions, the student will be able to verbalize or write the following:

1. The three factors that contribute to the development of foot problems in diabetics.
2. A minimum of three events that may cause trauma to the foot.
3. A minimum of five measures that can be taken to prevent foot problems.
4. Three rules in the selection and wearing of shoes for diabetics.

Goals

NURSE

To provide information on the following:

1. Neuropathies, vascular abnormalities and impaired defense mechanisms related to foot problems in the diabetic.
2. Foot deformities that may be a source of foot problems.
3. Footwear.
4. Daily care for prevention of foot lesions.

Contributing Factors

STUDENT

The skin is the first line of defense against infection. Any trauma that leads to a break in the skin can have serious consequences in the diabetic patient, especially if the trauma is related directly to the complications of diabetes that already are present. These complications cause nerve destruction, poor circulation, and problems with healing.

Neuropathies (Nerves)

The most common factor that contributes to the development of foot lesions is nerve involvement that causes decreased sensation to pain and temperature.

Examples

Burns may result from the patient's inability to distinguish temperatures that are either too hot (heating appliances, bath water, sunburn) or too cold (frostbite).

Blisters may result from the patient's inability to feel pain caused by pressure from a flaw or foreign object in a shoe or from a tightfitting shoe.

Ulcers occur at pressure points on the bottom of the foot, such as the ball of the foot, the heel, the bottom of the great toe, or the bottom of foot at base of the third toe. Calluses are the first manifestation of increased pressure on the skin, and, since ulcers often develop beneath thickened calluses, they should alert the patient (as well as those taking care of him or her) that something is wrong.

Muscle weakness and imbalance also may occur. This may result in either a clawfoot deformity (Fig. 8-7) or a hammertoe (Fig. 8-8). In both conditions the toe joints are "cocked up," making them very prominent and thus leading to pressure from the shoe on this area. If these conditions are not corrected by surgery or special shoes, ulcers eventually will develop.

Another problem related to nerve damage is a decrease in or lack of sweating, resulting in a "dry foot." This may lead to scaling and cracking of the skin, which allows bacteria and fungi to enter the broken area.

Vascular (Blood-Vessel) Abnormalities

One problem that diabetic patients develop is a narrowing of the large vessels at a faster rate than occurs in nondiabetics. This condition is called *atherosclerosis* and leads to a decreased blood supply to various parts of the body. Atherosclerosis is a slow process that can go on for years without causing symptoms. It consists of a buildup of fatty deposits along the inner walls of the arteries. Just like lime deposits that form in water pipes, atherosclerosis coats the inside of the arteries and gradually narrows them. The fatty buildup reduces the flow of blood through the arteries to important parts of the body. Small blood vessels in the foot also may narrow for a different reason but by the same process that affects the eyes and kidneys in diabetics. This causes an even greater decrease in circulation. Decreased blood flow to the feet may inhibit the delivery of nutrients to injured areas, thus causing ulceration, infection, or even gangrene.

Impaired Defense Mechanisms (Infections)

Another factor that contributes to the development of foot lesions in poorly controlled diabetic patients is the inability of the body to effectively neutralize invading bacteria. This is due not only to the inability of the blood to supply nutrition to the tissues, but also to an inability of the appropriate cells to fight infection properly. Thus, what starts out as a small infection can become much worse, sometimes very quickly.

NURSE

The majority of diabetic foot lesions result from local trauma (often unappreciated as a result of the neuropathy) in the presence of nutritional deficiencies

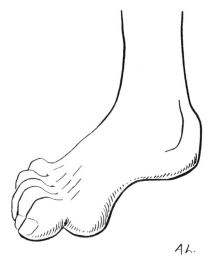

Figure 8-7. Illustration of clawfoot. (Reprinted with permission from Larson CB, Gould M: *Calderwood's Orthopedic Nursing.* CV Mosby, St. Louis, 1957, p. 511.)

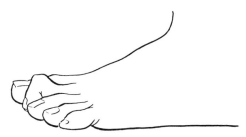

Figure 8-8. Illustration of hammertoe. (Reprinted with permission from Larson CB, Gould M: *Calderwood's Orthopedic Nursing.* CV Mosby, St. Louis, 1957, p.511.)

in the tissue that result from vascular insufficiency. This produces lowered resistance to infection and poor healing. Frequently, the end result of local trauma to the diabetic foot is gangrene. The prevalence of gangrene is 53 times higher in diabetic males and 71 times higher in diabetic females than in non-diabetic males and females, respectively.

Neuropathy

In addition to causing decreased appreciation of pain in some patients, sensory impairment of peripheral nerve function may paradoxically cause paresthesias, burning, and even hypesthesia (hypersensitivity to touch). Sensory neuropathy also interferes with the normal contraction and relaxation of ankle and calf muscles, which assist the body in adjusting to body weight. Inability of the sensory-deprived foot to make such adjustments results in excessive "pounding" of the foot on the ground with increased force. This can cause degeneration of foot or ankle joints secondary to repeated trauma. The result is a Charcot joint, named after the physician who first described it.

Motor nerve damage can cause weakness of foot muscles, primarily of the deep toe flexors and long extensors. This results in a deformity of the foot characterized by a protrusion of the ball of the foot, an elevated arch, and hammertoes. This deformity leads to calluses, skin breakdown, and ulcerations. Obesity, improperly fitting shoes, and coexisting sensory impairment can accelerate these conditions.

In autonomic neuropathy, sympathetic denervation interferes with normal sweating of the foot. This results in cracking of the skin, and fungi and bacteria normally present on the surface may infect the lesions and spread to the deep tissues.

Vascular Abnormalities and Impaired Defense Mechanisms

Disease of both the large and the small blood vessels (macroangiopathy and microangiopathy, respectively) are responsible for the complications of trauma-induced foot problems. In large-vessel disease, premature atherosclerosis can occur; in small-vessel disease, thickening of the structures surrounding the capillaries (the basement membrane) is often seen.

Vascular insufficiency may adversely affect host resistance to infection by

1. Decreasing blood flow to peripheral tissues, which impairs mobilization of the white blood cells for fighting the infection.
2. Decreasing the delivery of specific antibodies and other plasma factors necessary to fight the infection.
3. Decreasing oxygen tension in poorly perfused tissue, which sets the stage for multiplication of microaerophilic or anaerobic organisms (bacteria that proliferate in the absence of oxygen and that are very difficult to treat).

Infection is a double-edged sword in the diabetic patient. It interferes with the action of insulin, leading to poor control and the need for increased insulin dose. On the other hand, the normal body defenses against infection do not work well when the diabetic patient is uncontrolled. Persistence of the infection continues to inhibit the effectiveness of insulin, creating a vicious cycle. Therefore, prompt and vigorous treatment of infection is extremely important.

Prevention: Foot Care

STUDENT/NURSE

INSPECTION

1. Inspect pressure points (Fig. 8-9) daily for corns, calluses, blisters, or redness.
2. Inspect between toes for cracks, signs of fungus, blisters, or discoloration.
3. Inspect entire skin for dryness.

    If the patient's poor vision or obesity make inspection of the feet difficult, use a mirror. If the patient is not able to do the inspection, a family member or friend should perform the task.

Hygiene

1. Wash the feet with a mild soap as part of a daily shower or tub bath.
2. Patients who do not shower or bathe daily may clean the feet in a foot basin.
3. Water temperature must be comfortable (test with the elbow).
4. Dry carefully between the toes with a soft cloth.
5. If a foot basin is used, do not soak the feet longer than 10 minutes.

Toenails

1. Scrub the nails with a soft brush to soften them.
2. If the nails need cutting, use nail clippers, not scissors.

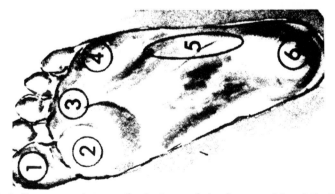

Figure 8-9. Pressure points on the bottom of the foot requiring daily inspection. (Reprinted with permission from Reed JK: Footwear for the diabetic. In *The Diabetic Foot*. CV Mosby, St. Louis, 1977, pp. 267-282.)

3. Keep the nails trimmed by using an emery board or a file with a blunt tip.
4. Trim the nails straight across; do not cut into corners.
5. Ingrown or thickened nails require special care and should not be self-treated.
6. Lubricate the cuticles with Vaseline or lanolin; then push them back with orange-wood stick.
7. Never trim nails with a knife or razor blade.

Skin

1. To prevent dryness, apply lanolin or other lubricating material daily (e.g., Alpha-Keri, Eucerin, Nivea).
2. Scrub gently with a soft brush, noncoarse pumice stone, or foot-cleansing sponge (e.g., a buff) to remove dead tissue.
3. Apply a small amount of talcum powder to remove excess moisture. Be alert to fungus infection, which will require special powders.
4. Burns

   a. Do not use hot water baths, heating pads, or other heating techniques to warm the feet.
   b. Be careful about placing the feet on or near heating registers, car heaters, or heat lamps.
   c. Avoid sunburn.

Corns and Calluses

Most ulcers that develop start under a corn or a callus on the pressure areas of the foot (Fig. 8-9). If the corn or callus is very pronounced or if discoloration develops, seek medical advice.

1. First soften the corn or callus by soaking the feet in a foot basin (no longer than 10 minutes).
2. Scrub corn or callus with a soft brush, pumice, or cleansing sponge.
3. Apply lubricating material.
4. Do not use any tools or commercial preparations for removal of corns or calluses (e.g., preparations that contain iodine, bichloride of mercury or phenol, or corn remedies, corn pads, or adhesives). Moleskin may be helpful in protecting the protruding parts of the foot.
5. If corns are caused by overlapping of toes, place a small amount of lamb's wool between them.

Shoes

Specific attention should be given to footwear to prevent trauma.

1. Protect feet by wearing shoes.

2. Special shoes may be needed for certain types of employment (e.g., construction or factory work). Adhere to the regulations on the job.

3. Shoe material should be pliable (leather is ideal) and should allow for evaporation of moisture and heat.

4. Break in new shoes gradually (maximum, 2 hours at a time) and then remove them to inspect the feet for any irritations.

5. Wear slippers only upon retiring at night and on arising in the morning; do not use them for total day wear.

6. Be careful when wearing sandals because the feet are not totally protected.

7. Inspect the insides of shoes (especially new ones) for rough ridges, exposed nails, or other protruding surfaces.

8. Rotate the use of at least two pairs of shoes to allow shoes to "dry out."

9. Seek medical advise if special shoes or foot appliances are necessary (e.g., for clawfoot deformities or hammertoes).

10. Shoes should be of proper fit, allowing for toe expansion and a snug heel fit.

Socks and Stockings

1. Socks, especially cotton ones, absorb moisture.

2. Socks or stockings that are too tight or have narrow elastic tops may decrease circulation. Buy knee-high or ankle-top stockings that have a wide elastic top. When putting on socks or stockings, allow enough space for toe expansion.

3. Never wear garters.

4. Socks or stockings should be changed at least once a day or as needed if they are wet with perspiration. They should be free of holes and, if they are repaired, there should be no uneven areas to irritate the skin.

Circulation

The following activities decrease circulation and should be avoided.

1. Cigarette smoking (extremely important).

2. Sitting with legs crossed at the knee.

3. Exposure to very high or very low temperatures.

Evaluation

Select the correct answer or answers to each question.

1. Circulatory problems involving the feet may occur in diabetics because

   a. the feet may swell due to increased blood sugar

   b. blood vessels in the feet may narrow in diabetes

    c. blood vessels in the feet become larger and stronger

    d. blood supply to the feet increases

2. With decreased nerve sensation to the feet, patients are apt to

    a. burn the feet with hot water

    b. injure the feet without feeling it

    c. develop pressure ulcers without feeling pain

    d. have thickening of the nails

3. Which of the following commercial foot products are harmful to the feet of a diabetic?

    a. corn plasters and corn removers

    b. foot sprays and soaks

    c. moleskin

    d. pumice stone

4. What features should a diabetic consider when selecting shoes?

    a. enclosed toe and heel

    b. shoes should be all leather

    c. avoid excessively high heels

    d. purchase shoes that have ample room and break them in slowly

5. Diabetics need to take special care of their feet because

    a. the feet may be less sensitive to pain, cold, heat, and pressure than the hands

    b. they have more corns and calluses than other people

    c. blood supply to the feet may be increased

    d. blood supply to the feet may be decreased

6. When a corn or callus develops, the diabetic should

    a. remove the source of rubbing or pressure

    b. keep calluses smooth and soft with lubricants

    c. trim the edges of corns or calluses

    d. inform doctor of corn or callus

7. Good ways to prevent foot problems are to

    a. always wear white socks

    b. bathe the feet daily

    c. inspect the feet daily

    d. wear the same shoes every day

8. When inspecting the feet, the diabetic should look for

    a. toenails that need trimming or that are ingrown

b. corns, calluses, and blisters

c. redness, cracks, and small blisters between the toes

d. open cuts and sores

EXERCISE

Exercise is an integral and essential part of diabetes management. The role of exercise was recognized 2,000 years ago in Rome and, in the preinsulin era, was recommended along with carbohydrate restriction to control blood sugar. Nowadays, the increased popularity of physical exercise and conditioning has precipitated an awareness of the importance of exercise in the treatment of diabetes.

The insulin-dependent diabetic requires education in preventing exercise-induced hypoglycemia as well as in the beneficial effects of exercise. Type 2 patients who do not take insulin can improve carbohydrate metabolism through exercise by two mechanisms. First, in obese patients, weight loss leads to increased effectiveness of insulin. Second, even without weight loss, exercise also enhances insulin action on tissues that normally respond to it.

Outcome Criteria (Student) and Goals (Nurse)

Objectives

STUDENT

Upon completion of the instructions, the student will have the following guidelines to assist in the development of an exercise program:

1. Benefits of exercise.
2. Types of exercise.
3. Components of a planned exercise program.
4. Prevention of hypoglycemia (in patients taking insulin).

Goals

NURSE

To provide information on the following:

1. Physiology of exercise.
2. Desired working heart rate.

3. Effects of exercise in uncontrolled diabetes.

4. Implications of exercise in patients with vascular complications.

Benefits

STUDENT/NURSE

Regular exercise is beneficial to everyone. Physical fitness through exercise is considered an important influence on reducing the risk factors that lead to coronary artery disease. The results of regular exercise are multiple. These include

1. Increasing the efficiency of the heart. Since diabetics may develop heart disease at an earlier age than nondiabetics, exercise that improves cardiovascular function (aerobic) is beneficial.
2. Indirectly increasing the efficiency of the lungs by circulating more oxygen with less effort.
3. Helping to handle stress by relieving physical tension. This promotes relaxation and sleep; fatigue lessens and the individual can accomplish more.
4. Helping to control weight by increasing tissue utilization of calories rather than storage as fat.
5. Decreasing hypertension by reducing stress and by making it easier for the heart to pump blood to all body tissues.
6. Reducing cholesterol and triglyceride concentrations, both of which are risk factors for heart disease.
7. Improving muscle and blood-vessel tone.
8. Helping insulin to control blood sugar more efficiently.

Physiology

STUDENT

No further information is required.

NURSE

The physiology of exercise is very complex and is not completely understood. The physiologic response to exercise is known to involve circulatory, metabolic, and hormonal regulatory mechanisms. The response also depends on the duration and intensity of the exercise. The circulatory system responds by increasing blood flow to muscles, which results in an increased oxygen supply. Since exercise requires an increased energy expenditure, circulating blood glucose levels must rise because suppliers of muscle glycogen (stored glucose) are limited.

In order to meet the energy demands of muscle, the following metabolic adjustments occur. The liver increases its output of glucose, mainly by breaking down stored glycogen (glycogenolysis). During short-term exercise, as the muscles use up the extra glucose produced by the liver, blood glucose levels usually remain the same. With prolonged exercise, free fatty acids produced by the breakdown of stored fat help to supply the energy needs of the muscle. The time at which fat metabolism supplies most of the energy needs depends on the level of exercise. With vigorous exercise, the shift to fat metabolism will take place within the first 30 minutes. If the exercise continues long enough, the liver eventually will produce new glucose from protein (gluconeogenesis). These metabolic changes are due in large part to increased secretion of the anti-insulin hormones (catecholamines, glucagon, growth hormone, and cortisol). The increased blood flow to muscle during exercise enables this tissue to receive a greater supply of circulating fuel sources (glucose and free fatty acids).

Types of Exercise

STUDENT/NURSE

Aerobic

Aerobic exercise refers to exercise that encourages the utilization of oxygen to meet the energy needs of muscles. This type of exercise promotes cardiovascular fitness by increasing the efficiency of the heart and by decreasing the resistance against which the heart has to work to pump blood throughout the body. This conditioning effect occurs over a period of weeks and is manifested by a decrease in both the resting and the exercise heart rate. Some examples of aerobic exercise are jogging, bicycling, swimming, walking, racquetball, jumping rope, aerobic calisthenics (active), tennis, and stationary running.

Anaerobic

Exercise is anaerobic if the energy demands of the muscles are supplied without utilization of oxygen. This type of exercise, (e.g., sprinting in running or swimming) conditions the muscle but does not produce cardiovascular benefits.

Exercise Prescription

STUDENT/NURSE

Three components of a prescription for aerobic exercise that must be considered are frequency, intensity, and duration.

Frequency

A minimum of three exercise sessions per week is essential. A schedule with less exercise results in loss of whatever adaptive benefits have already been gained.

Intensity

The intensity of exercise is reflected in the increase in heart rate. The goal of exercise is to achieve 70% to 85% of the maximal attainable heart rate. The maximal heart rate and the desired range are determined according to age and are summarized in Table 8-6 for individuals between the ages of 20 and 70 years.

The capacity to increase the heart rate during exercise is influenced not only by age, but also by the individual's physical condition. Exercise that exceeds 85% of the maximal heart rate may be harmful, and that which achieves <70% is not effective in developing cardiovascular fitness.

Table 8-6. Heart Rates (beats/min) to be Achieved During Exercise

Age	Maximum Rate	Desired Range (70% to 85% of maximum)
20	200	140–170
25	195	137–166
30	190	133–162
35	185	130–157
40	180	126–153
45	175	123–149
50	170	119–145
55	165	116–140
60	160	112–136
65	155	109–132
70	150	105–128

Duration

The duration of exercise should be 20 to 30 minutes of *continuous* activity. During this time the pulse should be maintained at 70% to 85% of the maximal heart rate (Table 8-6). This result may take several weeks or months to attain.

Starting a Program

Because cardiovascular complications, may occur, diabetic individuals over the age of 30 should be examined by a physician before starting an exercise program. An electrocardiogram or treadmill evaluation (stress test) may be required. All exercise programs should progress slowly, allowing several months to reach and maintain between 70% to 85% of the maximal heart rate appropriate for the patient's age.

Determining Heart Rate

1. *Resting pulse.* Before getting out of bed in the morning, count the pulse for a total of 1 minute.
2. *Exercising pulse.* After exercising steadily for 3 to 4 minutes, locate a pulse, count it for 10 seconds, and multiply it by 6.

How to Take a Pulse

The heart rate may be measured in one of three pulse areas: the carotid (side of neck), the radial (wrist), or the apical (over left chest). For carotid and radial pulses, place two fingers lightly either at the side of the neck just below jawbone or on the inside of the wrist. To take the apical pulse, place the palm of the hand over the left chest just above the left nipple.

Cardiovascular Problems

Persons with cardiac problems or who have risk factors for coronary heart disease (e.g., overweight, hypertension, diabetes) *must have their physician's approval* before they begin an exercise program.

General Guidelines for Exercise Programs

1. Select the exercise(s) to be done. Walking is the most natural, safest, and most economical exercise and is a good place to start before advancing to other forms of exercise. For some individuals, walking may be the only form of exercise in which they can indulge.
2. Select proper clothing and shoes. Clothing should not increase body temperature unnecessarily. Shoes should minimize strain and trauma on the joints and muscles.

3. Don't exercise during illness.
4. Avoid extremes in temperature and do not exercise on hot or smoggy days.
5. Do not exercise soon after a large meal.
6. Drink adequate amounts of water to replace fluids lost through perspiration.
7. Do not consume alcohol before or immediately after exercising.
8. Avoid marked fatigue (lightheadedness, difficulty in breathing, muscular pain).
9. The exercise session should last about 1 hour, which includes warm-up, aerobic exercise, and cooling down period.
10. Start the exercise session with a 5- to 10-minute warm-up period of stretching and flexibility exercises. Follow this with about 30 minutes of aerobic exercise, and finish with about 10 minutes of cooling down activity.
11. Breathe out (exhale) during the effort cycle.
12. If you experience pain in the chest, teeth, jaw, or arm, and/or irregular heart rate occurs, stop the exercise and report the symptoms to the physician.

Exercise for Type 1 Diabetics

STUDENT/NURSE

Diabetes Controlled

An insulin-dependent diabetic whose blood sugar levels are <300 mg/100 ml and who does not have long-term complications does not require a special exercise program or instructions except in the area of insulin reactions. The daily meals and insulin regimen should be planned carefully to provide the energy needed to maintain the usual daily activities and to allow for achievement and/or maintenance of ideal body weight. An unusual increase in physical activity, whether it be vigorous exercise or heavy physical labor, will increase the energy needs and require alterations in the diet in order to maintain a proper balance.

Exercise-Induced Hypoglycemia

In the insulin-dependent diabetic, increased exercise (unless accompanied by an adjustment in food intake and/or insulin dosage) may result in an insulin reaction (hypoglycemia). This occurs during increased exercise for three reasons.

1. There is an increased demand for glucose by the exercising muscle.
2. Exercise enhances the absorption of insulin from the site of injection into the blood stream. Recent studies demonstrate that exercise accelerates insulin absorption much more rapidly when it is injected into an exercising limb, especially the leg.
3. Exercising muscle responds more effectively to the insulin action.

Since the amount and kind of exercise cannot always be anticipated, it is generally recommended that food intake be increased rather than the insulin dose be decreased before the activity to avoid hypoglycemia. The following are some general considerations to keep in mind:

1. Increased exercise utilizes more calories and results in lowered blood sugar.
2. One to two hours after a light meal is a good time for exercise because the blood sugar is higher at this time.
3. If extra food is needed (in addition to scheduled meals and/or snacks), it should be eaten 15 to 20 minutes before the anticipated activity.
4. The peak action of NPH or Lente insulin occurs at ~10 to 16 hours after injection. Exercising at this time may necessitate a larger snack than usual before the exercise.
5. The use of regular insulin before eating may heighten the chances of hypoglycemia occurring 1 to 2 hours after a meal. The patient may need a larger snack at this time, too.
6. During periods of vigorous exercise, the patient may need additional food every 30 to 45 minutes.
7. All-day activities, such as skiing or backpacking, require planning. Be *overprepared* with extra food, and take plenty of carbohydrates that can be carried easily.
8. The potential for hypoglycemic symptoms can last several hours after exercise is completed. Thus, some diabetics may require additional food both after and before vigorous activity.
9. Always take a concentrated form of sugar with you to treat an insulin reaction. Some good sources and appropriate amounts are

    a. 4 cubes of sugar
    b. 6 to 7 Lifesavers
    c. 2 tablespoons of raisins
    d. 2 sugar packets
    e. 2 large marshmallows
    f. $\frac{1}{2}$ cup of orange juice
    g. $\frac{1}{2}$ cup of sweetened soft drink

If an insulin reaction occurs, take the concentrated sugar and wait 10 to 15 minutes. If the symptoms do not subside, repeat this treatment. Unless you will be eating a regularly scheduled meal within 30 to 45 minutes, follow the sugar with some complex carbohydrates (see chapter 3) and/or protein (e.g., cheese and crackers or a peanut butter sandwich).

The number of calories used in exercise depends upon the kind of exercise and its duration. Individual body size and exercise tolerance influence the determination. For this reason, only an estimate of the additional amount of carbohydrates and calories needed can be given. The caloric expenditures (calories per hour) of various exercises are given in chapter 3 (Table 3-20). These values are classified arbitrarily as light (50-199), moderate (200-299), marked (300-399), and vigorous (>400). Although the amount of supplemental calories and carbohydrates needed during exercise will vary among insulin-requiring patients, we recommend the following:

1. *Light and moderate activity*. These activities probably will not require additional food unless the activity is prolonged. If so, one fruit exchange every 30 to 45 minutes of continuous activity should be sufficient.

2. *Marked activity*. For these activities, approximately one half of the estimated caloric expenditure should be eaten before exercise. Snacks can include:

	Sample Menu
$\frac{1}{2}$ milk exchange	4 oz. nonfat milk
1 bread exchange	1 slice bread
1 meat exchange	1 oz. sliced chicken

or

1 fruit exchange	1 small orange
1 bread exchange	6 crackers
1 meat exchange	1 oz. low-fat cheese

An additional fruit exchange may be required every 30 to 45 minutes for continuous activity.

3. *Vigorous activity*. For these activities, approximately one half of the estimated caloric expenditure should be eaten before exercise. Snacks can include:

	Sample Menu
1 milk exchange	8 oz. nonfat milk
2 bread exchanges	2 slices bread
2 meat exchanges	2 oz. sliced turkey

or

1 fruit exchange	1 small apple
2 bread exchanges	1 whole bagel
2 meat exchanges	2 oz. low-fat cheese

One or two fruit exchanges may be required every 30 to 45 minutes for continuous activity.

These are only suggestions that attempt not only to prevent exercise-induced hypoglycemia in insulin-requiring patients, but also to limit unnecessary hyperglycemia due to ingestion of too many calories, especially of simple carbohydrates, for the amount of exercise performed. Patients may very well have to vary these recommendations according to their own experiences.

Uncontrolled Diabetes (Fasting Blood Sugar > 300 mg/100 ml)

In insulin-deficient diabetics, vigorous exercise may increase the level of blood sugar even further. This probably is a result of increased production of glucose by the liver (which occurs in both healthy individuals and controlled diabetics) that is not associated with an increase in glucose utilization because effective insulin is lacking. The rise in the antiinsulin hormones (adrenaline, glucagon, cortisol, and growth hormone) is greater in uncontrolled diabetes and contributes to the increase in blood sugar. Therefore, under these conditions, exercise may be more harmful than beneficial. *Exercise when the fasting blood glucose is >300 mg/100 ml may lead to even higher levels of glucose.*

Exercise for Type 2 Diabetes

STUDENT/NURSE

Type 2 diabetics tend to be obese and sedentary and lack a planned exercise program even though their lifestyle may be busy. A deliberate, planned, and graduated form of activity needs to be initiated even in older patients. Planning of individualized programs should include the following considerations:

1. The patient's physical limitations if any.
2. The patient's exercise interests (both past and present).
3. Community facilities available (e.g., YMCA/YWCA, senior citizens centers, community centers).
4. The patient's economic situation (walking is free!).

Although the presence of vascular disease may influence the type and duration of the exercise, a suitable program of aerobic exercise can be planned for most diabetic patients. For individuals whose physical limitations preclude aerobic exercise (even walking), consultation with a physical therapist to set up a program of passive and/or active exercises may be very helpful.

ANSWERS TO EVALUATIONS

A. Diabetic Syndrome (pp. 321–322)

    1. a, b
    2. a, d
    3. b, c
    4. a, b, c
    5. a, b, c, d
    6. a, c
    7. a, b, c, d

B. Insulin (pp. 339–340)

    1. c

    2. a

C. Oral Hypoglycemic Sulfonylurea Agents (p. 344)

    1. True

    2. True

    3. False

    4. b, c, f

D. Monitoring Diabetic Control (pp. 360–361)

    1. a, b, c

    2. c

    3. b, c

    4. b

    5. a, b, c

E. Diabetic Emergencies (pp. 375–376)

    1. a, d

    2. b, c, e, f

    3. a, b, d

    4. a

    5. c

    6. a, b, c, d, e

    7. a, b, c

F. Foot Care (pp. 383–385)

    1. b

    2. a, b, c

    3. a, b, d

    4. a, b, c, d

    5. a

    6. a, d

    7. b, c

    8. a, b, c, d

Appendix

Mechanical Aids

Insulin Needle Guide

A funnel-shaped opening that guides the needle into the rubber cap of the insulin bottle. Obtain from the American Foundation for the Blind, 15 W. 16th Street, New York, NY 10011.

Syringe Magnifiers

1. Monoject insulin-syringe scale magnifier. Available in 1-cc and 0.5 cc sizes. Fits all disposable insulin syringe brands. Magnification 2x for doubly accurate dosage. Catalog no. 8881-641005. Contact local Monoject representative or write Monoject, St. Louis, MO 63103.
2. Cemco Magnifier fits all disposable and glass insulin syringes. Order from Cemco, PO Box 21, Scanda, MN 55073.

Service Organizations

The American Foundation for the Blind
15 W. 16th St.
New York, NY 10011

A nonprofit organization that provides a wide variety of services, aids, and publications for the blind. Among their free publications are:

1. *Catalog of Publications.* A listing of all books, pamphlets, journals available from the organization.
2. *Catalog of Aids and Appliances for the Blind and Visually Handicapped.* Includes watches, alarm clocks, canes, kitchen aids, and devices that enable blind diabetics to measure and administer insulin.

The New York Association for the Blind
111 E. 59th St.
New York, NY 10022

This agency has an impressive range of services. Write for their list of books and pamphlets, available in inkprint or Braille. They record *Diabetes Forecast* in full. Cassette tapes are free on loan if you pick them up, or $1.50 per tape (there are usually three tapes per issue) if they are mailed to you. The association will record an issue for you free of charge if you send in 90 minutes' worth of blank tape. Another of its services is the Low-Vision Clinic, staffed by optometrists and ophthalmologists who work with insulin-dependent diabetics. They demonstrate different equipment available to the patient with low vision.

Library of Congress
Division of the Blind and Physically Handicapped
1291 Taylor St.
Washington, DC 20542

Provides materials for those who are unable to read or use standard printed materials because of visual impairment. Materials are available in Braille and large print and on cassettes, disks, and open-reel recordings. They can be both delivered to the patient's home and returned postage free. Cassette players and phonographs are loaned without charge to patients eligible to borrow talking books. The Library of Congress materials circulate through a network of 54 regional and 100 subregional libraries (local libraries with access to the resources of regional libraries). A wide selection of books and magazines is available to individuals of all ages. *Encore* is a bimonthly magazine of taped excerpts from selected publications (including *Diabetes Forecast*) of interest to blind and handicapped people. Bimonthly magazines with listings of new titles are available in large type and Braille and on cassettes.

Diabetes Forecast

American Diabetes Association, Inc.
2 Park Ave.
New York, NY 10016

National Diabetes Information Clearinghouse
805 15th St. NW, Suite 500
Washington, DC 20005

Provides monthly bibliographies and selected annotations on a variety of subjects, such as: Spanish language materials, careers, and employment. Some titles include *Spanish Language Materials, Employment,* and *Diabetic Educational Materials for Adults with Limited Reading Skills.*

Identification

Medic Alert Foundation International
PO Box 1009
Turlock, CA 95380

Supplies identification bracelets, necklaces, and wallet cards to identify individuals with chronic illnesses (e.g., diabetes) that may need immediate treatment or consideration in emergencies. Products are available for a small fee. A specific designation that the patient is taking insulin can be included on the identification.

Free Literature

Ames Co., Division of Miles Laboratories, Eckhart, In 46514

American Heart Association, local affiliates (exercise and nutrition)

American Diabetes Associations, local affiliates

Becton-Dickinson, Consumer Products, Rochelle Park, NJ 07662

Eli Lilly & Co., Indianapolis, In 46206

ER Squibb & Sons, Inc., Princeton, NJ 08540

The Upjohn Co., Kalamazoo, MI 49001

Monoject, 1831 Olive St., St. Louis, MO 63103

Bibliography

General

Krall L: *Joslin Diabetes Manual*, 11th ed. Lea and Febiger, Philadelphia, 1978

Nursing Skillbook: Managing Diabetes Properly. Intermed Communications, Inc, EW Jackson, Horsham, PA, 1978

Waife SO: *Diabetes Mellitus*, 8th ed. Eli Lilly & Co, Indianapolis, 1980

Patient Education

Peters V: Teaching learning strategies. Diabetes Educator 6:23-26, 1980

Redman BC: *Process of Patient Teaching in Nursing.* CV Mosby, St. Louis, 1972, pp 18-20

Diabetes Syndrome

Davidson MB: Diabetes mellitus and hypoglycemia. In *Endocrine Pathophysiology. A Patient-Oriented Approach.* Edited by Hershman JM. Lea and Febiger, Philadelphia, 1977, pp 193-208

Gebhardt M, Garnett W: Drugs affecting carbohydrate metabolism. In *Diabetes Mellitus*, 4th ed. Edited by Sussman KE, Metz RJS. American Diabetes Association, New York, 1975, pp 271-273

Classification

National Diabetes Data Group. Classification and diagnosis of diabetes mellitus and other categories of glucose intolerance. Diabetes 28:1039-1057, 1979

Complications

Coughlin RW, Patz A: Diabetic retinopathy. Diabetes Forecast 31:26-28, 1978

Danowski TS, Ohlsen P, Fisher E-R: Diabetic complications and their prevention or reversal. Diabetes Care 3:94-99, 1980

Insulin

Banting FG, Best CH, Collys JB, et al: Pancreatic extracts in the treatment of diabetes mellitus: preliminary report. Can Med Assoc J 12:141-146, 1922

Cahill G: *Insulin Physiology.* Medicon, USV Pharmaceutical Corp, New York, 1970, pp 27-41

Ferland L, Ehrlich M: Single-peak insulin in the treatment of insulin-induced fat atrophy. J Pediatr 86:741-743, 1975

Galloway JA: Insulin treatment for the early 80s. Facts and questions about old and new insulins and their usage. Diabetes Care 3:615-622, 1980

Hulst SGTh: Treatment of insulin-induced lipoatrophy. Diabetes 25:1052-1054, 1976

Kahn RC, Rosenthal AS: Immunologic reactions to insulin: insulin resistance and the autoimmune insulin syndrome. Diabetes Care 2:283-295, 1979

Kovisto V, Felig AP: Alterations in insulin absorption and in blood glucose control associated with varying insulin injection sites in diabetic patients. Ann Interm Med 92:59-61, 1980

Pital M: The subcutaneous injection. Am J Nurs 71:76-79, 1971

Oral Hypoglycemic Agents

Lebovitz H, Feinglos M: Sulfonylurea drugs: mechanism of antidiabetic action and therapeutic usefulness. Diabetes Care 1:189-198, 1978

Waife SO: Hypoglycemia due to insulin and the sulfonylurea agents. In *Diabetes Mellitus*, 8th ed. Eli Lilly & Co, Indianapolis, 1980, pp 140-149.

Monitoring Diabetic Control

Bernstein R: Blood glucose self-monitoring by diabetic patients: refinements of procedural technique. Diabetes Care 2:233-234, 1979

Bleicher S (ed): Symposium on home glucose monitoring. Diabetes Care 3:57-186, 1980

Cole R: The significance of hemoglobin A_{1c} in diabetes mellitus. In *Current Concepts*. The Upjohn Company, Kalamazoo, MI, 1978, pp 3-11

Guthrie D, Hinnen D, Guthrie RA: Single-voided vs. double-voided urine testing. Diabetes Care 2:269-271, 1979

Hamburger J, Richet G, Greenfeld JP: Organ physiology: structure and function of the kidney. WB Saunders, Philadelphia, 1971, pp 50-81

Home Urine Testing for the Diabetic: Instructional Aid for Diabetes Educators. Ames Co., Division of Miles Laboratories, Inc, Elkhart, IA, 1978

Malone J, Rosenbloom A, Gragic A, Weber T: The role of urine sugar in diabetic management. Am J Dis Child 130:1324-1326, 1976

Diabetic Emergencies

Clements RS, Vourganti B: Fatal diabetic ketoacidosis: major causes and approaches to their prevention. Diabetes Care 1:314-324, 1978

Kreisberg RA: Diabetic ketoacidosis: new concepts and trends in pathogenesis and treatment. Ann Intern Med 88:681-695, 1978

Mazzaferri EL: Endocrine and metabolic emergencies: heart and lung. J Crit Care 7:594-602, 1978

Wright AD, Penny ME: Beta blockers and hypoglycemia. Diabetes Care 3:204-205, 1980

Foot Care

Bagdade J: Infection in diabetes, implications of hyperglycemia. *Medical Information–Medical Education Communications Inc.* Pfizer, Inc, New York, 1972, pp 28-34

Bell ET: Atherosclerotic gangrene of lower extremities in diabetic and non-diabetic persons. Am J Clin Pathol 28:27–36, 1957

Levin ME, O'Neal LW: *The Diabetic Foot*, 2nd ed. CV Mosby, St Louis, 1977

Lippmann HI: Must loss of limb be a consequence of diabetes mellitus? Diabetes Care 2:432–436, 1979

Wagner W: The diabetic foot and amputation of the foot. In *DeVries Surgery of the Foot*, 4th ed. Edited by Mann RA. CV Mosby, St Louis, 1978, pp. 341–381

Exercise

Bierman J, Tookey B: *The Diabetic's Total Health Book*. JP Tarcher, Los Angeles, 1980, pp 94–121

Consolazia CF: Physiologic measurement of metabolic functions in man. McGraw-Hill, New York, 1963, pp 329–332

Cooper K: *The New Aerobics*. Bantam Books, New York, 1975.

Skyler JS: Diabetes and exercise: clinical implications. Diabetes Care 2:307–311, 1979

Chapter 9

Emotions: A Critical Factor in Diabetic Control

Wendy S. Citrin
Gary A. Kleiman
Jay S. Skyler

Patients with diabetes mellitus and their families may respond to the diagnosis, treatment, or complications of the disease with a variety of feelings, such as guilt, anger, anxiety, resentment, or challenge. The presence of diabetes changes one's self-image and creates internal and external conflicts related to a sense of loss, the demands of the treatment program, the fear or presence of debilitating complications, and the fear of shortened life. In addition, diabetes often serves as a focus for other problems and conflicts in life; in turn, the diabetes may be influenced by these life stresses. Indeed, emotional stress leads to secretion of a variety of hormones (epinephrine, norepinephrine, glucagon, growth hormone, cortisol) that, among their many biological effects, counteract the actions of insulin. This causes increased glycemia and lipolysis with ketonemia in insulin-dependent diabetes. Thus, emotional stress leads to disruption of metabolic control in patients who cannot compensate for the counterregulatory surge because they are incapable of incremental secretion of insulin.

In insulin-dependent diabetes mellitus (IDDM), glycemic control is maintained by a balance between the expenditure and availability of energy and the action of injected insulin necessary for effective utilization of energy. The three traditional components of therapy emerge from this equation: the *nutritional plan*, the *exercise prescription*, and the *insulin dosage*. Stress-induced secretion of counterregulatory hormones can disrupt this therapeutic balance. Dealing with a patient's emotional needs and problems is an equally important component of management. Not only do emotions directly affect glycemia (mediated via counterregulatory hormones), but emotional stress may result in alteration of eating habits, activity routine, or even adherence to the insulin regimen, thereby impairing glycemic control further. Moreover, emotions may be used in a positive sense to enhance treatment and thus become an integral component of therapy.

400

The purpose of this chapter is to discuss clinical strategies that we have found useful in helping diabetic patients to cope with their emotional responses. We base our approach on three fundamental premises. First, there is a bidirectional relationship between diabetes and life—diabetes affects life and life affects diabetes. Second, as a corollary to the first premise, our therapeutic program for diabetes should not compromise the patient's emotional well-being or life activities (e.g., educational, recreational, vocational); conversely, we must help the patient achieve a full life and attain emotional well-being without sacrificing diabetic control. Third, as already stated, emotions are an integral component of diabetes therapy. Indeed, often the most challenging aspect of diabetes management is helping the patient and family cope with the various emotional turmoils that emerge while watching for serious emotional problems that may require specific intervention.

Background

A work group at the recent National Conference on Behavioral and Psychosocial Issues in Diabetes (1) emphasized that certain events in the lives of individuals are predictable crises because they severely tax the patient's ability to cope. The onset of the diabetes is one such crisis. The first manifestations of a complication or the first experience with disability are other obvious crises, as is the recognition that, despite all efforts, diabetes cannot always be well controlled. Other predictable crises are related to transitions in the patient's life, such as marriage, pregnancy, career changes, moving, discrimination, bereavement, and so on.

A major predictable crisis may occur at the time of onset of IDDM. This event creates trauma in the life of the patient and his or her family that may be more powerful than the anxiety induced by other chronic diseases. Indeed, there is no other disease that requires such a lifelong commitment on the part of the patient: daily insulin injections, careful meal planning, balancing physical activity with variations in food intake and insulin, monitoring therapy. In addition, the patient labors under the threat of severe and devastating complications (both acute and chronic), the possibility of a shortened lifespan, and, if he or she is preoccupied with the incurability (at present) of the disease, a constant feeling of hopelessness. It is no surprise, then, that diabetic patients and their families often are overwhelmed and have difficulty adapting to the circumstances of the illness.

Conceptually, the reactions of a person who learns he or she has diabetes (or, at a later stage, who experiences a complication or confronts disability) may be seen as stages, akin to those described by Kübler-Ross for dying patients (2): (a) shock and denial, (b) anger and protest, (c) bargaining, (d) depression, and (d) either acceptance and growth or pathologic sequelae. Examples of this sequence appear in Table 9-1. The progression through these stages, however,

Table 9-1. Examples of Application of the Kübler-Ross Model to Diabetes

	Patient Response To	
Stage	New Diagnosis or Long-Term Management	Onset of Complications[a]
Shock and denial	Disregarding consistent food management	Disregarding reduced ability to drive car, particularly in bright sunlight or at night
Anger	Refusing to take insulin injection; consciously overeating	Wanting to change doctors
Bargaining	Agreeing to test urine, but not recording results	Agreeing to follow regimen only if complications are reversed
Depression	Reporting lethargy, fatigue, and feelings of pessimism and helplessness	Not attempting to maximize existing abilities (premature invalidism)
Adjustment	Keeping appointments; actively participating in management	Taking advantage of resources, e.g., Bureau of Blind Services

[a]Responses described use the example of diabetic retinopathy.

may not be smooth. At times the patient will regress and may fail to progress to the next stage, as with those who experience protracted depression. Occasionally, patients traverse the stages without adequate support systems (from self, family, and professionals) and have a disastrous pathologic outcome in lieu of achieving the anticipated acceptance and growth. The rate of progress through these stages varies and is influenced by a variety of interrelated factors, including the patient's personality structure, degree of maturity, and emotional response; the emotional and behavioral response of the patient's parents, spouse, family, and significant others; the family structure; and the adequacy of support systems offered by health professionals.

This conceptual framework may be helpful in understanding the patient's response. However, Giarratana-Oehler (3) questions whether anyone ever accepts or adjusts to a chronic disability. She argues that " 'acceptance' implies compliance and approval, and 'adjusted to' connotes something final and complete." Life, she points out, is a series of adjustments. She prefers the concept of "identity integration," which permits a person to express anger, depression, and frustration in constructive ways. Her point may be semantic, but it serves to emphasize that, after the initial adaptation period, the patient experiences a continuing series of conflicts and frustrations engendered merely by having diabetes. The challenge to therapists is to help patients deal with these conflicts and frustrations and express their emotions in a way that will minimize disruption of diabetic control.

Diabetes management imposes demands that alter the individual's lifestyle. The need to achieve balance among food, activity, insulin, and emotions requires coordination, is time consuming, and distracts from the spontaneous flow of life. The pressures imposed by the need to achieve physiologic regulation may result in psychic stress. Moreover, the attention required to balance food intake and activity results in exaggerated attention to the details of life. Conversely, relatively trivial life stresses are magnified because they may disrupt glycemic control. Thus, as the individual with diabetes goes through life, the details of life receive heightened importance.

Complications of diabetes impose additional stresses. Recognition of a complication can constitute a predictable crisis in the life of a diabetic patient. However, the manifestations of complications are quite varied, as is the degree of disability any given patient may suffer. For example, a substantial proportion of patients with advanced diabetic retinopathy may be legally blind but not functionally blind. Many may be able to maintain their usual employment, to read, or even to drive an automobile. Yet even though function is preserved, the emotional reaction to being legally blind may cripple the ability of some patients to function in life, since their negative perception of the disability is greater than is warranted by the actual impairment. Another example of the attitudinal component contributing to complications is the anticipation of impotence. This may become a self-fulfilling prophecy by producing sufficient anxiety to cause psychogenic impotence, which accounts for a substantial portion of impotence in the diabetic population.

Disability also may affect family relationships, since relatives must compensate for the disability, provide alternative sources of income, and help the patient live with the disability. Some complications may have a direct impact on specific family members, such as a spouse who is affected by impotence or a family member under consideration as a kidney donor. Thus, the attitudes of family members are important and must continually be considered.

The Therapeutic Relationship

The chronic nature of diabetes dictates that the therapeutic approach has both short-range and long-range goals, and the role of the patient and of the health professional differ accordingly.

The health-care system in the United States is such that patients and health professionals generally are more familiar and more comfortable handling acute problems with short-range solutions. In such circumstances the health professional assumes the dominant managerial role. The problems are concrete, usually unidirectional, perhaps crisis related, and have solutions that generally are straightforward and confined to the immediate situation. Goals are easily defined and are generally attainable. Ketoacidosis is an obvious example of such an acute type of problem. However, any intercurrent illness in a diabetic patient may also create an acute problem.

With acute problems, the patient usually assumes a relatively passive role. The health professional, however, may wish to emphasize to the patient the importance of some component of therapy or teach the patient more about diabetes in the hope of avoiding future calamities. Yet severe crises may induce fear in the patient. Although such fear may enhance motivation to learn how to avoid future crises, the emotional response to the existing crisis may block learning and thus prevent the patient from absorbing and integrating information. The astute professional recognizes the patient's fears and concerns and appreciates the complexities of providing detailed, long-range solutions but capitalizes on the situation by initiating a plan of action that can be sustained beyond the crisis period.

In contrast to the relationship between active professional and passive patient during acute crises, the long-term management of diabetes requires a partnership between patient and health professionals. The partners must build a foundation of communication to develop approaches to living with diabetes and dealing with its problems. The treatment process must be dynamic and ongoing, and be aimed at maintaining balance and control of the disease. Yet attempting to deal continually with a problem that will not go away may result in enormous frustrations for the patient. The struggle to live with diabetes requires health professionals who are sensitive to these frustrations, knowledgeable about the nature and dynamics of the patient's disease, responsive to the patient's needs and concerns, and willing and able to develop an appropriate and acceptable plan of action. The health professional must not only guide the patient by providing rational choices but be alert to the patient's reactions to life, diabetes, and the management plan. The patient assumes the active role in day-to-day management, while the health professional provides intermittent guidance, counseling, and support. This includes acknowledging the patient's frustrations.

Both the patient and health professional must adapt to their dual roles as partners in the management of a chronic disease that may be punctuated by acute crises. The active-passive relationship may be resumed during these crises. Moreover, life events may create episodic situations that require the development of special temporary interventions. If the professional fails to help orient the patient to the nature of their relationship, the patient may develop expectations of their interactions with the health professionals or of responses that may be appropriate to some situations and inappropriate to others (e.g., responsibility issues, time commitments). Further, and of paramount importance, the patient must appreciate that long-term management of diabetes involves all aspects of life and cannot be dealt with in a vacuum. As was emphasized earlier, diabetes affects life and life affects diabetes, with the problems of one magnifying those of the other.

Therapeutic Strategies

Emotions are an integral component in balancing the treatment of diabetes. Thus, health professionals need to recognize emotional stress and respond to the emotional needs of their patients. Moreover, health professionals can and should predict patient responses and take action to prevent and/or lessen emotional turmoil. Thus, just as the patient is given a dietary prescription, an exercise prescription, and an insulin prescription, he or she may be given a prescription for emotions. This prescription may include supportive, preventive, and/or therapeutic interventions.

Dialogue

A key prerequisite to successfully dealing with the emotional factor in diabetes is maintenance of open dialogue to encourage the patient to express feelings. All patients harbor feelings about diabetes and the limitations and regulations imposed by the disease, and must be able to express these feelings and ventilate their conflicts and frustrations. Such feelings must be accepted as natural and legitimate even if the resulting behavior (e.g., noncompliance, acting out) is intolerable. The patient's behavioral response to these feelings may need to be altered or channeled in another direction. It is not necessary (nor is it always possible) to analyze the dynamics of the patient's feelings and emotions. Rather, encouraging the patient to express feelings not only opens channels of communication and permits the health professional to understand how the patient is coping with diabetes and life, but it brings humanism to the therapeutic interaction and personalizes it by not being concerned solely with objective parameters (e.g., blood glucose measurements, glycosylated hemoglobin levels).

Central to a successful dialogue with the patient is the use of concrete communication and intervention skills. These may require the health professional to assume any of a number of roles, such as (a) positive reframer, (b) predictor, (c) role model/information giver, (d) emotional development planner, or (e) coordinator/coach.

As a *positive reframer*, the health professional communicates to the patient the positive aspects of any situation. For example, if the patient views having diabetes in solely a negative way, the professional may try to convey that successfully coping with diabetes is a challenge that offers the opportunity for personal growth, such as handling increased responsibility, increasing sensitivity, independence, and problem-solving capabilities, and making effective decisions.

As a *predictor*, the health professional predicts the nature and course of the diabetes, including the emotional aspects and the patient's response to the disease, in a time frame that is appropriate for the patient and family. The accurate prediction of the impact of emotional stress on diabetic control is as important as the accurate prediction of the impact of physical stress (e.g., intercurrent infection). For example, emotional stress may lead to anger, which in turn may be manifested by the patient's failure to comply with the routines of diabetes management. The health professional may wish to inform the patient that feelings of frustration or noncompliance may arise during times of stress. Merely predicting this possibility may actually lessen the likelihood of its occurrence by validating the feeling rather than by contending with the behavior.

Prediction may follow the Kübler-Ross scheme and may be related to the phenomenon of predictable crises noted earlier. For example, at the time a complication develops the health professional may tell the patient that he or she may go through a sequence of responses to the complication. Before the complication develops, we find it helpful to couple the prediction of the patient's response with a caveat that offers a positive viewpoint. For example, although it is possible for blindness to occur, it does so in only a small minority of diabetic patients and its risk can be lessened by maintaining careful diabetic control.

As a *role model/information giver*, the health professional creates an atmosphere conducive to learning—for example, by asking questions rather than by lecturing. This approach has the advantages of giving the patient a sense of control by allowing him or her to share in decision making and of increasing the patient's self-esteem with his or her growing mastery of diabetes management skills. Asking questions, together with other communication skills, provides a model approach that the patient can utilize in other life situations, such as dealing with family, friends, and associates. Once the professional is sure that the patient has mastered the concepts, he or she may then wish to identify other areas of concern. This permits the acknowledgment of goal completion and the setting of future goals. Yet the professional must also be a clear medical director. In this regard, the professional must be sure that the patient understands specific recommendations. Moreover, the professional may need to confront the patient on specific issues. Such confrontations should be honest and nonjudgmental, and the professional should display neither timidity nor authoritarianism. For example, a projective technique for confronting a patient suspected of fraudulently reporting urine test results might be as follows: "Why do you suppose you or a friend of yours might not want to be honest in recording results?" (4).

Another useful strategy for encouraging appropriate decision making is role reversal. For example, the health professional might ask the patient, "If you were the doctor, what would you say to me, the patient?" If the patient is blocked by his or her own case, it may be desirable either to project another one or to ask the patient to solve another patient's problem. These techniques are helpful in the patient's self-analysis and permit the patient to gain a sense of control and personal mastery. Even if the patient's choice of a solution is different from the therapist's own ideas, it may be desirable either to implement that plan (at least for a trial period) or to reframe the situation by providing additional information or asking more questions until the patient arrives at a more acceptable answer. For example, a patient who prefers to adjust food intake or activity rather than insulin dosage, as the physician suggests, may be permitted to do so.

As an *emotional development planner*, it is important for the health professional to devise an approach on the basis of the strengths and weaknesses of the individual patient and his or her family. In addition, factors such as personal and social development; cultural, ethnic, and religious background (e.g., some societies view overweight as healthy); financial status; and sexual development and reactions are important considerations in planning emotional development. The professional should proceed in a logical manner, as follows: recognize and predict problems, collect data from patient and family, assess the data, plan appropriate intervention strategies (or, for complex problems, provide referral information), evaluate outcome. The approach should be practical. For example, permitting and planning for unusual food intake (with appropriate administration of compensatory insulin or increase in physical activity) can help the patient avoid potential eating disorders and the accompanying loss of both diabetic and emotional control. Such planning also eliminates expectations of perfection and prevents unplanned eating binges from sabotaging control.

Each patient's personality structure influences his or her response to diabetes therapy. Therefore, the health professional may wish to assess the patient's personality style in order to reinforce assets, limit the negative extremes of these assets, and create new coping mechanisms. Table 9-2 illustrates how some personality styles might be assessed in this manner.

As *coordinator/coach*, the health professional is responsible for helping the patient learn to manage diabetes on a daily basis, for ensuring that the patient has available appropriate therapy for any problems, and for monitoring the progress of the disease and its therapy. Health professionals differ in their ability both to handle and solve emotional problems and to foster the patient's emotional growth. Each professional must establish his or her appropriate place on the continuum from direct provision of services to referral. Excesses on either end of the continuum (omnipotence or "dumping") are inappropriate. Thus, professionals probably will attempt to solve some problems and refer others for appropriate intervention. The professional will select a role on the basis of his or her background and interests in dealing with emotional issues; the cost to the professional in time, energy, and emotional expenditure; and how effectively and comprehensively the professional can deal with the problem. Table 9-3 gives a sample dialogue that illustrates several of the points discussed above.

Specific Interventions

In helping patients learn to cope with diabetes and to lessen the frequently disruptive impact of life events on diabetic control, the health professional may use any of a number of specific intervention strategies that mental health

Table 9-2. Examples of Strategies Based on Patient's Personality Style

Personality Style	Intervention		
	Supportive[a]	*Preventive*[b]	*Therapeutic*[c]
Compulsive	Patient will be organized in care procedure.	Physician should help patient to relax expectations of perfection in care by predicting fluctuations regardless of quality of management.	Patient should create self-taught statements that prohibit negative self-image when control is less than perfect.
Demanding	Patient will get needed attention from physician, community agencies.	Patient should be shown how his or her demands may alienate family or physician or overwhelm self. Physician should discuss how patient can get good care without causing alienation.	Patient should be taught to be more independent through self-analysis rather than through decision making by family or physician.
Laissez-faire	Patient will be less likely to experience either stress-induced loss of control or stress due to loss of control	Patient should be encouraged to recognize that lack of attention to diabetes management may have adverse outcomes.	Patient should be taught to introduce new tasks gradually and successively and at a comfortable pace.

[a]Consists of positive reframing and reinforcement of the patient's assets.
[b]Consists of deemphasizing extremes of behavior that hinder diabetic control.
[c]Consists of creating new mechanisms for coping with diabetes.

Table 9-3. Sample Dialogue Illustrating Roles and Communication Skills for the Physician

Dialogue		Role and Skill
Patient:	"My sugars are still high. *You're* not helping me."	
Doctor:	"I know how frustrated you are with not being in good control."	Role model (listening and reflecting supportively)
Patient:	"Well, wouldn't you be?"	
Doctor:	"Yes, I think I might be, too."	
Patient:	"Well, at least I'm normal."	
Doctor:	"Yes, your feelings are normal. You have to expect that, no matter how perfect you attempt to be, there will be times when your glycemic control will waiver."	Predictor (validating patient's feelings and anticipating the course of management)
Patient:	"Well, what should I do now?"	
Doctor:	"The first step to solving problems is voicing your feelings, as you have just done. I'm glad to hear you express this annoyance."	Positive reframer (communicating positive aspects of the problem)
	"Let's take a look at the records and see if we can trace what factors are involved."[a]	Coordinator/coach (helping patient plan concrete solution)

[a]At this point, the patient no longer is distracted from the real issues by blaming doctor. Having vented his or her feelings, the patient may be more receptive to solving the problem.

specialists have utilized extensively for other problems. Some of these intervention strategies, along with some potential advantages of each for diabetes management, are outlined in Table 9-4. Many of these intervention strategies are helpful in facilitating general coping with diabetes, while others are useful in helping the patient cope with specific problems related to their disease.

Emotional Reactions of Diabetic Patients

Emotional reactions may occur in response to the diabetes itself, to failure at attaining diabetic control, or to effects from other spheres of life. Having diabetes in itself may lead to feelings of inferiority related to loss of independence or control (e.g., the need for help when hypoglycemic reactions occur or if vision

Table 9-4. Strategic Interventions That are Useful for Improving Patient's Emotional Response to Diabetes

Intervention	Description	Examples of Advantages
Relaxation training	Behavioral therapy techniques used to counteract tension or anxiety	Reduces effects of stress on blood glucose during family argument or before examination
Successive approximation	Division of a comprehensive goal into smaller, more workable goals	Offers intellectual information in discrete units, e.g., emotional adjustment to diabetes will occur in stages, with grief as the first response
Cognitive therapy/restructuring	Method of using intellectual and verbal processes to deal with feelings of inadequacy	Helps patient to plan ahead to avoid impulsive eating behavior, possibly by taking supplemental insulin prior to a party. Helps to improve patient's self-image in relation to poor results of urine test; patient can learn that "my urine records are not indicators of personal badness or goodness; therefore, when my records reflect imperfect control, I don't have to lie about the results."
Parenting skills	Method for single parent or husband and wife to develop concrete decision making, and communication skills in unit separate from their children; any orientation may be effective as long as they agree on the nature of the discipline	Helps parents of diabetic children to be confident in insisting that child follow guidelines
Marital interaction	Extension of parenting skills. Men and women actualize their roles by strengthening existing interaction or creating new outlets	Helps alleviate strains of managing a diabetic child; helps develop good communication that is essential to reducing stress when one partner in marriage has diabetes

Self-reinforcement	System for changing or strengthening behavior patterns through self-reward	Fosters statements of self-praise in relation to achieving/maintaining control ("I really liked how I didn't eat anything extra at the party"); encourages concrete self-reward that the patient decides he or she deserves ("I will treat myself to a concert now that I have begun to test regularly again")
Exercise	Regular, disciplined outings for reducing stress and increasing well-being	Encourages running as an antidepressant, source of improved body image and self-concept
Concrete services	Community agencies that offer various aspects of physical care	Provide transportation services to lessen family's financial burden or reduce family responsibility; Bureau of Blind Services, United Way, Visiting Nurse, Hot Meals on Wheels, etc.
Systematic desensitization	Behavior therapy technique that teaches relaxation and gradual and successive management of learned concepts/ideas or concrete management behavior	Helps to reduce fears of blood being drawn or injections given; helps patient to adjust slowly to accepting diabetes and its management
Booster group session	Periodic meetings to review intellectual and emotional viewpoints and to remotivate patients by allowing self-expression and providing emotional support	Serves as a socially acceptable outlet for expressing feelings about being diabetic; encourages self-esteem through mutual support, regardless of level of control achieved
Role play	Simulation of a problem situation by patient and/or family in order to reduce the anxiety surrounding it or to try alternative approaches to it	Allows the patient to rehearse his or her reaction to a problem situation

Table 9-4. (continued)

Intervention	Description	Examples of Advantages
Buddy system	Matching of patient with another patient in a similar circumstance or with a patient successful in adjusting to diabetes management	Prevents isolation, reinforces growth a patient and family have already achieved; serves as a booster session for patient and/or family to encourage continued growth and good compliance
Hypnotherapy	Technique for controlling phobias, pain, habits, or attitudes by utilizing the subconscious mind	Reduces phobias of self-injection in newly diagnosed patients; reduces pain resulting from complications (e.g., neuropathy)
Group-process formats	Supportive, prophylactic, and therapeutic approach to teaching and growing	Offers some of the healing and change-producing qualities inherent in group learning or therapy and relevant to diabetes control; imparts information, instills hope, universality, altruism, corrective recapitulation of primary family, etc.
Assertiveness training	Learning to identify and express both positive and negative needs, expectations, disappointments, and anger to family, health professionals, peers, and work systems	Helps patient to overcome shyness about scheduling eating times during school or work; helps patient to handle questions about his or her disease without becoming irritated with friends, coworkers, etc.
Self-help group with professional guidance	Method of helping patients balance their relationship with their disease	Reduces patients feelings of isolation through identification with others; introduces means of catharsis and exchange of creative ideas for solving problems; encourages effective interaction; fosters greater self-esteem through

		expertise in diabetes management; introduces "generalization" principle of learning, which involves application of new skills in other areas by behavior simulation in group
Diabetes camp	Extension of self-help group; beneficial properties for teaching, improved body image, and interactional skills	Teaches physical agility for building good body image; teaches patient to cope with the need for exercise and its relaxing effects on emotions
Positive reframing	Technique of salvaging and stating positive aspects of a situation	Illuminates what the crisis of diabetes has done for individual or family; refocuses attention from loss of control to present efforts to maintain control; suggests that positive thoughts lead to positive self-concept and possibly to better diabetic control
Humor	Device for approaching sensitive material through catharsis and improving interactional skills	Helps to break stalemates by providing a flexible perspective of a situation; stresses that laughter changes physiologic state by lessening anxiety or tension

is impaired, concern over living alone), financial problems (e.g., medical bills, insurance, limitations to employment), and altered or decreased sexual response (e.g., the effects of vaginal monilial infections from chronic hyperglycemia on desire and comfort, neurogenic impotence, psychogenic impotence resulting from fear of neurogenic impotence). Other feelings in this category include guilt from being a burden to one's family, resentment from being "different," depression from worrying what will happen next, and hostility from feeling that the diabetes is a "punishment." The patient also may feel disappointment when he or she fails to achieve diabetic control. Yet failure to achieve control may result from (*a*) unrealistic expectations on the part of health professionals, the patient, or the family; (*b*) deliberate noncompliance, as a sign of either depression or a need for attention; or (*c*) ungoverned emotional stress that exacerbates hyperglycemia. Effects from other spheres of life may lead to emotional trauma and thus disrupt control. Any of these or other emotional reactions may ultimately have the same manifestations: a sad patient with uncontrolled hyperglycemia. Thus, it is important to assess the problem carefully and seek out the patient's feelings before designing an intervention strategy.

Objective data may contribute to the evaluation and assessment of emotional problems. For example, we have found that a marked discrepancy between diabetic control, as determined by levels of glycosylated hemoglobin, and diabetic control, as reflected by results of urine glucose tests, often is a sign of emotional problems in dealing with diabetes (4). Indeed, there may be a number of mechanisms responsible for such discrepant results. In the scheme shown in Table 9-5, the diabetic patient may respond either to personal expectations or to those of family, peers, or health professionals. Thus, seeking perfection may be either an individual or a family characteristic. Resentment can be seen as either the patient's own resentment toward the disease or the resentment of family or medical professionals who impose demands concerning diabetes management. In order to understand the origin of discrepant results and to choose appropriate action, health professionals often must deal with the family unit. Health professionals may need to display great sensitivity to these important issues and may need to alter even their own behavior.

Identification of the underlying mechanism responsible for discrepant results (Table 9-5) involves a carefully conducted interview that is nonjudgmental and solicits patient interpretation of the "meaning" of the discrepancy between the glycosylated hemoglobin level and the urine glucose results. Role playing or role reversal may be used in the assessment process. An honest exchange should be promoted, but from the standpoint of self-understanding rather than confession. Often, face-saving gestures may be used, e.g, reviewing urine testing procedures, using new Clinitest tablets, or agreeing to careful testing practices for one week. This allows the patient time to reflect on the circumstances and may permit a more fruitful interchange at the next encounter.

The underlying mechanism defines the patient's needs and concerns and dictates in large part the corrective action. With appropriate guidance, the patient

Table 9-5. Underlying Mechanisms Responsible for Discrepant Test Results

Underlying Mechanism	Feeling[a]	Behavioral Response
Seeking perfection	I want to be 100% okay	Therefore, I record results as being 100% okay
Seeking approval	I want you to be pleased and proud of me	Therefore, I give you results that make you pleased and proud
Seeking independence	I want to be in charge	Therefore, I give you results that show what I want you to see
Avoiding punishment	I don't want you to punish me	Therefore, I give you results that won't make you think I deserve punishment
Avoiding confronta-tation (criticism)	I don't want you to question or accuse me	Therefore, I give you results that encourage you to leave me alone
Avoiding judgment	I don't want to hear that I'm bad	Therefore, I give you results that won't elicit negative comments from you
Avoiding depression	I don't want to pay attention to diabetes and feel sad	Therefore, I won't do the tests so that I won't have to face sadness
Expressing denial	I don't have diabetes	Therefore, I need not do the tests
Expressing resent-ment or anger	I hate diabetes; I hate how you make me deal with diabetes	Therefore, I won't do what you ask me to do
Expressing guilt	I cheated	Therefore, I'll hide the cheating

[a]"You" refers to the health professional.

should set the goals for change. The expectations must be realistic and must be met over a planned time frame. Goals may be staggered, and the patient may reach the ultimate objective in successive steps. A diary of the patient's feelings and alternative actions is often a useful adjuvant in defining issues and developing strategies. The patient should be encouraged to work through the process, with the health professional assuming an educative, supportive, and facilitative role rather than an executive or authoritative one. This approach also encourages the patient to learn responsible decision making and to improve self-understanding. Many of the interventions outlined previously (Table 9-4) may be helpful in solving the problem.

This discussion indicates that different underlying mechanisms may result in the same behavioral outcome, that assessment is crucial to therapy, and that a variety of intervention strategies may be useful. Discussing the problem with the patient is therapeutic in itself. For example, a patient may be reporting fraudulent urine results because he or she is tired of striving for good control. In order to encourage good long-term control, the health professional should routinely acknowledge the difficulty of always having to face the burdens of diabetes and should support the patient's need to "take a vacation" from the demands of diabetic control. Acceptance of the patient's struggle, or at least acknowledgment of the patient's need to be relieved of the responsibilities, might be sufficient to help the patient continue these tasks without actually taking the vacation. If ventilation or acknowledgment of frustrations do not fulfill the patient's need, the health professional and the patient can control the loss of control paradoxically by specifically authorizing the vacation. The agreement may state that "for one week, your spouse will give you your injections and test your urine while you are on vacation." As a result, the patient may feel that his or her emotions have been accepted and validated. This solution returns the patient's sense of control and, perhaps, a sense of well-being and a desire for fulfilling positive interactions through his or her own efforts. Indeed, the feeling of well-being simply from having arrived at a solution very often cancels out the need to perform the exercise. Table 9-6 gives another illustration of how a diabetes-related emotional problem can be dealt with by the problem-oriented ("SOAP") system.

Dealing with Life Situations. By its nature, diabetes magnifies the problems of daily living; in turn, the problems of daily living magnify the patient's preoccupation with diabetes. The diabetic individual experiences the same emotions as does the nondiabetic individual, but perhaps with more intensity and frequency and certainly with additional considerations. For example, for the diabetic, the fears associated with the first day of school or a new job are intensified by the additional fears of "Will I be able to leave a meeting in time to avoid a reaction?" "Will having a reaction jeopardize my position or alienate co-workers or friends?" These concerns demonstrate the importance of predicting and planning constructively rather than abandoning good control to reduce fears. For instance, teaching a patient assertive communication skills will enable him or her either to excuse himself or herself from the meeting comfortably and self-confidently (rather than manipulatively or embarrassingly) at the time of need or to inform others of the needs before beginning work.

The strategies outlined earlier in this chapter include the learning of skills that are useful in dealing with many life situations. A preventive prescription for any diabetic patient might include some of these strategies.

Table 9-6. Example of the Use of the Problem-Oriented System (SOAP) in Dealing with an Emotional Response to Diabetes

Subjective

Patient cannot remember facts of management, forgets to bring records, reports constant fatigue, fights often with spouse.

Objective

Discrepancy between patient's intellect and ability to absorb facts.

Assessment

Patient needs to work through grief reaction to diagnosis prior to handling details of management; emotions block absorption of information.

Plan
1. Encourage assertive and direct handling of feelings, when appropriate, rather than passive forgetfulness, repression, or fatigue.
2. Introduce individual and family buddy system to reinforce support and provide model for adjustment.
3. Institute six-week group of multifamily therapy to work through grief response with other families. May reduce fighting through experience of group setting; can help patient handle overwhelming feelings and offer concrete ideas for better exchanges.
4. Marital therapy may be indicated later if emotional stress is not starting to dissipate. Failure to respond to intervention may indicate preexisting interactional problems.

Resources

Identification of existing support in the form of clinical services and emotional therapy is useful to the diabetic patient. In addition, it may be useful to create new support systems in a given practice, clinic, or community. Such systems might include self-help groups guided by a professional; "matching" diabetic families in a buddy system; enlisting the aid of a psychological social worker or other counselor as part of the diabetes management team; training diabetologists in specific psychological manipulations that are applicable to diabetes management; utilizing all available community or distant resources, and enlisting therapists for referral of complex problems.

Conclusions

Diabetic patients and their families have the same emotional needs as all persons. In addition, the burdens of diabetes both impose additional demands that magnify the problems of daily living and serve to focus on issues and outcomes related to other aspects of life. The impositions that diabetes place on the individual can be summarized by the following questions (5):

1. How do diabetic patients adapt to their illness—to both the fact of having diabetes and to the daily burdens imposed by it?
2. How do they adapt to the risk of complications?
3. When complications occur, how do diabetic patients adapt to both the complications and their treatment? How does the patient's family adapt?
4. When complications create disability, what can the health professional do to help maintain the patient as a functioning, productive member of society?

More research is needed to develop better approaches to understanding these problems and defining solutions for them.

A number of clinical strategies are available today that help patients to ventilate their feelings so that unexpressed emotions have appropriate outlets rather than lead to internal stress and thereby disrupt diabetic control. These clinical strategies also may permit patients to cope better with diabetes and adapt to its burdens. Implementing these strategies involves encouraging the patient to express feelings; evaluating and assessing the reasons for the patient's reactions, symptoms, and feelings; and developing a plan to deal with the problems. It is important that the patient be involved in the development of this plan. The process is a dynamic one, and the patient recognizes and learns both generalized approaches and specific solutions.

The role of emotions is an integral part of diabetes management. Emotions affect the diabetic's responses at all levels: to the disease itself, to its treatment, and to the impact of life events. In addition, emotional stress disrupts diabetic control. The emphasis of this chapter has been the importance of recognizing the patient's emotions as a factor in diabetes management and the development of clinical strategies to deal with these emotions.

Acknowledgments

The research reported in this chapter was supported by the Health Program Office, and the Division of Children's Medical Services, Department of Health and Rehabilitative Services, State of Florida; and the Diabetes Research Institute Foundation, Miami, FL.

References

1. Hamburg BA, Lipsett LF, Inoff GE, Drash AL (editors): *Behavioral and Psychosocial Issues in Diabetes. Proceedings of the National Conference.* NIH Publication No 80-1993. US Government Printing Office, Washington, D.C. 1980

2. Kübler-Ross E: *On Death and Dying.* Macmillan, New York, 1969
3. Giarratana-Oehler J: Personal and professional reactions to blindness from diabetic retinopathy. New Outlook for the Blind 70:237-239, 1976
4. Citrin W, Ellis GJ, Skyler JS: Glycosylated hemoglobin: a tool in identifying psychological problems? Diabetes Care 3:563-564, 1980
5. Skyler JS: Living with complications. In *Behavioral and Psychosocial Issues in Diabetes. Proceedings of the National Conference.* Edited by Hamburg BA, Lipsett LF, Inoff GE, Drash AL. NIH Publication No 80-1993. U.S. Government Printing Office, Washington, DC, 1980, pp 167-181

Additional Reading

Anderson BA, Auslander WF: Research on diabetes management and the family. A critique. Diabetes Care 3:696-702, 1980

Baker L, Minuchin S, Milman L, et al: Psychosomatic aspects of juvenile diabetes mellitus: a progress report. Mod Probl Paediatr. 12:332-343, 1975

Hauser ST, Polletts D: Psychological aspects of diabetes mellitus: a critical review. Diabetes Care 2:227-232, 1979

Minuchin S, Rosman BL, Baker L: *Psychosomatic Families.* Harvard University Press, Cambridge, 1978

Moos, RH. (Ed.): *Coping with Physical Illness.* New York, Plenum, 1977

Skyler JS: Diabetes in adolescence: the forgotten years. In Podolsky, S. *Clinical Diabetes: Modern Management.* Edited by Podolsky S. Appleton-Century-Crofts, New York, 1980, pp 463-479

Wishner WJ, O'Brien MD: Diabetes and the family. Med Clin North Am 62:849-856, 1978

Yalom ID: *The Theory and Practice of Group Psychotherapy.* Basic Books, New York, 1970

Chapter 10

Hypoglycemia

Hypoglycemia is a biochemical abnormality, not a disease. An abnormally low glucose concentration can be caused by a number of factors, such as drugs, tumors, altered gastrointestinal anatomy, and failure of both endocrine and nonendocrine tissues. Hypoglycemia even occurs along with impaired glucose tolerance and infection, situations that have classically been associated with elevated glucose levels. This chapter will describe a practical approach to the often confusing subject of hypoglycemia.

One major problem is how to define hypoglycemia, i.e., what concentration of glucose is abnormally low? An important consideration is whether whole-blood or plasma glucose concentrations are being measured. As explained in chapter 1, the glucose concentration in plasma or serum is 15% higher than in whole blood. The conditions under which the blood sample is drawn are also important. For instance, a plasma glucose concentration of 54 mg/100 ml is abnormal after an overnight fast but not 4 hours after a carbohydrate-rich meal or an oral challenge with dextrose. For reasons that will be discussed, we define hypoglycemia by the criteria listed in Table 10-1.

In essence, the clinical approach to a patient with possible hypoglycemia involves the documentation of a low glucose concentration and systematic efforts to determine what condition is responsible for the low concentration. In making this determination, it is important to ascertain whether hypoglycemia occurs in the fasting or the fed state. Do the symptoms develop when the patient misses breakfast (or other meals), or do they routinely occur after the patient eats (especially after ingestion of large amounts of simple carbohydrate)? This distinction is important because, with few exceptions, fasting and fed (or reactive) hypoglycemias are caused by different conditions. Furthermore, the causes of fasting hypoglycemia are often more serious, and consequently a more diligent workup is usually required than with fed hypoglycemia. Therefore, the distinguishing of

Table 10-1. Criteria for Definition of Hypoglycemia

Glucose Concentration (mg/100 ml)	Condition of Patient	
	Fasted	Fed[a]
Plasma	<60	<50
Whole blood	<50	<40

[a]After ingestion of glucose or meals.

fed from fasting hypoglycemia simplifies considerably the differential diagnosis and alerts the physician to the potential gravity of the situation. So that the pathophysiology of the various types of hypoglycemia can be understood, normal fasted (1) and fed (2) glucose homeostasis will now be described.

Normal Glucose Homeostasis

Fasting State

Metabolic homeostasis after an overnight fast is depicted in Figure 10-1. During a short fast, only a few tissues require glucose. The most important obligate glucose consumer is the brain, which utilizes most of the available glucose (125 to 150 g/day). The red blood cells are the next most avid glucose consumers, but utilize a much smaller amount (35 to 50 g/day) than does the central nervous system. Platelets, leukocytes, peripheral nerves, and the renal medulla also require glucose during a short fast; as a group, however, these tissues consume only half as much glucose as the red blood cells. All other tissues utilize predominantly free fatty acids, which are produced by the breakdown of adipose tissue triglycerides. A small amount of the energy required by these tissues is provided by ketone bodies, which are produced from the hepatic catabolism of free fatty acids.

The liver is the sole source of glucose production during short fasts. Glucose is produced through two separate pathways: glycogenolysis and gluconeogenesis. Glycogenolysis is the breakdown of glycogen, the storage form of glucose. Approximately half of the carbohydrates contained in meals are stored as hepatic glycogen. Hepatic glycogen is slowly hydrolyzed and released as glucose in order to maintain stable levels of glucose in plasma during periods when an individual is not eating. After an overnight fast, ~75% of hepatic glucose is produced by glycogenolysis. Gluconeogenesis is the synthesis of new glucose from noncarbohydrate precursors. There are three major gluconeogenic substrates (Fig. 10-1). One is lactate, an end product of the glucose utilized by the peripheral tissues. The second category of substrate is made up of the amino acids, which are

PRECURSORS   GENERATOR   CONSUMERS

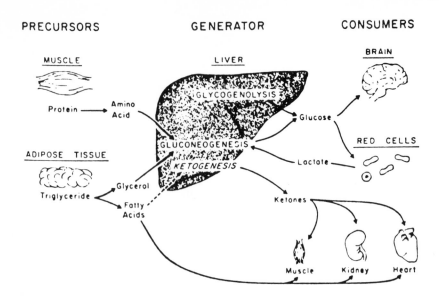

Figure 10-1. Glucose homeostasis after an overnight fast. (Reprinted with permission from Arky RA: Pathophysiology and therapy of the fasting hypoglycemias. DM, February 1968, pp 1-47.)

supplied by muscle tissue. The most important of the gluconeogenic amino acids is alanine. A transamination pathway in muscle facilitates the conversion of pyruvate, another product of glucose metabolism, into alanine, which is released and delivered to the liver. The final substrate for gluconeogenesis is glycerol, the other product (along with free fatty acids) of triglyceride hydrolysis. Thus, gluconeogenic precursors are derived from the catabolism of glucose (lactate and pyruvate), protein (glucogenic amino acids other than alanine), and fat (glycerol). The rate-determining step for gluconeogenesis seems to be the amount of substrate presented to the liver. Although only 25% of hepatic glucose production derives from gluconeogenesis after an overnight fast, the contribution from glycogen decreases considerably soon thereafter, and gluconeogenesis becomes dominant as the period of fasting lengthens.

Because powerful mechanisms defend the plasma glucose concentration even during a prolonged fast, the obligate glucose consumers can continue to function normally. Figure 10-2 depicts the changes in a number of substrates and hormones during total caloric deprivation for several days. The glucose level decreases initially by 15 to 20 mg/100 ml and then usually stabilizes. However, in some normal-weight individuals (especially females) undergoing a prolonged fast, glucose concentrations may fall to values as low as 35 to 40 mg/100 ml without the development of symptoms of hypoglycemia (3). After the initial decrease, glucose levels remain constant. This stability reflects the equilibrium

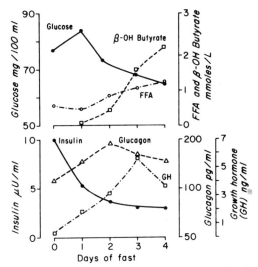

Figure 10-2. Changes in certain substrates and hormones during fasting. (Reprinted with permission from Ensinck JW, Williams RH: Disorders causing hypoglycemia. In *Textbook of Endocrinology*, 5th ed. Edited by Williams RH; WB Saunders, Philadelphia, 1974, pp 627-659.)

between hepatic glucose production (which is solely dependent on gluconeo-genesis) and peripheral glucose utilization. Insulin concentrations uniformly fall to low levels and remain there.

An important metabolic alteration occurs after several weeks of starvation. If degradation of muscle protein were to continue in order to supply the gluco-genic amino acids, the depletion of protein would become severe. To counteract such a continued drain, the brain adapts so that ketone bodies can be utilized for energy in place of glucose. Since glucose concentrations remain steady, the decrease in utilization of this substrate by peripheral tissues is matched by a con-comitant fall in hepatic glucose production (or gluconeogenesis); hence, muscle protein is conserved. With regard to the workup of a patient with fasting hypo-glycemia, the important point is that glucose concentrations decrease modestly in association with a profound drop in insulin levels during total starvation.

Fed State

As described in chapter 3, a normal diet includes both simple (mono- and disac-charides) and complex (polysaccharides) carbohydrate. The simple form, which constitutes approximately half of the total carbohydrate in the typical American diet, is quickly absorbed either directly or after rapid hydrolysis to glucose and the other constituent sugar in the small intestine. The complex form, composed mainly of polymers of glucose, is hydrolyzed and absorbed more slowly. The rising concentration of glucose in the bloodstream stimulates insulin secretion by the beta cell of the pancreas into the portal vein. The newly released insulin traverses the liver first, where ~50% is degraded on each passage. The remainder escapes into the general circulation, in which its half-life is ~5 to 10 minutes. The hormone binds to specific receptors in the three insulin-sensitive tissues—liver, muscle and adipose tissue; there, it may exert an effect for 1 to 2 hours after the initial binding.

Dietary carbohydrate is disposed of as follows. Initially, 75% to 80% is taken up by the liver, but after several hours some of this amount is released and metabolized by the peripheral tissues. Therefore, 3 hours after the ingestion of oral carbohydrate, ~55% is retained in the liver, 25% has been utilized by the obligate glucose consumers, only 15% has been deposited in muscle and fat, and <5% remains unmetabolized in the extracellular fluid.

Postprandial changes in concentrations of glucose and insulin, as measured in one study, are shown in Figure 10-3. Blood samples were taken each hour from subjects fed three meals at the indicated times. Each meal consisted of 600 calories, of which 40% were carbohydrate, 20% protein, and 40% fat. Approximately half of the carbohydrate was in the simple form. All subjects

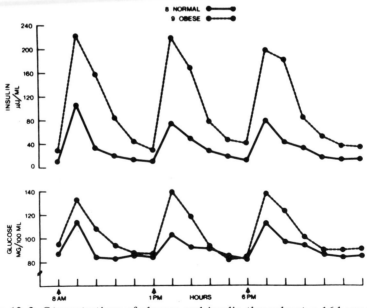

Figure 10-3. Concentrations of glucose and insulin throughout a 16-hour period in subjects who had normal carbohydrate tolerance and ate three identical meals. (Reprinted with permission from Genuth SM: Plasma insulin and glucose profiles in normal, obese, and diabetic persons. Ann Intern Med 79:812–822, 1973.)

were considered to have normal carbohydrate metabolism, but glucose concentrations were higher in the obese individuals, whose weights ranged from 169% to 315% of their ideal body weights. Glucose values peaked 1 hour after a meal and had returned to basal levels 3 to 4 hours later. The glucose elevations were modest, especially in lean subjects. Insulin concentrations followed a similar pattern, peaking 1 hour after a meal and returning to baseline levels by 3 to 4 hours. The hyperinsulinemia that characterizes obesity is well demonstrated by these results.

Hormonal Response to Hypoglycemia

Glucoreceptors in the hypothalamus initiate certain hormonal responses to low concentrations of glucose or to rapidly falling concentrations that are not yet in the hypoglycemic range. The released hormones stimulate potent metabolic mechanisms that prevent glucose concentrations from dropping to dangerously low levels. The four hormones secreted in response to hypoglycemia are depicted in Figure 10-4; in the study illustrated, hypoglycemia was artificially induced by an iv insulin tolerance test. The nadir of glucose concentrations is reached 20 minutes after injection of insulin. Secretion of epinephrine, norepinephrine, and glucagon quickly increases, whereas that of cortisol and growth hormone

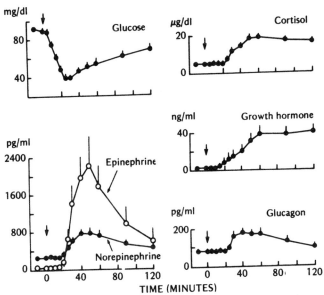

Figure 10-4. Hormonal responses to hypoglycemia induced by insulin (0.15 U/kg) in 6 normal subjects. (Reprinted with permission from Cryer PE: *Diagnostic Endocrinology*. Oxford University Press, London, 1976, p 183.)

increases more slowly. Secretion of the later two hormones is sustained, whereas concentrations of the catecholamines and glucagon return almost to basal levels 2 hours after the administration of insulin.

In response to hypoglycemia, glucose concentrations are increased by the following mechanisms. A signal emanating from the hypothalamus increases the activity of the sympathetic nervous system; this increase is reflected by increased levels of norepinephrine in plasma. The sympathetic nerve endings in the liver stimulate hepatic glycogenolysis. Although epinephrine secreted by the adrenal medulla was also thought to cause hepatic glycogenolysis, the studies upon which this precept was based used pharmacologic (not physiologic) amounts of epinephrine; therefore, this conclusion is probably not valid. However, epinephrine does affect hepatic glycogenolysis indirectly by stimulating the secretion of glucagon. Epinephrine also directly increases glucose concentrations by increasing hepatic gluconeogenesis and inhibiting the utilization of glucose by muscle. This hormone further counteracts hypoglycemia by blocking insulin secretion. Glucagon stimulates both hepatic glycogenolysis and gluconeogenesis, but has no effect on the utilization of glucose by peripheral tissues. Cortisol increases hepatic gluconeogenesis and inhibits peripheral glucose utilization. The major effect of growth hormone is to block peripheral glucose utilization. This hormone may also increase hepatic gluconeogenesis. There is a 1- to 2-hour lag period before growth hormone begins to act, and its effect may last for 4 to 6 hours.

Thus, the response to hypoglycemia is finely orchestrated (Table 10-2). The activation of the autonomic nervous system and of epinephrine and glucagon secretion is quick and has a rapid effect that is soon dissipated. The secretion of cortisol and growth hormone is delayed, and the effect of growth hormone is even further delayed because of the lag period before it begins to work. Thus, antihypoglycemic factors start to exert their effects almost immediately after hypothalamic recognition of a low or rapidly falling glucose concentration and continue to operate until 4 to 6 hours later.

Signs and Symptoms of Hypoglycemia

The signs and symptoms of hypoglycemia (Table 10-3) fall into two categories: adrenergic (those caused by increased activity of the autonomic nervous system) and neuroglucopenic (those caused by depressed activity of the central nervous system). Since the hypothalamic glucoreceptors can sense a rapid fall in glucose concentrations, a subject may show adrenergic signs and symptoms at a time when glucose levels are only mildly decreased, normal, or even high (i.e., if the patient is a diabetic who has recently taken regular insulin). If glucose concentrations fall slowly enough, however, the autonomic nervous system may not be activated, and only the neuroglucopenic signs and symptoms will appear. Many of the latter are similar to some of the signs and symptoms of cerebral hypoxia. They develop only in the presence of low glucose level, and not simply with

Table 10-2. Hormonal Responses to Hypoglycemia

| Hormone | Onset of | | Effects |
	Secretion	Action	
Epinephrine	Rapid	Rapid	Inhibits glucose utilization by muscle; increases hepatic gluconeogenesis; stimulates glucagon secretion; inhibits insulin secretion
Glucagon	Rapid	Rapid	Increases hepatic glycogenolysis; increases hepatic gluconeogenesis
Cortisol	Delayed	Probably immediate	Increases hepatic gluconeogenesis; inhibits glucose utilization by muscle
Growth hormone	Delayed	Delayed	Inhibits glucose utilization by muscle; increases hepatic gluconeogenesis(?)

rapidly changing concentrations. Although the signs and symptoms of hypoglycemia vary widely among subjects, the pattern in an individual patient tends to be similar during each episode. It cannot be emphasized too strongly that hypoglycemia does not cause allergies, alcoholism, drug addition, depression, sexual dysfunction, chronic fatigue, poor concentration, behavioral problems, and other such maladies. Although mental deterioration and even schizophrenia have been reported to be possible permanent sequelae of hypoglycemia, such an association is extremely rare and is found only after repeated and profound hypoglycemic episodes.

Fasting Hypoglycemia

Because the onset of fasting hypoglycemia is often gradual, the adrenergic component of the signs and symptoms is minimal or absent in many cases. Fasting hypoglycemia is usually persistent and requires glucose administration for reversal. The differential diagnosis of hypoglycemia in adults is described in Table 10-4. Hypoglycemia can occur both in the fasting state and after meals in three situations: adrenal insufficiency, the presence of insulinomas, and the presence of autoantibodies to insulin. All of the other factors and conditions listed in Table 10-4 cause *either* fasting *or* postprandial hypoglycemia. This fact underscores the importance of determining whether the signs and symptoms occur in the

Table 10-3. Signs and Symptoms of Hypoglycemia

Adrenergic[a]	Neuroglucopenic[b]
Weakness	Headache
Sweating	Hypothermia
Tachycardia	Visual disturbances
Palpitations	Mental dullness
Tremor	Confusion
Nervousness	Amnesia
Irritability	Seizures
Tingling of mouth and fingers	Coma
Hunger	
Nausea[c]	
Vomiting[c]	

[a]Caused by increased activity of the autonomic nervous system; may be triggered by a rapid fall in the glucose concentration.

[b]Caused by decreased activity of the central nervous system; require an absolutely low level of glucose.

[c]Unusual.

fasted state or after a meal in a patient with suspected hypoglycemia. This distinction is also helpful in cases involving adrenal insufficiency or insulinomas, because in these instances fasting hypoglycemia is much more prominent than postprandial hypoglycemia, which is usually not evident. Whether fasting hypoglycemia predominates in patients with autoantibodies to insulin cannot be determined because the evidence is so limited. Although exact prevalence figures are not available, the factors and conditions associated with fasting hypoglycemia are listed in the table in their general order of frequency.

Drugs

Drugs that can potentiate the hypoglycemic effect of the sulfonylurea agents were discussed in chapter 5 (Table 5-2). Other drugs that can cause hypoglycemia are listed in Table 10-5. Drugs that are listed as rarely associated with hypoglycemia have been implicated in only one or two patients. Drugs described as uncommonly associated with hypoglycemia have been reported to induce this condition in many more patients. Drug-induced hypoglycemia is often associated

Table 10-4. Differential Diagnosis of Hypoglycemia in Adults

Fasting	Fed (Reactive)
Drugs[a]	Hyperalimentation
Ethanol	Impaired glucose tolerance
Non-β-cell tumors	Idiopathic reactive
Hepatic failure	Adrenal insufficiency[b]
Adrenal insufficiency	β-cell tumors (insulinomas)[b]
β-cell tumors (insulinomas)	Insulin autoantibodies[c]
Renal failure	
Insulin autoantibodies	
Insulin receptor autoantibodies	
Sepsis	
Congestive heart failure	

[a]Includes factitious hypoglycemia.
[b]Although fed hypoglycemia occasionally occurs, fasting hypoglycemia predominates.
[c]Experience is too limited too determine which form of hypoglycemia predominates.

Table 10-5. Drugs Associated with Hypoglycemia[a]

Common	Uncommon	Rare
Insulin	Salicylates	Oxytetracycline
Sulfonylurea agents	Propranolol	Propoxyphene[b]
	Monoamine oxidase inhibitors	Para-aminobenzoic acid
		Chlorpromazine plus orphenadrine[c]

[a]Citations for case reports can be found in (4).
[b]Patient took 3 to 4 times the usual daily dose (130 mg every 3 hours).
[c]This case report can be found in (5), not as originally reported in (4).

with restricted food intake, hepatic and/or renal disease, ethanol intake (see next section), old age, or a combination of these factors (4). Insulin is obviously the drug most commonly associated with hypoglycemia, and the sulfonylurea agents are the next most common. The other drugs listed in the table usually cause hypoglycemia by potentiating the effects of insulin or the sulfonylurea agents, although salicylates, monoamine-oxidase inhibitors, propranolol (6), and propoxyphene have also been reported to induce hypoglycemia by themselves (4). In addition, the combination of chlorpromazine and orphenadrine (a substituted derivative of diphenhydramine) was associated with hypoglycemia in one patient (5). Paraaminobenzoic acid was stated to cause hypoglycemia in two patients (4), but no details were given in the original report. Salicylates and monoamine oxidase inhibitors lower glucose concentrations by increasing insulin secretion. The effect of propranolol is probably mediated by an enhancement of peripheral glucose utilization. The mechanisms whereby the other drugs contribute to hypoglycemia are unknown.

Seltzer (4) stresses that the treatment of drug-induced hypoglycemia must not be discontinued too soon. Hypoglycemic relapse can be difficult to prevent by means of oral carbohydrate ingestion, especially if the inciting drug was a sulfonylurea agent or a monoamine oxidase inhibitor. Therefore, after the initial bolus of 50 ml of 50% glucose, 10% dextrose in water should be infused at a rate sufficient to keep the glucose concentration above 100 mg/100 ml. If the first liter of this solution (usually given over a 6-hour period) fails to achieve this goal, infusion should be continued at the same rate and the glucose level monitored every 3 to 4 hours until hyperglycemia develops. Seltzer (4) suggests the addition of 100 mg of hydrocortisone (or its equivalent), and 1 mg of glucagon to each bottle. With increasing hyperglycemia, these drugs (if used) can be discontinued and the patient gradually weaned from iv glucose. The necessary duration of continuous glucose infusion is unpredictable in an individual patient. The usual period is 2 to 3 days for cases secondary to treatment with sulfonylurea agents, although a few patients have required infusion for over a week.

In factitious hypoglycemia, an unusual form of drug-induced hypoglycemia, emotionally disturbed patients surreptitiously take insulin or sulfonylurea agents. These individuals are usually females in health-related occupations (7) or relatives of diabetics who are legitimately taking these drugs. Patients with factitious hypoglycemia often undergo extensive medical testing, and even repeated laparotomies with eventual total pancreatectomy, without divulging the true nature of their hypoglycemia (7, 8). The major diagnostic problem is to distinguish factitious hypoglycemia from beta-cell tumors of the pancreas; the biochemical hallmark of the latter condition is a low glucose concentration with a relatively high insulin concentration. Since administration of insulin and sulfonylurea agents also cause this combination of low glucose and high insulin levels, differentiation between the two conditions may seem difficult at first glance. Fortunately, newer techniques for measuring antibodies to insulin, connecting (C–) peptide, and metabolites of the sulfonylurea agents permit the identification of patients with factitious hypoglycemia once the proper diagnosis is suspected.

Daily administration of insulin to diabetics over a period of several months causes the production of IgG insulin-binding antibodies (see chapter 4). Therefore, the presence of these antibodies in a patient in whose case factitious hypoglycemia is suspected (and who is not an insulin-dependent diabetic) provides fairly good evidence for the diagnosis (7, 9). However, both false-positive and false-negative results can be obtained. If the length of exposure to exogenous insulin is insufficient to generate insulin-binding antibodies, the result may be falsely negative. Conversely, a few patients with hypoglycemia who have never been treated with exogenous insulin seem to acquire antibodies to insulin spontaneously, as will be discussed later. These patients will have a false-positive result, but such cases are extremely rare.

The measurement of C-peptide should reliably distinguish between factitious hypoglycemia and beta-cell tumors. As discussed in chapter 4, in insulin synthesis, a single polypeptide chain is formed and aligns the appropriate amino acids for disulfide bonding (the result of which is proinsulin), with subsequent cleavage to insulin plus the C-peptide (Fig. 4-3). Insulin and C-peptide are secreted in equimolar amounts. However, because the C-peptide is only minimally degraded by the liver, its half-life is much longer than that of insulin. Consequently, C-peptide concentrations are proportionately higher than insulin levels after secretion from the β-cells. On the other hand, commercial insulin preparations do not contain the C-peptide. Therefore, a combination of low concentrations of glucose and C-peptide with high concentrations of insulin assures the diagnosis of factitious hypoglycemia secondary to administration of exogenous insulin, whereas a combination of low glucose concentrations with high insulin and C-peptide levels usually indicates secretion of endogenous insulin. Since surreptitious administration of sulfonylurea agents also results in the latter combination of concentrations, measurement of the appropriate compounds in serum or urine (7, 8) is necessary in order to rule out this cause of factitious hypoglycemia.

Ethanol

Ingestion of ethanol is associated with hypoglycemia much more frequently than the relatively small number of case reports (10, 11) would suggest. It has been estimated (4) that ethanol ingestion is the most common cause of "profound, disabling and lethal hypoglycemic coma in children and adults alike." Alcoholic hypoglycemia may be seen in one or two patients per month in emergency rooms of large city hospitals. Concomitant intake of ethanol has been noted in many of the reported cases of drug-induced hypoglycemia (4). In vitro experiments suggest that alcohol causes hypoglycemia by interfering with hepatic gluconeogenesis (10). The mechanism is related to the oxidation of ethanol to acetaldehyde and subsequently to acetate. Both reactions involve the reduction of diphosphopyridine nucleotide (NAD), and the resultant increase in the ratio of NADH (the reduced form) to NAD provides an unfavorable intracellular environment for gluconeogenesis. In addition, ethanol seems to inhibit the release of alanine, an important gluconeogenic precursor, from muscle.

Studies with normal volunteers also suggest that ethanol causes hypoglycemia in vivo by interfering with gluconeogenesis (Fig. 10-5). After an overnight fast, a 4-hour infusion of ethanol has little effect on glucose concentrations. In fact, little effect would be expected since, as discussed earlier, ~75% of hepatic glucose production at this time results from glycogenolysis. After a 72-hour fast, however, when gluconeogenesis is the sole source of circulating glucose, the same infusion lowers glucose levels by 30%.

Therefore, alcoholic hypoglycemia is more likely under circumstances of restricted food intake. This condition often occurs in malnourished chronic alcoholics, but may also develop in heavy weekend drinkers or even in social drinkers who miss meals. It should be stressed that ethanol decreases glucose concentrations in patients with normal liver function. Children are particularly sensitive to this effect of alcohol. Clinically, the neuroglucopenic signs and symptoms predominate in alcoholic hypoglycemia. The adrenergic response is often

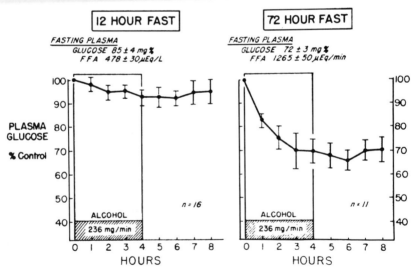

Figure 10-5. Plasma glucose response to ethanol in fasted healthy subjects. The response is expressed as a percentage of the glucose concentration before infusion, which was considered 100%. FFA, free fatty acids. (Reprinted with permission of the *New England Journal of Medicine* from Arky RA, Freinkel N: V. Alcohol infusion to test gluconeogenesis in starvation, with special reference to obesity. N Engl J Med 274:426–433, 1966.)

diminished or absent, possibly because of the gradual decrease in glucose levels (since glucose utilization is not increased) and/or a depletion of catecholamine stores after repeated exposure to ethanol.

Prompt diagnosis and treatment are important. The failure to recognize this syndrome may be responsible for the high associated mortality: $\sim$25% in children and 10% in adults. Glucagon therapy is usually not effective because glycogen stores are already depleted. In contrast to drug-induced hypoglycemia, alcoholic hypoglycemia may not require long-term continuous iv administration of glucose after the initial response to such therapy. Relapses can usually be prevented by the ingestion of modest amounts of carbohydrate.

Non-β-Cell Tumors

A number of non-β-cell tumors are associated with hypoglycemia (12). Relatively rare, large, mesenchymal tumors account for approximately one half to two thirds of the cases reported. The tumors weigh at least 1 kg and are located in the thorax, retroperitoneal space, or pelvic area. These mesenchymal tumors, many of which are benign, include mesotheliomas, fibrosarcomas, neurofibromas, neurofibrosarcomas, spindle cell sarcomas, leiomyosarcomas, and rhabdomyosarcomas. The next most common cause of tumor hypoglycemia is the hepatocellular carcinoma (hepatoma); this type accounts for $\sim$20% to 25% of cases of hypoglycemia associated with tumors. Adrenal carcinomas, gastrointestinal tumors, and lymphomas account for 5% to 10% each. Most other tumors have occasionally been associated with hypoglycemia. Of these remaining types, kidney tumors, lung tumors, anaplastic carcinomas, and carcinoid tumors are most commonly associated with hypoglycemia.

The mechanism(s) whereby any of these non-β-cell tumors causes hypoglycemia have not been agreed upon. Although it is commonly held that glucose requirements of the large mesenchymal tumors eventually exceed the ability of the liver to produce glucose and thereby lead to hypoglycemia, good evidence for this sequence of events is lacking. Indeed, in the few studies in which glucose kinetics was evaluated under such circumstances, hepatic glucose production was found to be decreased. Immunoreactive insulin has been extracted from a few of the involved tumors. However, in view of (a) recent evidence that extracts of most normal tissues contain immunoreactive insulin, (b) normal or low concentrations of insulin in the plasma of these patients, and (c) failure to demonstrate the actual release of insulin (by arteriovenous differences across the tumor at surgery), it can be asserted that few if any of these cases of hypoglycemia are caused by tumor secretion of the same hormone contained in the pancreatic β-cell.

A likely explanation (in my view) for many cases of tumor hypoglycemia is the synthesis and release of certain polypeptide growth factors that also have hypoglycemic properties (13). It has been known for many years that most of the insulinlike activity of plasma measured in vitro was not attributable to insulin, since very little of this activity was neutralized or suppressed by antibodies to the hormone. The material responsible for these findings was termed nonsuppressible insulinlike activity, or NSILA. Recent work has identified two compounds of relatively small molecular weight that are soluble in ethanol and are designated NSILA-S. A compound of greater molecular weight that precipitates in alcohol has been isolated and is designated NSILA-P

Independent of this line of investigation, another group of compounds with growth-promoting properties has been found in the circulation and has been termed somatomedins (SM) (14). It is interesting that the somatomedins also have some insulinlike activity and that the NSILA compounds have growth-promoting effects to variable degrees. Because of these properties, the two compounds of smaller molecular weight (NSILA-S) have been renamed insulinlike growth factors (IGF).

These compounds in human plasma and their metabolic activities are listed in Table 10-6. Many of their effects have also been demonstrated in vivo. Their effect on glucose metabolism would explain many of the biochemical findings

Table 10-6. Polypeptides Found in Human Plasma That Have Insulinlike Activities and Growth-promoting Properties[a]

| Peptide | Metabolic Effects[b] | |
	Insulinlike	Growth-Promoting
IGF-1	Amino acid transport[c]	Amino acid transport
IGF-2	Sugar transport[c]	Ribonucleic acid synthesis
NSILA-P	Glycogen synthesis[c]	Deoxyribonucleic acid synthesis
SM-A	Protein synthesis	Protein synthesis
SM-C	Glucose oxidation; lipid synthesis;[c] inhibition of lipolysis;[c] increased glucose turnover;[d] hypoglycemia[d]	Collagen synthesis; mitogenic activity; growth of animals[d]

Abbreviations: IGF, insulinlike growth factor (formally called nonsuppressible insulinlike activity, soluble in ethanol, or NSILA-S); NSILA-P. nonsuppressible insulinlike activity, precipitable in ethanol; SM, somatomedin.

[a]Adapted with permission of the *New England Journal of Medicine* from Phillips LS, Vassilopoulou-Sellin R: Somatomedins. N Engl J Med 302:371–380, 438–445, 1980; all effects are in vitro unless designated otherwise.

[b]Peptides differ in their ability to influence individual pathways, but all share both kinds of metabolic effects.

[c]Also occurs in vivo.

[d]Occurs only in vivo.

in patients with tumor hypoglycemia. Some evidence for their involvement in this syndrome does exist. Insulinlike activity has been demonstrated in the extracts of many of these tumors. More important, increased amounts of IGF (13) and NSILA-P (15) have also been found in the plasma of affected patients; levels of IGF were elevated in the majority of a small series of subjects. A refinement of assay techniques and a much clearer understanding of the relation between these compounds will be required to substantiate this hypothesis further.

The diagnosis of tumor hypoglycemia can be difficult if hypoglycemia is the initial manifestation of the neoplasm. The differential usually includes only β-cell tumors, adrenal insufficiency, and factitious hypoglycemia, since the other causes of fasting hypoglycemia (Table 10-4) are easily ruled out. Differentiation from β-cell tumors and factitious hypoglycemia requires a fast (usually, only a short fast can be tolerated), with concomitant monitoring of glucose and insulin concentrations. Evaluation of the pituitary-adrenal axis is also simple and will be described later. In many instances, however, the tumor is already known to be present. This is usually the case with the large mesenchymal tumors and often with many other types since hypoglycemia is a relatively late manifestation.

Adrenal carcinomas deserve special mention from a diagnostic standpoint. Although rare (16), they are commonly represented among neoplasms associated with hypoglycemia. Some patients show endocrine manifestations (other than hypoglycemia) secondary to these tumors; many others present with intra-abdominal masses, and the diagnosis is made at surgery. In endocrine tests, the majority of patients with these tumors are found to have increased urinary 17-ketosteroid values (sometimes >40 to 50 mg per day). Therefore, adrenal carcinoma should be suspected in a patient with fasting hypoglycemia and elevated urinary levels of 17-ketosteroids. Recently, serum dehydroepiandrosterone (DHEA) sulfate concentrations have been shown to correlate well with urinary 17-ketosteroid excretion. Therefore, very high circulating levels of DHEA sulfate may possibly characterize patients with adrenal carcinoma.

The treatment of tumor hypoglycemia is often difficult. If large amounts of the tumor (especially the large mesenchymal tumors) can be surgically removed, long-term remissions from hypoglycemia are likely. Effective radio- or chemotherapy also increases glucose concentrations. However, in many cases, therapy directed at the tumor is not successful and specific treatment for hypoglycemia is necessary. Frequent feedings are the obvious first choice but are often not effective. Continuous iv administration of glucose is not practical for any length of time. Diazoxide and streptozotocin are usually ineffective, as one might expect from their mechanisms of action (see β-Cell Tumors [Insulinomas]). Administration of glucocorticoids is sometimes helpful because it stimulates hepatic gluconeogenesis and to some extent inhibits peripheral glucose utilization. The initial dose should be the equivalent of 15 to 20 mg of prednisone, with fairly rapid increases if no effect is detectable. Although neither our experiences nor the published experiences of others with this form of treatment for tumor hypoglycemia are extensive, if a dose equivalent to 60 to 80 mg of prednisone is reached and no effect is noted, the dose should probably be tapered off rapidly in order to avoid adrenal suppression and dependence on exogenous glucocorticoid. If the patient is given glucocorticoid therapy for less than a month, the hypothalamic-pituitary-adrenal axis usually returns to normal.

Hepatic Failure

Death from hepatic failure is very common, but associated hypoglycemia is distinctly unusual. This is because the liver has a tremendous capacity to produce glucose and hypoglycemia ensues only when the liver is severely compromised. The diagnosis is obvious, since the patient has all of the clinical and laboratory stigmata of hepatic failure. Although treatment is simple (i.e., support of the glucose concentration with iv dextrose until the liver regenerates the capacity to maintain appropriate levels itself), hypoglycemia in this situation is a serious prognostic sign, indicating that there is little functioning hepatic tissue left. Indeed, the capacity of the liver to produce glucose may be restored and the patient still succumb to the other complications of hepatic failure.

Adrenal Insufficiency

The mechanism whereby adrenal insufficiency leads to fasting hypoglycemia is straightforward. Cortisol is necessary to support gluconeogenesis; in its absence, hepatic glucose production is significantly impaired, whether adrenal failure is primary or secondary. Although a deficiency of growth hormone sometimes causes hypoglycemia in children, the absence of this hormone in adults is not associated with hypoglycemia. Patients with pituitary destruction who are receiving adequate replacement doses of glucocorticoids do not experience difficulties maintaining normal glucose concentrations.

The diagnosis of adrenal insufficiency usually is also straightforward once it is considered. A simple diagnostic method is to collect urine for a 24-hour period and to measure 17-hydroxysteroids. Recently, the measurement of free cortisol in urine has become popular, but few relevant data have been published concerning adrenal insufficiency. Two stimulation tests—with either Cortrosyn (the 1-24 amino acid sequence of adrenocorticotropic hormone [ACTH]) or metyrapone (Metopirone)—are available. If treatment is deemed imperative, the Cortrosyn test should be performed before administration of a glucocorticoid because a reliable assessment of the pituitary-adrenal axis will be extremely difficult after such treatment. The test, which can be completed within 1 hour, involves the iv or im injection of 0.25 mg of Cortrosyn; blood samples for measurements of plasma cortisol levels are obtained before injection and 60 and 120 minutes afterward. A normal response is classically defined as a baseline value of at least 5 μg/100 ml *and* an increase of >7 μg/100 ml *and* a maximal level of >18 μg/100 ml. Some endocrinologists feel that any increase of >10 μg/100 ml constitutes a normal response regardless of baseline and maximal levels. In some patients, however, plasma cortisol levels may increase by <7 μg/100 ml over a relatively high base-line value. Therefore, if any value is >20 μg/100 ml, adrenal insufficiency is essentially ruled out.

A metyrapone stimulation test is useful if secondary adrenal insufficiency is suspected. Furthermore, although a chronically suppressed adrenal gland will not usually respond normally to one dose of Cortrosyn, it may do so if ACTH secretion has been decreased for only a short period. Thus, the Cortrosyn test may yield a normal result in cases of secondary adrenal insufficiency of recent onset. Since the result of the metyrapone stimulation test will also be abnormal in cases of primary adrenal insufficiency, this test serves to evaluate both primary and secondary adrenal impairment. Metyrapone blocks 11-hydroxylation in the adrenal cortex, which is the final step in the synthesis of cortisol (compound F). The release of ACTH is not inhibited by its immediate precursor, 11-deoxy-cortisol (compound S). Therefore, the brain senses a low cortisol level and secretes more ACTH, which stimulates the adrenal cortex to synthesize more compound S. Compound S can now be measured separately in the plasma, and its accumulation signals a normal pituitary-adrenal response to metyrapone.

Metyrapone (0.25-mg tablets) is given by mouth at 11 PM or 12 PM, and a plasma sample is collected at 8 AM the next day. For patients weighing >50 kg, the dose is 3.0 g; for those weighing <50 kg, the dose is 2.0 g. A normal response consists of a concentration of compound S of >7 to 8 μg/100 ml (regardless of the concomitant compound F value). A valid abnormal response of <7 to 8 μg/100 ml requires that the cortisol level be <5 μg/100 ml. This latter value proves that the 11-hydroxylation step was adequately blocked and the patient was unable to mount a satisfactory compound S response. A concentration of 11-deoxycortisol that is below normal in the presence of a compound F level of >5 μg/100 ml signifies that the blockade was not complete. In this instance, either the test must be repeated (with a higher dose of metyrapone if a 2.0-g dose was used) or an alternative diagnostic approach must be used. An abnormal response does not enable one to distinguish between primary and secondary adrenal insufficiency.

Some patients may experience nausea and occasionally vomiting secondary to metyrapone. These symptoms are recognized adverse reactions to the drug and do not represent acute adrenal insufficiency, which, to the best of our knowledge, has not been reported under these circumstances.

The treatment of the hypoglycemia associated with adrenal insufficiency is straightforward. In addition to the bolus of iv glucose, the patient should be given 100 mg of hydrocortisone over an 8-hour period. Gluconeogenesis will be restored quickly, and hypoglycemia should cease to be a problem. Whether or not further glucocorticoids are administered will depend on the other symptoms of adrenal insufficiency. Hypoglycemia is not a problem in patients receiving chronic replacement doses of glucocorticoids. Even in situations where increased stress calls for more exogenous glucocorticoids but they are not administered, hypoglycemia will not occur. Apparently, amounts of glucocorticoids that approximate baseline secretion rates from the adrenal cortex are sufficient to support hepatic glucose production and to prevent hypoglycemia, even under stressful circumstances.

β-Cell Tumors (Insulinomas)

Insulinomas, or β-cell tumors, encompass at least five pathologic entities in adults: single adenomas, multiple adenomas, islet cell carcinomas, microadenomatosis, and hyperplasia (17). Nesidioblastosis seems to be confined to infants and children. Approximately 80% of the β-cell tumors are single benign adenomas, and 10% are multiple benign lesions (adenoma, microadenomatosis, and hyperplasia). A large percentage of the multiple type are part of the syndrome of multiple endocrine adenomatosis, Type 1. This familial syndrome, inherited in an autosomal dominant manner and also called Wermer's syndrome, is characterized by multiple tumors of the parathyroid, pancreas, and pituitary glands. Associated neoplasms occurring less often in this syndrome are adrenal cortical adenomas, thyroid adenomas, or multiple lipomas.

Insulinomas are small tumors (usually <2 cm in diameter) located with equal frequency in the tail, body, and head of the pancreas. Women develop insulinomas more commonly than do men. These tumors usually become manifest between the ages of 30 and 50 years; patients almost invariably present clinically with fasting hypoglycemia. Although insulinomas are rare tumors, the correct diagnosis is extremely important because they are usually curable and because, if they remain undiagnosed for long periods, they may result in permanent neuropsychiatric sequelae. Because the glucose level usually drifts down slowly in affected patients, adrenergic signs and symptoms (Table 10-3) are often lacking, and the presence of hypoglycemia may thus be obscured. Patients with insulinomas tend to present with the more confusing neuroglucopenic signs and symptoms, which can include visual difficulties, transient neurologic syndromes, mental confusion, convulsions, and personality changes. Weight gain is common in these patients because chronic hyperinsulinemia and hypoglycemia lead to excessive caloric intake and fat deposition.

The diagnosis of a β-cell tumor is usually not difficult once it is considered. The cardinal rule in the evaluation of glandular function is to stimulate the gland if hypofunction is suspected and to suppress it if hyperfunction is suspected. The most physiologic test to suppress insulin secretion is fasting. Characteristic changes in the relation between glucose and insulin concentrations during total caloric deprivation are the most reliable diagnostic criteria for insulinomas and will be found in almost every patient who is tested appropriately. In normal subjects, levels of both glucose and insulin fall during starvation (Fig. 10-2). In some individuals, especially women, plasma glucose concentrations commonly decrease asymptomatically to values as low as 30 to 35 mg/100 ml after 24 to 72 hours without food (3). However, the relation between glucose and insulin is relatively unchanged since the hormone levels fall in parallel.

After an overnight fast, plasma glucose concentrations are ~80 mg/100 ml, and serum insulin levels range as high as 20 to 25 μU/ml in nonobese normal subjects. The ratio of whole-blood glucose (mg/100 ml) to insulin (μU/ml) after an 8- to 12-hour fast, as measured once in each of 30 normal subjects and repeatedly before and after surgery in three patients with insulinomas, is shown in Figure 10-6. Only three of the values in the normal subjects were <2.5, whereas all of the ratios in the three surgical patients were <2.5 before surgery and >2.5 after surgery (18). In obese but otherwise normal subjects, the glucose-to-insulin ratio may be <2.5 after an overnight fast, since hyperinsulinemia is the rule in these patients. However, as fasting proceeds, the fall in insulin concentrations is proportionally greater than the decrement in glucose levels. Thus, although the glucose-to-insulin ratio in obese individuals and in a few lean subjects

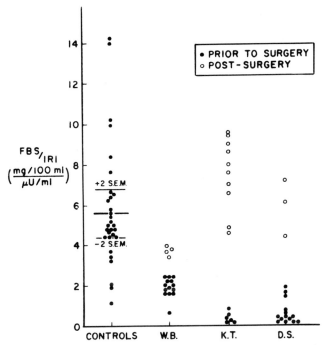

Figure 10-6. Ratio between whole-blood glucose concentrations (mg/100 ml) and immunoreactive insulin (IRI) levels (μU/ml) in samples from 30 normal subjects and 3 patients with β-cell tumors. FBS, fasting blood sugar; SEM, standard error of the mean. (Reprinted with permission from Grunt JA, Pallotta JA, Soeldner JS: Blood sugar, serum insulin and free fatty acid interrelationships during intravenous tolbutamide testing in normal, young adults and in patients with insulinoma. Diabetes 19:122–126, 1970.)

may be <2.5 after an overnight fast, this value will increase as starvation continues. An additional distinguishing feature is that obese subjects usually maintain glucose concentrations of >50 mg/100 ml during prolonged starvation.

Therefore, the most reliable way to diagnose a β-cell tumor is simply to extend the overnight fast until the patient becomes symptomatic. Blood samples for glucose and insulin determinations are drawn after the overnight fast and then every 4 hours. Approximately two thirds of the patients will experience hypoglycemic symptoms within the first 24 hours of food deprivation. Another one quarter or so will become symptomatic during the second 24 hours of starvation. A third day of fasting is required in <5% of patients who harbor insulinomas. Some authorities (17) recommend 2 hours of vigorous exercise at the end of a 3-day fast in asymptomatic patients in a final effort to precipitate hypoglycemic symptoms. In patients whose β-cell tumors secrete only small amounts of insulin (or in those with other types of fasting hypoglycemia), exercise will cause a further drop in glucose concentrations. The relation between glucose and insulin concentrations after exercise will distinguish between patients with insulinomas and those with other causes of fasting hypoglycemia. In normal subjects or in those with fed hypoglycemia, glucose levels will remain stable or increase in response to exercise.

The glucose and insulin concentrations during the morning after an overnight fast in a patient subsequently proven to have an insulinoma are depicted in Figure 10-7. The glucose levels gradually drifted down after 10 AM, while the insulin levels slowly rose. The glucose-to-insulin ratio simultaneously fell to <2.5, and the patient experienced symptoms at noon. It should be emphasized that insulin concentrations are usually not elevated very much, if at all, during fasting in patients with insulinomas. Levels remain constant or rise slightly instead of falling (Fig. 10-7). However, the relation of insulin levels to the prevailing glucose concentrations is clearly abnormal, and the diagnosis of a β-cell tumor is easily established (if factitious hypoglycemia has been excluded).

Two other relations between fasting concentrations of glucose and insulin have been suggested as means by which to discriminate between patients with islet cell tumors and those with fasting hypoglycemia stemming from other causes. (In this discussion, the values given are for plasma glucose concentrations.) One (19) is simply the inverse ratio—i.e., the insulin-to-glucose ratio. Values of >0.3 during a fast are considered abnormally high and establish the diagnosis of an insulinoma. The other (20) is an "amended" insulin-to-glucose ratio: (insulin × 100)/(glucose − 30). The rationale for amending the insulin-to-glucose ratio in this manner is that at a plasma glucose concentration of 30 mg/100 ml, plasma insulin levels should be approaching 0. The upper limit of normal for the amended ratio is 50 (19, 20). A whole-blood glucose-to-insulin ratio of <2.5 is comparable to an insulin-to-plasma glucose ratio of >0.30.

In practice, any one of the three relations discussed should serve equally well in the evaluation of patients with fasting hypoglycemia. The utility of the insulin-to-glucose ratio is shown in Figure 10-8. The 12 control subjects were

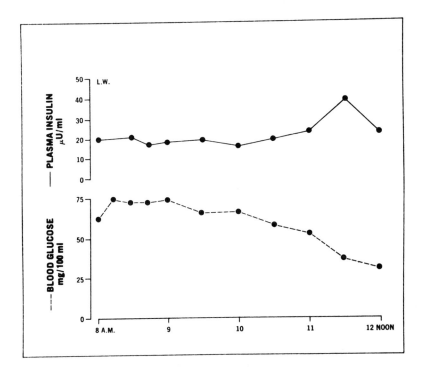

Figure 10-7. Concentrations of glucose and insulin in a patient with an insulinoma during the morning after an overnight fast that commenced at midnight. (Reprinted with permission from Conn JW, Pek S: *Current Concepts: On Spontaneous Hypoglycemia.* Upjohn, Kalamazoo, MI, 1970, pp 7–33.)

women whose glucose concentrations fell to ≤35 mg/100 ml during 72 hours of fasting. Nevertheless, their insulin-to-glucose ratios all decreased, and in 11 of the 12 this value fell considerably. In contrast, the insulin-to-glucose ratios increased in 6 patients with verified insulinomas during the 10 to 36 hours in which they were able to fast. The fasting data shown in the figure are for the times at which the glucose concentration was lowest.

One specialized test can be very helpful in confirming or occasionally even establishing the diagnosis of an insulinoma. As discussed in chapter 4, insulin is synthesized via a single-chain precursor called proinsulin. Enzymes cleave the proinsulin molecule into insulin and the C-peptide, both of which remain stored in the granules of the normal β-cell (Fig. 4-3). At the time of secretion, both insulin and the C-peptide are released along with a small amount of intact proinsulin. The antibodies used to measure plasma insulin also react with proinsulin (but not with the C-peptide). Therefore, the insulin concentration that is measured is really the sum of the concentrations of insulin and proinsulin. Under

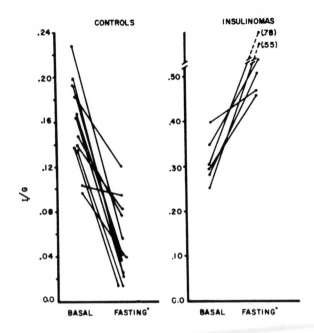

Figure 10-8. Plasma insulin (μU/ml)-to-glucose (mg/100 ml) ratios (I/G) at the beginning of a fast (basal) and at the nadir of the glucose concentration. (Reprinted with permission from Merimee TJ, Tyson JE: Hypoglycemia in man. Pathologic and physiologic variants. Diabetes 26:161–165, 1977.)

normal circumstances, proinsulin constitutes <20% of the fasting insulin concentration. After secretion is stimulated, the percentage of immunoreactive insulin that is actually proinsulin falls even further.

In most neoplasms, the normal mechanisms that control the synthesis and release of polypeptides and proteins are compromised, and abnormal amounts and patterns emerge. This alteration in β-cell tumors leads to elevated levels of proinsulin in the fasting samples of most patients. In Figure 10-9, the normal range for 10 control subjects is enclosed in the rectangles, and each dot represents a patient who was subsequently proven to have an insulinoma. The higher the percentage of proinsulin, the more likely the β-cell tumor is to be malignant. An occasional patient with an insulinoma ($\sim$1%) does not manifest hypoglycemia after 72 hours of fasting. In this situation, the diagnosis can be established by the high proportion of proinsulin in a sample obtained after an overnight fast (21).

Special techniques must be used for the separate measurement of proinsulin. The prohormone and insulin are separated on the basis of their different molecular weights before the immunoassay is applied. This measurement can be

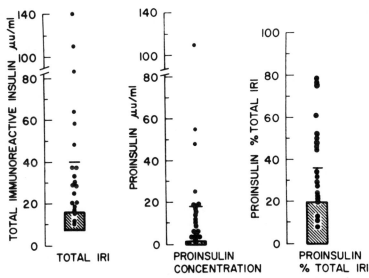

Figure 10-9. Fasting plasma concentrations of total immunoreactive insulin (IRI), proinsulin, and proinsulin expressed as a percentage of total IRI. (Reprinted with permission from Sherman BM, Pek S, Fajans SS, et al: Plasma proinsulin in patients with functioning pancreatic islet cell tumors. J Clin Endocrin Metab 35:271-280, 1972.)

made in only a few centers around the country. Dr. Arthur Rubenstein* at the University of Chicago is willing to measure proinsulin in fasting samples from patients in whom the existence of a β-cell tumor is suspected.

Finally, in the extremely rare situation in which an insulinoma develops in an insulin-requiring diabetic (22), the secretion of endogenous insulin can be monitored by measurement of the levels of C-peptide, since this polypeptide is not contained in commercial insulin preparations.

Preoperative localization of a diagnosed insulinoma is extremely helpful to a surgeon because of the small size of this type of lesion. Pancreatic arteriography correctly identifies a β-cell tumor ~50% of patients. (Microadenomatosis and hyperplasia do not give discrete tumor blushes, and the smaller tumors may also be missed.) However, removal of a tumor localized by arteriography does not guarantee a successful outcome, since multiple tumors occur in ~10% of all cases. Inaccuracies involved in the localization of insulinomas by arteriography have led to the use of more sophisticated techniques, in which the vessels

---

*Dr. Rubenstein requests that the physician consult with him regarding the patient *before* sending the sample for measurement of proinsulin. His address is: Department of Medicine, University of Chicago, 950 East 59th Street, Chicago, Illinois 60637.

draining various parts of the pancreas are catheterized via a transhepatic approach and samples are collected for measurement of insulin concentrations. Much higher levels of insulin are found in the veins draining the tumor. This diagnostic technique, which has been helpful in localizing small β-cell tumors or areas of hyperplasia that were not seen on arteriography or palpated during previous surgery (17), obviously requires the resources of a specialized center. Unfortunately, noninvasive techniques for localizing insulinomas, such as ultrasound, radioactive scans, and computerized axial tomography, are rarely helpful.

No stimulatory tests are recommended for the diagnosis of an insulinoma. In the past, stimulation of insulin secretion by administration of iv tolbutamide, iv glucagon, and/or oral leucine was suggested for this purpose. However, many false-negative results and even some false-positive results occur in these tests. There is no rationale for an oral glucose tolerance test in a patient in whom an insulinoma is suspected (or, for that matter, in a patient with any other type of fasting hypoglycemia). To reiterate, simple measurement of glucose and insulin concentrations during a fast establishes the diagnosis in almost every case. An increased proportion of immunoreactive insulin in a fasting sample that is actually proinsulin is seen in >80% of patients with β-cell tumors (Fig. 10-9) and either confirms the diagnosis or occasionally establishes it. If the percentage of proinsulin in a sample is increased, it is essential to rule out other conditions in which a high proportion of the prohormone may be seen—i.e., cirrhosis, hypokalemia, renal failure, pheochromocytoma, thyrotoxicosis, and familial hyperproinsulinemia.

Removal of a single adenoma is curative. However, hypoglycemia and hyperinsulinemia may persist after surgery because of the failure to locate a small adenoma; the incomplete removal of multiple adenomas, microadenomatous growths, or hyperplasias; or the presence of metastatic tumors. In this situation, medical therapy is indicated, and oral diazoxide (Proglycem) is usually employed. This preparation should not be confused with iv diazoxide (Hyperstat), which is administered as a bolus in order to lower markedly elevated blood pressure.

Diazoxide is a nondiuretic benzothiadiazine that causes hyperglycemia in normal subjects and animals. Its primary mechanism of action is the direct inhibition of insulin secretion from the pancreatic β-cell. It also stimulates the adrenal medulla to secrete epinephrine, which in turn impairs the release of insulin and blocks peripheral glucose utilization. Some evidence indicates that diazoxide also blocks hepatic glucose production directly. The usual dose is 100 mg given 3 or 4 times a day. Occasionally, patients may respond to somewhat higher doses. If no response is seen within 2 to 3 weeks, therapy with the drug should be discontinued. Adverse reactions may include nausea, vomiting, sodium retention (for treatment of which a diuretic is usually necessary), rash, increased lanugo hair growth, unexplained tachycardia, hyperuricemia, eosinophilia, and thrombocytopenia. Hyperglycemia reflects a good clinical response and indicates that the dose must be decreased. Patients treated with oral diazoxide require careful follow-up since this therapy occasionally precipitates diabetic ketoacidosis.

Approximately half of all patients treated respond to oral diazoxide (23). A few patients with β-cell tumors respond to diphenylhydantoin (Dilantin) (24), chlorpromazine (25), and propranolol (26).

The drug of choice for metastatic islet cell carcinoma is streptozotocin (27), an experimental antibiotic isolated from *Streptomyces achromogenes*. This drug localizes in normal and neoplastic β-cells and destroys them, thereby effecting both objective tumor regression and amelioration of hypoglycemia. Approximately 50% of the patients so treated respond, and the average response is a doubling of the median survival time. Streptozotocin is given iv; the recommended schedule is 1 g/m^2 of body surface area weekly for 4 weeks. Most of the drug is excreted by the kidneys. Its use is associated with a significant degree of toxicity, which frequently includes nausea, vomiting, and hepatic and renal dysfunction. Mild hematologic toxicity occurs in ~20% of treated patients. The first sign of renal toxicity is proteinuria, which is often followed by renal insufficiency. The adverse renal reactions may limit further treatment. In view of the serious toxicity associated with this drug, only patients with metastatic and unresectable tumors should receive it. Patients refractory to streptozotocin occasionally respond to L-asparaginase (28), doxorubicin (Adriamycin) (29), or mithramycin (30).

Renal Failure

Hypoglycemia accompanying renal failure is being increasingly recognized (31). A clear-cut picture of the setting in which this syndrome is most likely to occur has not yet emerged, however. Insulin requirements have long been known to decrease in diabetics with progressive uremia, and this decrement can be rapid in patients with acute renal failure (32). However, fasting hypoglycemia occurs in uremic diabetics who either are taking sulfonylurea agents or are controlled with dietary therapy alone; it has also been reported in uremic nondiabetics. The relation of the hypoglycemic episodes to dialysis is variable (29). Although poor dietary intake has been associated with many of the reported cases (31), some patients are clearly well fed (33). Most authors suggest that impairment of hepatic gluconeogenesis underlies the hypoglycemia, and inadequate delivery of alanine, an important gluconeogenic precursor, to the liver has been demonstrated in one patient (34). However, some patients remain hypoglycemic despite the iv administration of large amounts of glucose (33); this finding points toward enhanced glucose utilization in this situation. Although these patients are sometimes seriously ill, hypoglycemia does not characterize a terminal illness (31).

Therefore, hypoglycemia seems to be specific for a minority of patients experiencing chronic renal failure, although the circumstances of its appearance have been difficult to define. Hypoglycemia deserves serious consideration in uremic patients who present with dysfunction of the central nervous system. The goal of treatment should be to support glucose concentrations with iv dextrose until they spontaneously stabilize at normal levels. Because hypoglycemia in this situation tends to recur, careful follow-up is important.

Insulin Autoantibodies

In recent years, the spontaneous development of hypoglycemia for no apparent reason has been described in a few patients. During their workups, extremely elevated "insulin" concentrations were noted. Upon further testing, autoantibodies to the insulin molecule were measured in the plasma of these patients; this finding accounted for the spuriously high values for insulin allegedly found in the radioimmunoassay (35). None of these patients had ever received exogenous insulin. One patient developed hypoglycemia while being treated for Graves' disease (36). Another patient had rheumatoid arthritis (35). These cases suggest that the insulin autoantibody syndrome may be associated with the general syndromes of autoimmunity. The mechanism involved in the hypoglycemia is probably related to the binding of large amounts of endogenous insulin, with the subsequent release of free insulin at inappropriate times. Although most of the patients had both fasting and postprandial hypoglycemia, a few seemed to experience postprandial episodes only (35).

Treatment of these patients with glucose is usually sufficient since the hypoglycemic attacks seem self-limited. Therapy with immunosuppressive agents may be a reasonable alternative if the hypoglycemia became difficult to manage.

Insulin Receptor Autoantibodies

As described in chapter 4, an occasional patient (usually female) has a syndrome of insulin resistance and acanthosis nigricans associated with the following conditions in various combinations: obesity , hirsutism, amenorrhea, polycystic ovaries, and certain immunologic features, such as elevated erythrocyte sedimentation rates, high titers of antinuclear and anti-DNA antibodies and decreased complement levels. Affected patients also have autoantibodies to the insulin receptor (not to the insulin molecule). The presence of these antibodies accounts for insulin resistance in these patients, since insulin is unable to exert its action at the critical initial step of binding. A few of these patients inexplicably manifest recurrent hypoglycemia (37).

Sepsis

Hypoglycemia is not considered to be clinically associated with infection. Classically, in fact, insulin antagonism and hyperglycemia have been described in conjunction with infection. However, a recent report (38) describes nine patients in whom hypoglycemia was associated with overwhelming sepsis. In five of these patients, another factor (ethanol ingestion or chronic renal failure) was implicated. In the other four, no cause for hypoglycemia other than sepsis was found. With regard to possible mechanisms, it has long been known that the administration of endotoxin to animals causes hypoglycemia, probably through an inhibition of hepatic gluconeogenesis. However, some of the patients described were infected with gram-positive organisms. Sepsis-related hypoglycemia may not be rare, since three additional cases were seen by the authors in the period between the submission of the manuscript and its publication.

Congestive Heart Failure

A few patients with congestive heart failure have developed fasting hypoglycemia (39). Common features have included weight loss, anorexia, low cardiac output, and only mild hepatic dysfunction. In such instances, hypoglycemia is postulated to be secondary to decreased delivery of gluconeogenic substrates to the liver as a result of poor appetite and diminished hepatic blood flow. In view of the extremely high prevalence of congestive heart failure and the mere handful of reported cases of associated hypoglycemia, this association is probably quite rare.

Fed (Reactive) Hypoglycemia

In contrast to the signs and symptoms of fasting hypoglycemia, those of fed (reactive) hypoglycemia are predominantly adrenergic. Their onset is characteristically rapid. The neuroglucopenic component is unusual in reactive hypoglycemia. This type of hypoglycemia is transient and is usually reversed by normal hormonal responses (Table 10-2). Administration of exogenous glucose will hasten, but is not necessary for, the abatement of the adrenergic signs and symptoms.

The differential diagnosis (2, 40, 41) of fed hypoglycemia is described in Table 10-4. As discussed earlier, two of the six causes listed (adrenal insufficiency and insulinomas) cause predominantly fasting hypoglycemia. This is probably true also for a third cause, the presence of autoantibodies to insulin, although there are too few reported cases on which to base a firm conclusion. The remaining three diagnoses listed must be considered when a patient gives a history suggestive of postprandial hypoglycemia only: hyperalimentation, impaired glucose tolerance, and idiopathic reactive hypoglycemia.

The patterns of glucose and insulin concentrations in these three conditions after an oral challenge with dextrose are depicted in Figure 10-10. Alimentary hyperglycemia is an older name for what is now called hyperalimentation, early diabetes is now called impaired glucose tolerance (as discussed in chapter 1), and functional hypoglycemia has recently been renamed idiopathic reactive hypoglycemia. Each curve in the figure represents data from a separate patient. The characteristic pattern for hyperalimentation hypoglycemia consists of very high initial glucose concentrations and relatively early hypoglycemia (after 2 to 3 hours). Both impaired glucose tolerance and idiopathic reactive hypoglycemia are associated with later hypoglycemia (after 3 to 5 hours). Abnormally high glucose levels in the early part of the oral glucose tolerance test obviously define impaired glucose tolerance, whereas normal early concentrations characterize idiopathic reactive hypoglycemia. However, as discussed in detail in chapter 1,

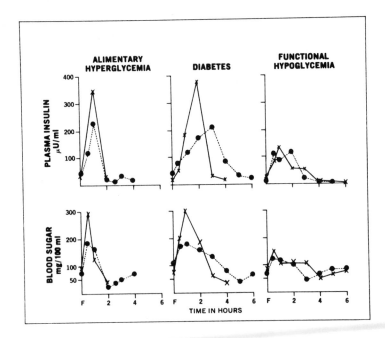

Figure 10-10. Late hypoglycemia following oral glucose load (100 g). Characteristic glucose and insulin concentrations in the three common types of fed (reactive) hypoglycemia. Data from two patients with each condition are shown. (Reprinted with permission from Yalow RS, Berson SA: Dynamics of insulin secretion in hypoglycemia. Diabetes 14:341-350, 1968.)

the results of the oral glucose tolerance test are not reliably reproducible in any individual patient, and in repeated tests the "type" of postprandial hypoglycemia may vary (2, 4, 1). Thus, a single oral glucose tolerance test may be inadequate grounds on which to decide what kind of fed hypoglycemia is involved. With this caveat in mind, the three common types of fed hypoglycemia will now be discussed separately. However, since the treatment given is similar for all three types, therapy will be described generally, with individual differences for each condition noted.

Hyperalimentation

The conventional setting for reactive hypoglycemia caused by hyperalimentation is in a patient who has undergone gastric surgery. The normal relation between the stomach and the small intestine is altered so that entry of the gastric contents into the duodenum is not delayed by the pyloric sphincter. This rapid entry into the duodenum increases the rate of absorption of glucose from the small intestine into the systemic circulation and accounts for the early hyperglycemia.

These high glucose levels trigger an enhanced insulin response (Fig. 10-10), which subsequently causes hypoglycemia. However, rapid gastric emptying may not be the sole explanation. Patients who have undergone antrectomy (removal of the lower part of the stomach) are much less likely to become hypoglycemic (42) although food enters the duodenum quickly. This observation suggests a role for one or more of the gastrointestinal hormones that amplify glucose-stimulated insulin secretion.

The situation is further complicated by the occasional patient who has all of the characteristics of reactive hypoglycemia secondary to hyperalimentation but who has not had gastrointestinal surgery. In one such patient with rapid gastric emptying (demonstrated by intubation studies), reactive hypoglycemia was reversed with large amounts of an anticholinergic agent that slowed gastric emptying (43). In another small group of patients who had not undergone gastric surgery and who had the typical pattern of hyperalimentation, the role of gastric emptying was normal (as shown by radioisotope methodology) but the rate of glucose absorption from the duodenum was increased (44). These patients were helped by phenformin, which inhibits the intestinal trasnport of glucose. (Phenformin is an antidiabetic drug recently removed from the market by the FDA because of its propensity to induce lactic acidosis.) Thus, reactive hypoglycemia secondary to hyperalimentation probably represents more than one disorder and involves various alterations in the factors governing gastric emptying, carbohydrate absorption, intestinal hormone secretion and action, and glucose-stimulated insulin release. It is hardly surprising that abnormalities in this complex process leading to clinical problems are much more likely in patients who have undergone gastrointestinal surgery than in other individuals.

Impaired Glucose Tolerance

The prompt insulin response (with maximal levels at 1 hour and a return toward normal at 2 hours) after a 600-calorie meal containing 60 g of carbohydrate was depicted in Figure 10-3. The same pattern of insulin secretion occurs during an oral glucose tolerance test in normal subjects. This normal pattern contrasts with the insulin response in patients with reactive hypoglycemia caused by impaired glucose tolerance, as shown in the middle panel of Figure 10-10. In the two patients described, insulin concentrations were maximal at 2 hours or later. The conventional explanation for the late hypoglycemia is that high levels of insulin several hours after a meal cause glucose concentrations to become abnormally low because the influx of carbohydrate from the intestinal tract is not available at this time to buffer the effect of the hormone. Although insulin secretion in patients with impaired glucose tolerance and reactive hypoglycemia is delayed compared with that in normal subjects, many individuals with abnormal glucose tolerance have delayed insulin responses without late hypoglycemia (45). Therefore, other unidentified factors may also play a role.

The natural history of patients with impaired glucose tolerance and reactive hypoglycemia is not known. In view of the slow and inconstant progression of abnormal glucose tolerance to overt diabetes (see chapter 1), it might be helpful to know whether patients with associated reactive hypoglycemia would be more or less likely than others to undergo this development. Unfortunately, no data on this point are available. Reactive hypoglycemia does not seem to occur in patients with fasting hyperglycemia.

Idiopathic Reactive Hypoglycemia

Idiopathic reactive hypoglycemia is not a well-defined entity. The characteristic glucose pattern, as depicted in the right panel of Figure 10-10, consists of normal early concentrations and later low levels. The two subjects described in the figure had a normal insulin response. However, many patients with idiopathic reactive hypoglycemia manifest either excessive (46) or delayed (45) insulin secretion. Since others of these individuals clearly have a normal insulin response (45, 46), idiopathic reactive hypoglycemia may be a heterogeneous disorder. Preliminary evidence suggests that some of the affected patients may be abnormally sensitive to insulin (47).

The classification of idiopathic reactive hypoglycemia as a discrete, bona fide clinical entity involves a number of problems, some of which have already been mentioned. Because the results of an oral glucose tolerance test in a single individual are not reliably reproducible, is the diagnosis legitimate one week but not the next? The large amount of simple carbohydrate used in the oral glucose tolerance test is certainly not physiologic; thus, the question arises of whether a diagnosis based on the results of this test is a valid explanation for symptoms occurring under different conditions. In addition, a disparity often exists between the numbers generated in glucose tolerance tests and the symptoms experienced by the patient involved (48). A partial explanation of this discrepancy may be that symptoms correlate with a rapid drop in glucose concentrations (as documented by continuous blood sampling) and the glucose nadir is sometimes missed in intermittently obtained samples (49). Of more serious concern in the establishment of a clinically relevant entity is that many patients who have idiopathic reactive hypoglycemia according to biochemical criteria do not experience symptoms compatible with this diagnosis in their daily lives (46). Conversely, the many patients with alleged symptoms of hypoglycemia who have severe personality disorders (as judged by intensive psychiatric interviews and Minnesota Multiphasic Personality Inventory testing) cannot be distinguished by the results of the oral glucose tolerance test (50). That is, there is no correlation between their glucose tolerance, their alleged symptoms, and the severity of their personality disorder.

In spite of these considerations, there do seem to be a few patients who have idiopathic reactive hypoglycemia and who routinely have symptoms when they ingest large amounts of simple carbohydrates. In my view, four criteria must be met before this diagnosis can legitimately be made: (a) Decreased glucose concentrations must be documented (see Table 10-1). (b) Signs and symptoms must occur at the time of hypoglycemia. (c) Signs and symptoms must improve markedly shortly after the patient eats. (d) The pattern just described must be regular in occurrence. The first point raises the additional question of what value defines postprandial hypoglycemia. Low glucose concentrations after an oral challenge with dextrose are relatively common in normal populations. The results in 285 women are summarized in Table 10-7 (48). A glucose tolerance test was done for adult female participants in a health survery. The prevalence of "hypoglycemia" was almost 1 in 3 among younger, more obese women; approximately 1 in 5 among younger, relatively thin females; 1 in 10 among older obese subjects; but only 1 in 50 among older thin individuals.

A high prevalence of low glucose levels during an oral glucose tolerance test is not limited to females. Fariss (51) measured glucose concentrations 2 hours after the ingestion of 100 g of dextrose in almost 5,000 recent inductees into the U.S. Army. The results are shown in Figure 10-11. Approximately 2% had plasma glucose concentrations below 40 mg/100 ml. Plasma glucose levels were between 40 and 49 mg/100 ml in another 7% and between 50 and 59 mg/100 ml in 16%. Thus, one quarter of healthy young men had plasma glucose concentrations below 60 mg/100 ml 2 hours after oral glucose challenge! The prevalence of low glucose values would certainly have been much higher if values at later times had also been included. Since relatively low glucose concentrations after an oral dextrose challenge are so common, values below 50 mg/100 ml in plasma and below 40 mg/100 ml in whole blood were considered to signify possible reactive hypoglycemia (Table 10-1).

It must be stressed, however, that the mere presence of a suitably low glucose concentration during a glucose tolerance test is not a sufficient basis on which to make the diagnosis of idiopathic reactive hypoglycemia. For physiologic relevance, the signs and symptoms of hypoglycemia should be present at this time. Furthermore, these signs and symptoms should be relieved quickly (within

Table 10-7. Prevalence of Reactive Hypoglycemia[a] During an Oral Glucose Tolerance Test in Healthy Women, by Age and Weight

| | Prevalence Among Those Weighing | |
Age	> 145 lbs	< 146 lbs
> 45 years	18.8% (n=122)[b]	2.3% (n=43)
< 46 years	31.0% (n=58)	11.3% (n=62)

[a]Defined as a whole-blood glucose concentration below 59 mg/100 ml from the second to the fifth hour after challenge with oral glucose (1.75 g/kg).
[b]The total number tested was 285.

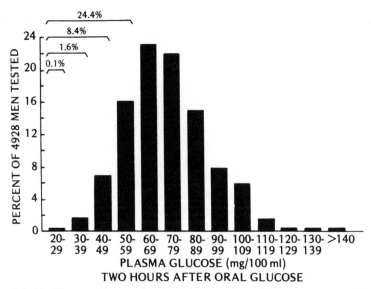

Figure 10-11. Plasma glucose levels 2 hours after challenge with a 100-g oral glucose load in overtly healthy, young adult men. The results are expressed as the percentage falling into each glucose range listed on the horizontal axis. The cumulative frequency of the lower values is shown in the upper left part of the figure. (Reprinted with permission from Cryer PE: *Diagnostic Endocrinology*. Oxford University Press, London, 1976, p 192.)

10 to 20 minutes) when the patient eats simple carbohydrates. Finally, whatever the pathophysiologic basis for idiopathic reactive hypoglycemia, this condition should cause symptoms after the ingestion of relatively large amounts of simple carbohydrates in a fairly predictable pattern if the patient continues to eat inappropriately. If all of these criteria are fulfilled, a diagnosis of idiopathic reactive hypoglycemia is justified.

In my experience, few individuals meet these criteria. Typically, a patient gives a vague history that includes some of the following: tiredness, lethargy, anxiety, weakness, depression, mental dullness, headache, paresthesia, loss of vitality, irritability, and a "trembly" feeling inside. It is usually difficult to obtain a clear description of these symptoms; rather, the history is characterized by its vagueness. There is no clear relation between food intake and either the onset or the relief of symptoms. Patients often wake up with symptoms, many of which improve only slowly (several hours) after eating. Other patients complain of the onset of symptoms within 30 to 60 minutes of eating. Unfortunately, these individuals are usually convinced that they are "hypoglycemic" and that they will improve if only the correct diet and/or vitamin and/or mineral and/or other nostrum is prescribed.

This situation has been termed the syndrome of nonhypoglycemia (52). It is the result of the superficial similarlity between the symptoms of anxiety and those of hypoglycemia, the high prevalence of low glucose values during a glucose tolerance test, the high prevalence of anxious individuals in our society, and misattribution. The last term refers to the patient's (and sometimes the physician's) desire to attribute functional complaints to a biochemical abnormality rather than confront the social or personal situation that is usually the basis for the symptoms. In an occasional patient, misattribution may delay the diagnosis of serious organic pathology that is the real cause of the problem.

One other situation should be mentioned with regard to the diagnosis of idiopathic reactive hypoglycemia. Patients whose oral glucose tolerance tests give "flat" results are sometimes considered to have fed hypoglycemia. However, a flat glucose tolerance test result is seen in ~20% of the normal population (Table 10-8) (53) and simply reflects the efficiency of the normal homeostatic mechanisms in disposing of an oral glucose load.

In summary, bona fide idiopathic reactive hypoglycemia does occur but in relatively few individuals, according to the criteria listed earlier in this section. If this diagnosis is suspected, a 5-hour oral glucose tolerance test, with sampling every 30 minutes and at the time of symptoms, should be performed. If 75 g of dextrose is used, the glucose values obtained every half hour during the first 2 hours will also provide data useful in the diagnosis of impaired glucose tolerance or diabetes mellitus (see chapter 1).

Miscellaneous Associations

The association of two other conditions with fed hypoglycemia has been described briefly (40). Hypoglycemia in 4 patients with hypothyroidism was reversed by thyroid hormone replacement. Five patients with reactive hypoglycemia reportedly had a partial deficiency of a rate-determining gluconeogenic enzyme, fructose-1,6-diphosphatase.

Treatment

The mainstay of treatment for fed hypoglycemia is diet. The most important element in the dietary prescription is the avoidance of simple or refined carbohydrates (40, 41). Patients who truly suffer from reactive hypoglycemia usually make this discovery for themselves. Since ~50% or more of the calories in the usual American diet are derived from carbohydrate and half of the carbohydrate calories are in the simple form (see chapter 3), there is much potential for decreasing simple carbohydrate intake. For obese individuals, a weight reduction diet is important. If the reduction of simple carbohydrate intake is not entirely effective, the next step is to limit carbohydrate intake to 35% to 40% of the total number of calories ingested. This decrease should be effected by increasing

Table 10-8. Prevalence of Flat[a] Glucose Tolerance Test Results in Healthy Women, by Age and Weight.

Age	Prevalence Among Those Weighing	
	< 146 lbs	*> 145 lbs*
< 46 years	28.0% (n=107)[b]	15.9% (n=44)
> 45 years	26.1% (n=23)	15.2% (n=33)

[a]defined as an increase in whole-blood glucose concentrations of <20 mg/100 ml at 0.5, 1, 2, 3, 4, or 5 hours after an oral glucose challenge (1.75 g/kg).
[b]The total number tested was 207.

the protein content of the diet whenever possible because of the deleterious effects of high fat intake (i.e., increased plasma lipid levels that are associated with an increased risk of atherosclerosis). Should this dietary change not alleviate the symptoms, food intake should be divided into multiple smaller feedings—e.g., three meals a day interspersed with three snacks. Limits on the intake of simple carbohydrates are effective in the majority of patients. A reduction in total carbohydrate intake takes care of the problem in most of the remaining cases. Multiple small feedings are usually not necessary except in patients with hyperalimentation, in whom this dietary approach is often used.

Finally, one last dietary caveat should be mentioned. Alcohol potentiates fed hypoglycemia (54) and should obviously be avoided in patients who remain symptomatic when it is included in their diet. There is no solid evidence that caffeine-containing beverages in modest amounts potentiate fed hypoglycemia. Any symptoms of jitteriness, irritability, and "hyper" feelings stem from the direct effects of caffeine and not from changes in glucose homeostasis. Therefore, coffee and tea do not have to be excluded from diets of patients with reactive hypoglycemia.

Several drugs are available for the few patients in whom dietary therapy is not effective. Anticholinergic agents are helpful, probably because they act to delay gastric emptying and to slow down intestinal motility. High doses (30 mg of Pro-Banthine) given 45 minutes before an oral glucose tolerance test were uniformly effective in alleviating both hypoglycemia, and its symptoms in 6 patients (55). However, the adverse reactions—of blurred vision, dry mouth, and urinary retention—can be very disturbing. Smaller doses (7.5 mg given 30 minutes before each meal) have been reported to be effective and much better tolerated (41).

Some patients for whom dietary changes were allegedly ineffective responded to treatment with diphenylhydantoin (Dilantin) (56). This treatment (200 mg, 3 times a day) resulted in both objective and subjective improvement, as assessed in oral glucose tolerance tests. The insulin response was also inhibited by the drug, as was expected (see chapter 1). Therefore, diphenylhydantoin may be most helpful in patients who are refractory to dietary therapy and whose reactive hypoglycemia is associated with enhanced insulin secretion.

Propranolol, an agent that blocks the β-adrenergic nervous system, increased the glucose nadir and abolished symptoms after an oral glucose challenge in patients with hypoglycemia secondary to hyperalimentation (57). Insulin secretion was unchanged by this drug. A dose of 10 mg was given by mouth 30 minutes before the oral glucose tolerance test. Propranolol may be more effective in treating symptoms than in reversing hypoglycemia; some patients remained hypoglycemic after administration of the agent.

Sulfonylurea agents have been used in the treatment of patients with reactive hypoglycemia associated with impaired glucose tolerance. However, it seems prudent first to try dietary therapy, which alleviates symptoms in the vast majority of patients. If this type of treatment proves ineffective, and especially if the 1- to 2-hour postprandial glucose concentration is elevated despite the prescribed diet, treatment with an oral hypoglycemic agent is recommended (see chapter 5).

A recent surgical approach has been successful for treatment of patients with hyperalimentation and reactive hypoglycemia whose severe symptoms were refractory to dietary therapy (58). A reverse jejunal segment (10 cm) was placed just below either the gastric outlet or the ligament of Treitz. When the small intestinal segment was reversed, antiperistalsis occurred, delaying the arrival of ingested carbohydrate at the absorptive surfaces of the small intestine. This delay, in turn, impaired the rapid entry of glucose into the bloodstream. Such surgical therapy was uniformly successful in correcting hypoglycemia and alleviating its disabling symptoms in a small group of patients.

Practical Summary

Hypoglycemia is a biochemical abnormality, not a disease entity per se, and can be caused by a number of different conditions. In the evaluation of patients, it is important to distinguish the hypoglycemia that occurs in the fasting state from that which is seen after eating. These two types of hypoglycemia are usually caused by different conditions. Fasting hypoglycemia is more serious, requiring not only treatment that will restore normal glucose levels but often sophisticated investigation in order to determine the cause. Treatment can be difficult. Fed hypoglycemia is usually a more benign, self-limited process, with causes that are easier to identify and treatment that is simpler.

The definition of hypoglycemia is a major problem. Although we use the criteria listed in Table 10-1, the mere documentation of a low glucose concentration is not an adequate basis for the diagnosis of hypoglycemia since values lower than those listed are sometimes measured in normal individuals. For instance, during fasting (especially in female subjects), plasma glucose levels often fall below 40 mg/100 ml, and after an oral dextrose challenge, plasma glucose concentrations below 50 mg/100 ml are common. Therefore, other factors associated with low glucose values are necessary before a diagnosis of hypoglycemia is tenable. In addition to the signs and symptoms of hypoglycemia, these factors include the ingestion of alcohol, certain disease processes, and the use of any of several drugs that can lower glucose levels.

Falling glucose concentrations stimulate the secretion of four contra-hypoglycemic hormones: epinephrine, glucagon, cortisol, and growth hormone. The patterns of secretion and mechanisms of action of these hormones are listed in Table 10-2. In addition, the activation of the sympathetic nervous system releases norepinephrine, which stimulates hepatic glycogenolysis.

The sign and symptoms of hypoglycemia (Table 10-3) fall into two categories: adrenergic, which are caused by activation of the sympathetic nervous system and can be secondary to a rapid decrease in glucose concentrations, and neuroglucopenic, which are caused by a depressed central nervous system and require an absolutely low concentration of glucose to become manifest. In fed hypoglycemia, adrenergic signs and symptoms always develop, but the neuroglucopenic component is much less common. In fasting hypoglycemia, neuroglucopenic signs and symptoms usually predominate; in fact, if the glucose concentration falls slowly enough, the adrenergic component may not develop at all. Although hypoglycemic signs and symptoms vary widely among subjects, the pattern in a given patient tends to be similar during each episode.

The differential diagnosis of hypoglycemia in the adult patient is described in Table 10-4. Hypoglycemia can occur both in the fasting state and after meals in only three conditions: adrenal insufficiency, the presence of insulinomas, and the presence of autoantibodies to insulin (a very rare situation). All of the other conditions and factors listed in Table 10-4 cause *either* fasting *or* fed hypoglycemia. Even in the three situations in which the two types occur together, fasting hypoglycemia predominates. *This fact underscores the importance of determining whether the signs and symptoms occur in the fasted state or following a meal in a patient with suspected hypoglycemia.*

Fasting Hypoglycemia

The conditions and factors causing fasting hypoglycemia are listed in Table 10-4 in their general order of frequency. The first two—drugs and ethanol—are fairly common causes, while the rest are unusual or rare. Of the drugs (Table 10-5), insulin is obviously the most common cause, and the sulfonylurea agents are the next most common. Although they themselves do not cause hypoglycemia, certain drugs (chapter 5, Table 5-2) can potentiate the hypoglycemic effects of the sulfonylurea compounds. The other drugs listed in Table 10-5 often cause hypoglycemia in the presence of insulin or the sulfonylurea agents, although salicylates, monoamine oxidase inhibitors, propranolol, and propoxyphene (in large doses) lower glucose levels by themselves.

Treatment of drug-induced hypoglycemia must not be discontinued too soon. After the initial bolus of 50 ml of 50% dextrose, 10% dextrose in water must be infused at a rate sufficient to maintain glucose concentrations above 100 mg/100 ml. The length of the period for which this therapy is necessary cannot be predicted for any given individual; many patients require 2 to 3 days of treatment (especially if a sulfonylurea agent was the culprit).

Factitious hypoglycemia results from the surreptitious administration of insulin or sulfonylurea agents. The affected patients are usually emotionally disturbed females in health-related occupations or relatives of diabetics for whom these drugs have been legitimately prescribed. The major problem in the diagnosis of factitious hypoglycemia is to distinguish it from the presence of insulinomas—a condition that stems from increased endogenous insulin secretion. The biochemical characteristics of both conditions are low glucose concentrations and elevated insulin levels. If the patient is suspected of injecting insulin, C-peptide concentrations should be measured because this peptide is secreted by the pancreatic β-cell but is not found in commercial insulin preparations. High levels of C-peptide therefore signify increased endogenous insulin release, while low values signify exogenous administration.

Ethanol ingestion is a common cause of hypoglycemia. The oxidation of ethanol in the liver generates cofactors that interfere with hepatic gluconeogenesis. Therefore, alcohol-induced hypoglycemia is more likely in a setting of restricted food intake. In many patients drug-induced hypoglycemia is associated with alcohol ingestion. Ethanol ingestion may cause hypoglycemia even in patients with normal liver function who miss a meal or two. Children are particularly sensitive. Ethanol ingestion can even potentiate postprandial hypoglycemia. Clinically, the neuroglucopenic signs and symptoms usually predominate, whereas the adrenergic signs and symptoms are diminished or absent. Delays in the diagnosis of alcoholic hypoglycemia may be responsible for the high mortality reported in both children (25%) and adults (10%).

A number of *non-β-cell tumors* are associated with hypoglycemia. The most common cause of tumor hypoglycemia are large mesenchymal tumors (mesotheliomas, fibromas, and sarcomas of various tissues) located in the thorax, retroperitoneal space, or pelvic area. Hepatocellular carcinomas (hepatomas) are the next most common causes of tumor hypoglycemia, and adrenal carcinomas, gastrointestinal carcinomas, and lymphomas follow. Many other neoplasms have occasionally been associated with hypoglycemia; the most common of these are kidney neoplasms, lung neoplasms, anaplastic carcinomas, and carcinoid tumors.

The pathogenesis of tumor hypoglycemia is obscure. This type of hypoglycemia is not caused by the secretion of insulin but may result from the release of polypeptide growth factors with insulinlike activity (Table 10-6). Diagnosis involves the location and identification of the tumor. Treatment ideally should be directed at the neoplasm. Extirpation of the tumor (even if only partial) is frequently helpful in ameliorating hypoglycemia. If surgery, irradiation, or chemotherapy does not increase glucose levels, specific treatment for hypoglycemia must be utilized. Such therapy includes frequent feedings and possible administration of glucocorticoids. Obviously, iv administration of glucose will be effective but is not a long-term solution.

Although *hepatic failure* is very common, associated hypoglycemia is distinctly unusual because of the tremendous capacity of the liver to produce glucose. Thus, hypoglycemia in this situation is a poor prognostic sign. Treatment consists of support of plasma glucose concentrations until hepatic regeneration occurs.

The impairment of hepatic gluconeogenesis because of a lack of glucocorticoids in *adrenal insufficiency* (primary or secondary) can cause hypoglycemia. In adults, a deficiency of growth hormone is not associated with hypoglycemia. The diagnosis of adrenal insufficiency is usually not difficult (once it is considered) and can be made by measurement of 24-hour urinary 17-hydroxysteriods or by means of a stimulation test with either Cortrosyn (the 1-24 amino acid sequence of ACTH) or metyrapone (Metopirone), an 11-hydroxylase inhibitor in steroid synthesis. Treatment is simple and consists of glucocorticoid replacement, with high doses initially and physiologic amounts after 1 to 2 days.

Although *β-cell tumors (insulinomas)* are rare, their correct diagnosis is extremely important. Insulinomas are potentially curable but, if unrecognized over long periods, can lead to devastating neuropsychiatric sequelae. The most reliable method of diagnosis is the measurement of glucose and insulin concentrations every 4 hours throughout a fast. Approximately two thirds of patients with insulinomas will experience hypoglycemic symptoms within 24 hours of food deprivation. Most of the rest will become symptomatic during the second 24 hours of starvation. Fewer than 5% will require a third day of fasting. Glucose (mg/100 ml)-to-insulin (μU/ml) ratios of <2.5 (Fig. 10-6) or insulin (μU/ml)-to-glucose (mg/100 ml) ratios of >0.3 (Fig. 10-8) during the fast are abnormal and serve to establish the diagnosis of an insulinoma. The other recommended test is the measurement of the percentage of proinsulin in the total immunoreactive insulin concentration in a sample taken after an overnight fast. Values of $>20\%$ are abnormal and confirm the diagnosis (Fig. 10-9). A very high proportion of proinsulin suggests that the tumor may be malignant. Provocative tests (stimulation by tolbutamide, leucine, and glucagon) are usually not helpful and may even be confusing. Glucose tolerance tests are worthless in evaluating a patient for a possible insulinoma (or for any other type of fasting hypoglycemia).

Preoperative localization of a diagnosed tumor is helpful to a surgeon because of the small size of these neoplasms (often <2 cm). Tumors can be localized successfully in $\sim$50% of cases. (Microadenomatosis and hyperplasia do not give discrete tumor blushes, and smaller tumors are likely to be missed.) Removal of a tumor localized by arteriography does not guarantee a successful outcome since multiple tumors occur in $\sim$10% of all cases. Inaccuracies in the localization of insulinomas by arteriography have led to the use of more sophisticated techniques, in which the vessels draining various parts of the pancreas are catheterized via a transhepatic approach and samples are collected for measurement of insulin concentrations. Much higher levels are found in the veins draining the tumor.

This diagnostic technique, which has been helpful in localizing small β-cell tumors or areas of hyperplasia that were not seen on arteriography or palpated at a previous surgery, obviously requires the resources of a specialized center. Unfortunately, noninvasive techniques for localizing insulinomas, such as ultrasound, radioactive scans, and computerized axial tomography, are rarely helpful.

If hypoglycemia and hyperinsulinemia persist after surgery, medical therapy is indicated. Of patients requiring treatment, approximately half will respond to diazoxide, a nondiuretic benzothiadiazine that inhibits insulin secretion. The oral preparation, Proglycem, should not be confused with Hyperstat, the iv formulation administered as a bolus in the treatment of markedly elevated blood pressure. The dose is 100 to 200 mg taken 3 or 4 times per day. Adverse reactions include nausea, vomiting, sodium retention (for reversal of which a diuretic is usually necessary), rash, increased lanugo hair growth, unexplained tachycardia, hyperuricemia, eosinophilia, and thrombocytopenia. Occasionally the affected patients become hyperglycemic, and in rare instances they develop ketoacidosis. Of patients who do not respond to diazoxide, a few will respond to diphenylhydantoin (Dilantin), propranolol, or chlorpromazine.

The drug of choice for metastatic islet cell carcinoma is streptozotocin, an experimental antibiotic isolated from *Streptomyces achromogenes*. This drug localizes in normal and neoplastic β-cells and destroys them, thereby causing both objective tumor regression and amelioration of hypoglycemia. Approximately 50% of patients will respond to this drug, and the average response is a doubling of the median survival time. Streptozotocin is given iv, with a recommended dosage schedule of 1 g/m^2 of body surface area weekly for 4 weeks. Most of the drug is excreted by the kidneys. Its use is associated with a significant degree of toxicity, which frequently includes nausea, vomiting, and hepatic and renal dysfunction. Mild hematologic toxicity occurs in ~20% of treated patients. The first sign of renal toxicity is proteinuria, which is often followed by renal insufficiency. The adverse renal reactions may limit further treatment. In view of the serious toxicity caused by this drug, it should be used only in patients with metastatic and unresectable tumors. Patients refractory to streptozotocin occasionally respond to L-asparaginase, doxorubicin (Adriamycin), or mithramycin.

The remaining conditions and factors listed in Table 10-4 have only rarely been cited as causes of fasting hypoglycemia. Fasting hypoglycemia is occasionally seen in cases of *chronic renal failure* in both diabetic and nondiabetic patients. No clear relation to nutritional status and/or dialysis has been discerned. Preliminary evidence suggests that hepatic gluconeogenesis may be impaired in these patients. A few patients who clearly have never been exposed to exogenous insulin have nevertheless been reported to have antibodies to insulin. The mechanism behind the hypoglycemia in this syndrome of *insulin autoantibodies* is probably related to the binding of large amounts of endogenous insulin, with the subsequent release of free insulin at inappropriate times. As described in chapter 4, an occasional patient (usually female) with *insulin receptor autoantibodies* (as opposed to antibodies directed against the insulin molecule) has the syndrome of insulin resistance and acanthosis nigricans associated with the following conditions in various combinations: obesity, hirsutism, amenorrhea, polycystic ovaries, and certain other immunologic features, such as increased erythrocyte sedimentation rates, high titers of antinulcear and anti-DNA antibodies, and decreased complement levels. A few of these patients inexplicably manifest recurrent hypoglycemia at various times. Finally, hypoglycemia has been noted in a few patients with either *sepsis* or *congestive heart failure*.

Fed (Reactive) Hypoglycemia

There are three common types of postprandial hypoglycemia. One is associated with hyperalimentation, the second is associated with impaired glucose tolerance, and the third (termed idiopathic reactive hypoglycemia) occurs for no apparent reason. The characteristic glucose and insulin patterns for these three types of fed hypoglycemia are depicted in Figure 10-10, in which each curve represents an individual patient.

Nearly all cases of *hyperalimentation* hypoglycemia (formerly called alimentary hyperglycemia) seen are in patients who have undergone gastric surgery. The rapid emptying of food into the small intestine leads to very high glucose concentrations soon after the patient eats, and these high glucose levels stimulate an excessive insulin response. This enhanced insulin secretion causes hypoglycemia within 2 to 3 hours. An occasional patient who has not undergone surgery may have this type of hypoglycemia.

In *impaired glucose tolerance* (formerly called early, chemical, or latent diabetes; see chapter 1), glucose concentrations are elevated during the initial several hours after a meal and fall to abnormally low levels after 3 to 5 hours. This pattern may be caused by a delay in insulin secretion, with the late peak causing hypoglycemia at a time when no more carbohydrate is entering the circulation from the gastrointestinal tract. (Normally, insulin levels peak by 1 hour after oral ingestion of carbohydrate, as shown in Fig. 10-3.)

Patients with *idiopathic reactive hypoglycemia* (formerly called functional hypoglycemia) have normal glucose concentrations during the initial several hours after oral ingestion of carbohydrate but manifest hypoglycemia later (usually after 3 to 5 hours). Although the subjects whose results are depicted in the right panel of Figure 10-10 had normal insulin responses, many other such patients have excessive and/or delayed insulin secretion. Thus, this disorder may be heterogeneous.

There are several major problems in the diagnosis of idiopathic reactive hypoglycemia. The results of the oral glucose tolerance test in a given individual are not reliably reproducible. Therefore, the question arises of whether the diagnosis is legitimate at one time but not at another. The large amount of simple carbohydrate used in the oral glucose tolerance test is certainly not physiologic and raises the question of whether a diagnosis made on the basis of this test is a valid explanation for symptoms occurring under different conditions. In addition, a disparity often exists between the numbers generated in glucose tolerance tests and the symptoms experienced by the patient involved. Of more serious concern in the establishment of a clinically relevant entity is the fact that many patients who have idiopathic reactive hypoglycemia according to biochemical criteria do not have symptoms compatible with this diagnosis in their daily lives. In other patients who allegedly have hypoglycemic symptoms, there is no correlation between the results of the oral glucose tolerance test and these symptoms. In addition, the symptoms of which these patients complain do not routinely occur several hours after eating and are usually not relieved quickly by the ingestion of simple carbohydrates.

In spite of these considerations, there do seem to be a few patients who have idiopathic reactive hypoglycemia and who routinely have symptoms when they ingest large amounts of simple carbohydrates. In my view, four criteria must be met before this diagnosis can legitimately be made. (*a*) Decreased glucose concentrations must be documented. However, since low glucose values after an oral challenge with dextrose are so common in the normal asymptomatic population (Table 10-7 and Fig. 10-11), a glucose concentration that meets the criteria for fed hypoglycemia, as listed in Table 10-1, is not a sufficient basis for the diagnosis of idiopathic reactive hypoglycemia. (*b*) For physiologic relevance, the signs and symptoms of hypoglycemia should be present at the time of hypoglycemia. (*c*) Furthermore, these signs and symptoms should be relieved within a short period (10 to 20 minutes) after the patient eats simple carbohydrates. (*d*) Finally, whatever its pathophysiologic basis, idiopathic reactive hypoglycemia should cause symptoms after the ingestion of relatively large amounts of simple carbohydrates in a fairly predictable pattern if the patient continues to eat inappropriately.

One other situation should be mentioned with regard to the diagnosis of idiopathic reactive hypoglycemia. Patients whose oral glucose tolerance tests give "flat" results are sometimes considered to have fed hypoglycemia. However, a flat glucose tolerance test result is seen in ~20% of the normal population (Table 10-8) and simply reflects the efficiency of the normal homeostatic mechanisms in disposing of an oral glucose load.

In summary, bona fide idiopathic reactive hypoglycemia does occur but in relatively few individuals, according to the four criteria listed earlier. If this diagnosis is suspected, a 5-hour oral glucose tolerance test, with sampling every 30 minutes and at the time of symptoms, should be performed. If 75 g of dextrose is used, the glucose values obtained every half hour during the first 2 hours will also provide data useful in the diagnosis of impaired glucose tolerance or diabetes mellitus (see chapter 1).

The association of two other conditions with fed hypoglycemia has been described briefly. Hypoglycemia in 4 patients with hypothyroidism was reversed by thyroid hormone replacement. Five other patients with reactive hypoglycemia reportedly had a partial deficiency of a rate-determining gluconeogenic enzyme, fructose-1,6-diphosphatase.

The treatment of fed hypoglycemia is mainly dietary. The most important element is the avoidance of simple or refined carbohydrates, a maneuver which patients who truly suffer from postprandial hypoglycemia usually discover for themselves. In obese patients, weight reduction is important. If limits on intake of simple carbohydrate do not satisfactorily resolve the problem, the next step is to decrease the amount of dietary carbohydrate to 35% to 40% of the total caloric intake. (In the usual American diet, over 50% of calories are in the form of carbohydrate, and approximately half of these carbohydrate calories are ingested in the simple form; see chapter 3.) Should this dietary change not relieve the symptoms, the allotted caloric intake should be divided into six feedings. Alcohol potentiates postprandial hypoglycemia in some patients, and its consumption should be decreased or eliminated if it is implicated.

If dietary therapy fails, several drugs have been found to be helpful in selected patients. These drugs include anticholinergic agents; Pro-Banthine (7.5 mg given 30 minutes before each meal), which presumably slows gastric emptying; Dilantin (100 to 200 mg given 3 times a day), whose effectiveness is presumably related to the inhibition of insulin secretion; and propranolol (10 mg before meals), which may blunt the symptoms rather than reverse the hypoglycemia. Finally, a few patients with hyperalimentation hypoglycemia refractory to dietary therapy have been successfully treated by placement of a reversed jejunal segment (10 cm) high in the duodenum. The resulting antiperistalsis presumably slows the entry of food into the distal small intestine, and this delay inhibits the rapid entry of glucose into the circulation.

References

1. Cahill GF, Jr: Starvation in man. N Engl J Med 282:668–682, 1970
2. Freinkel N, Metzger BE: Oral glucose tolerance curve and hypoglycemias in the fed state. N Engl J Med 280:820–828, 1969
3. Merimee TJ, Tyson JE: Stabilization of plasma glucose during fasting. Normal variations in two separate studies. N Engl J Med 291:1275–1278, 1974
4. Seltzer HS: Drug-induced hypoglycemia. A review based on 473 cases. Diabetes 21:955–966, 1972
5. Buckle RM, Guilleband J: Hypoglycemic coma occurring during treatment with chlorpromazine and orphenadrine. Br Med J 4:599–600, 1967
6. Skinner DJ: Uses of propranolol. N Engl J Med 293:1205, 1975
7. Service JF, Palumbo PJ: Facititial hypoglycemia. Three cases diagnosed on the basis of insulin antibodies. Arch Intern Med 134:336–340, 1974
8. Jordan RM, Kammer J, Riddle R: Sulfonylurea-induced factitious hypoglycemia. A growing problem. Arch Intern Med 137:390–393, 1977
9. Scarlett JA, Mako ME, Rubenstein AH, et al: Factitious hypoglycemia. Diagnosis by measurement of serum C-peptide immunoreactivity and insulin-binding antibodies. N Engl J Med 297:1029–1032, 1977

10. Freinkel N, Arky RA, Cohen AK, Alcohol hypoglycemia. IV. Current concepts of its pathogenesis. Diabetes 14:350-361, 1965

11. Madison LL: Ethanol-induced hypoglycemia. In *Advances in Metabolic Disorders*, vol 3. Edited by Levine R, Luft R. New York, Academic Press, 1968, pp 85-109

12. Laurent J, Debry G, Floquet J: *Hypoglycaemic Tumours*. Excerpta Medica, Amsterdam, 1971, pp 87-159

13. Megyesi K, Kahn CR, Roth J, Gorden P: Hypoglycemia in association with extrapancreatic tumors: demonstration of elevated plasma NSILA-S by a new radioreceptor assay. J Clin Endocrinol Metab 38:931-934, 1974

14. Phillips LS, Vassilopoulou-Sellin R: Somatomedins. N Engl J Med 302:371-380, 438-445, 1980

15. Plovnick H, Ruderman NB, Aoki T, et al: Non-β-cell tumor hypoglycemia associated with increased nonsuppressible insulin-like protein (NSILP). Am J Med 66:154-159, 1979

16. Hutter AM, Jr, Kayhoe DE: Adrenal cortical carcinoma. Clinical features of 138 patients. Am J Med 41:572-580, 1966

17. Fajans SS, Floyd JC, Jr: Diagnosis and medical management of insulinomas. Annu Rev Med 30:313-329, 1979

18. Grunt JA, Pallotta JA, Soeldner JS: Blood sugar, serum insulin and free fatty acid interrelationships during intravenous tolbutamide testing in normal young adults and in patients with insulinoma. Diabetes 19:122-126, 1970

19. Fajans SS; Floyd JC, Jr: Fasting hypoglycemia in adults. N Engl J Med 294:766-772, 1976

20. Turner RC, Oakley NW, Nabarro JDN: Control of basal insulin secretion, with special reference to the diagnosis of insulinomas. Br Med J 2:132-135, 1971

21. Rayfield EJ, Pulini M, Golub A, et al: Nonautonomous function of a pancreatic insulinoma. J Clin Endocrinol Metab 43:1307-1311, 1976

22. Sandler R, Horwitz DL, Rubenstein AH, Kuzuya H: Hypoglycemia and endogenous hyperinsulinism complicating diabetes mellitus. Application of the C-peptide assay to diagnosis and therapy. Am J Med 59:730-736, 1975

23. Stefanini P, Carboni M, Patrassi N, et al: Problems of the management of insulinomas. Review of 132 cases treated with medical measures. Acta Diabet Lat 11:71-77, 1974

24. Brodows RG, Campbell RG: Control of refractory fasting hypoglycemia in a patient with suspected insulinoma with diphenylhydantoin. J Clin Endocrinol Metab 38:159-161, 1974

25. Federspil G, Casara D, Stauffacher W: Chlorpromazine in the treatment of endogenous organic hyperinsulinism. Diabetologia 10:189-191, 1974

26. Scandellari C, Zaccaria M, De Palo C, et al: The effect of propranolol on hypoglycemia. Observations in five insulinoma patients. Diabetologia 15:297-301, 1978

27. Broder LE, Carter SK: Pancreatic islet cell carcinoma. II. Results of therapy with streptozotocin in 52 patients. Ann Intern Med 79:108-118, 1973

28. Sadoff L: Control of hypoglycemia with L-asparaginase in a patient with islet cell cancer. J Clin Endocrinol Metab 36:334-337, 1973

29. Eastman RC, Come SE, Strewler GJ, et al: Adriamycin therapy for advanced insulinoma. J Clin Endocrinol Metab 44:142-148, 1977

30. Kiang DT, Frenning DH, Bauer GE: Mithramycin for hypoglycemia in malignant insulinoma. N Engl J Med 299:134-135, 1978

31. Peitzman SJ, Agarwal BN: Spontaneous hypoglycemia in end-stage renal failure. Nephron 19:131-139, 1977

32. Weinrauch LA, Healy RW, Leland OS, Jr, et al: Decreased insulin requirement in acute renal failure in diabetic nephropathy. Arch Intern Med 138:399-402, 1978

33. Frizzell M, Larsen PR, Field JB: Spontaneous hypoglycemia associated with chronic renal failure. Diabetes 22:493-498, 1973

34. Garber AJ, Bier DM, Cryer PE, Pagliara AS: Hypoglycemia in compensated chronic renal insufficiency. Substrate limitation of gluconeogenesis. Diabetes 23:982-986, 1974

35. Goldman J, Baldwin D, Rubenstein AH, et al: Characterization of circulating insulin and proinsulin-binding antibodies in autoimmune hypoglycemia. J Clin Invest 63:1050-1059, 1979

36. Hirata Y, Tominaga M, Ito J-I, Noguchi A: Spontaneous hypoglycemia with insulin autoimmunity in Graves' disease. Ann Intern Med 81:214-218, 1974

37. Flier JS, Bar RS, Muggeo M, et al: The evolving clinical course of patients with insulin receptor autoantibodies: spontaneous remission or receptor proliferation with hypoglycemia. J Clin Endocrinol Metab 47:985-995, 1978

38. Miller SI, Wallace RJ, Jr, Musher DM, et al: Hypoglycemia as a manifestation of sepsis. Am J Med 68:649-654, 1980

39. Block MB, Gambetta M, Resnekov L, Rubenstein AH: Spontaneous hypoglycaemia in congestive heart-failure. Lancet 2:736-738, 1972

40. Hofeldt FD: Reactive hypoglycemia. Metabolism 24:1193-1208, 1975

41. Permutt MA: Postprandial hypoglycemia. Diabetes 25:719-733, 1976

42. Breuer RI, Moses H, III, Hagen TC, Zuckerman L: Gastric operations and glucose homeostasis. Gastroenterology 62:1109-1119, 1972

43. Veverbrants E, Olsen W, Arky RA: Role of gastrointestinal factors in reactive hypoglycemia. Metabolism 18:6-12, 1969

44. Permutt MA, Kelly J, Bernstein R, et al: Alimentary hypoglycemia in the absence of gastrointestinal surgery. N Engl J Med 288:1206-1210, 1973

45. Hofeldt FD, Lufkin EG, Hagler L, et al: Are abnormalities in insulin secretion responsible for reactive hypoglycemia? Diabetes 23:589-596, 1974

46. Luyckx AS, Lefebvre PJ: Plasma insulin in reactive hypoglycemia. Diabetes 20:435–442, 1971

47. Goldman J: Increased responsiveness to insulin and receptor-effector coupling in functional hypoglycemia. Clin Res 28:393, 1980

48. Jung Y, Khurana RC, Corredor DG, et al: Reactive hypoglycemia in women. Results of a health survey. Diabetes 20:428–434, 1971

49. Hadji-Georgopoulos A, Schmidt MI, Margolis S, Kowarski AA: Elevated hypoglycemic index and late hyperinsulinism in symptomatic postprandial hypoglycemia. J Clin Endocrinol Metab 50:371–376, 1980

50. Ford CV, Bray GA, Swerdloff RS: A psychiatric study of patients referred with a diagnosis of hypoglycemia. Am J Psychiatry 133:290-294, 1976

51. Fariss BL: Prevalence of post-glucose-load glycosuria and hypoglycemia in a group of healthy young men. Diabetes 23:189-191, 1974

52. Yager J, Young RT: Non-hyperglycemia is an epidemic condition. N Engl J Med 291:907-908, 1974

53. Nolan S, Stephan T, Khurana RC, et al: Low profile (flat) glucose tolerances. Am J Med Sci 264:33–39, 1972

54. O'Keefe SJD, Marks V: Lunchtime gin and tonic. A cause of reactive hypoglycaemia. Lancet 1:1286–1288, 1977

55. Permutt MA, Keller D, Santiago J: Cholinergic blockade in reactive hypoglycemia. Diabetes 26:121-127, 1977

56. Stambaugh JE, Tucker DC: Effect of diphenylhydantoin on glucose tolerance in patients with hypoglycemia. Diabetes 23:679-683, 1974

57. Leichter SB, Permutt MA: Effect of adrenergic agents on postgastrectomy hypoglycemia. Diabetes 24:1005-1010, 1975

58. Fink WJ, Hucke ST, Gray TW, et al: Treatment of postoperative reactive hypoglycemia by a reversed intestinal segment. Am J Surg 131:19-22, 1976

Index

Metropolitan Transportation Planning